Neuroanatomical Tract-Tracing Methods 2

Recent Progress

Neuroanatomical Tract-Tracing Methods 2

Recent Progress

Edited by

Lennart Heimer and László Záborszky

University of Virginia Medical Center
Charlottesville, Virginia

Plenum Press • New York and London

Library of Congress Cataloging in Publication Data

Neuroanatomical tract-tracing methods, 2: recent progress / edited by Lennart
Heimer and László Záborszky.

    p.   cm.

  Includes bibliographies and index.

  ISBN 0-306-43165-3

  1. Neural circuitry — Research — Methodology. 2. Neuroanatomy — Research —
Methodology. 3. Immunohistochemistry. 4. Immunocytochemistry. I. Heimer, Lennart. II. Záborszky, László, 1944-   . III. Title: Neuroanatomical tract-tracing
methods, two.

  [DNLM: 1. Histocytochemistry — methods. 2. Nervous System — anatomy &
histology. 3. Neural Pathways. WL 102 N49451]

QP363.3.N45   1989

591.4′8′0724 — dc20

DNLM/DLC   89-16045

for Library of Congress   CIP

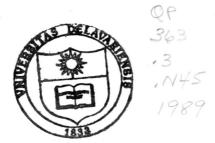

Cover art courtesy of Peter Somogyi,
MRC Anatomical Neuropharmacology Unit,
Oxford, United Kingdom

© 1989 Plenum Press, New York
A Division of Plenum Publishing Corporation
233 Spring Street, New York, N.Y. 10013

Printed in the United States of America

Contributors

JØRN CARLSEN Department of Gastroenterology C, Copenhagen County Hospital, DK-2730 Herlev, Denmark

HOWARD T. CHANG Department of Anatomy and Neurobiology, College of Medicine, University of Tennessee, Memphis, Tennessee 38163

BIBIE M. CHRONWALL School of Basic Life Sciences, Division of Structure and Systems Biology, University of Missouri, Kansas City, Missouri 64108

TAMÁS F. FREUND MRC Anatomical Neuropharmacology Unit, University Department of Pharmacology, Oxford OX1 3QT, United Kingdom; *present address:* First Department of Anatomy, Semmelweis University Medical School, H-1450 Budapest, Hungary

WILLIAM A. GEARY II Department of Neurology, University of Virginia Medical Center, Charlottesville, Virginia 22908

CHARLES R. GERFEN Laboratory of Cell Biology, National Institute of Mental Health, Bethesda, Maryland 20892

LENNART HEIMER Departments of Otolaryngology and Neurosurgery, University of Virginia Medical Center, Charlottesville, Virginia 22908

CINDA HELKE Department of Pharmacology, Uniformed Services University of the Health Sciences, Bethesda, Maryland 20814

TOMAS HÖKFELT Department of Histology, Karolinska Institute, Stockholm, Sweden

STEPHEN T. KITAI Department of Anatomy and Neurobiology, College of Medicine, University of Tennessee, Memphis, Tennessee 38163

CSABA LERANTH Section of Neuroanatomy and Department of Obstetrics and Gynecology, Yale University School of Medicine, New Haven, Connecticut 06510

MICHAEL E. LEWIS Cephalon Inc., West Chester, Pennsylvania 19380

R. LONG Clinical Neuroscience Branch, National Institute of Mental Health, Bethesda, Maryland 20205

JESUS LUNA Department of Anatomy and Cell Biology, Division of Neurobiology, University of Cincinnati College of Medicine, Cincinnati, Ohio 45267

JOHN H. McLEAN Department of Anatomy and Cell Biology, Division of Neurobiology, University of Cincinnati College of Medicine, Cincinnati, Ohio 45267

TERESA A. MILNER Department of Neurology and Neuroscience, Division of Neurobiology, Cornell University Medical College, New York, New York 10021

ENRICO MUGNAINI Department of Psychology, University of Connecticut, Storrs, Connecticut 06269–4154

THOMAS L. O'DONOHUE† J. D. Searle and Co., CNS Research, St. Louis, Missouri

MIKLÓS PALKOVITS First Department of Anatomy, Semmelweis University Medical School, H-1450 Budapest, Hungary, and Laboratory of Cell Biology, National Institute of Mental Health, Bethesda, Maryland 20892

G. RICHARD PENNY Department of Anatomy and Neurobiology, College of Medicine, University of Tennessee, Memphis, Tennessee 38163

VIRGINIA M. PICKEL Department of Neurology and Neuroscience, Division of Neurobiology, Cornell University Medical College, New York, New York 10021

BRITA ROBERTSON Clinical Neuroscience Branch, National Institute of Mental Health, Bethesda, Maryland 20205, and Department of Anatomy, Karolinska Institute, Stockholm, Sweden

PAUL E. SAWCHENKO Developmental Neurobiology Laboratory, The Salk Institute, San Diego, California 92138

JAMES S. SCHWABER Neurobiology Group, E. I. duPont de Nemours and Co., Inc., Wilmington, Delaware 19858

MICHAEL T. SHIPLEY Department of Anatomy and Cell Biology, Division of Neurobiology, and Department of Neurosurgery, University of Cincinnati College of Medicine, Cincinnati, Ohio 45267

LANA R. SKIRBOLL Clinical Neuroscience Branch, National Institute of Mental Health, Bethesda, Maryland 20205

PETER SOMOGYI MRC Anatomical Neuropharmacology Unit, University Department of Pharmacology, Oxford OX1 3QT, United Kingdom

KARL THOR Department of Pharmacology, Uniformed Services University of the Health Sciences, Bethesda, Maryland 20814

G. FREDERICK WOOTEN Department of Neurology, University of Virginia Medical Center, Charlottesville, Virginia 22908

LÁSZLÓ ZÁBORSZKY Department of Otolaryngology, University of Virginia Medical Center, Charlottesville, Virginia 22908

† Deceased.

Preface

This book is dedicated to Alf Brodal, Walle J. H. Nauta, and János Szentágothai, all of whom we have had the privilege to know as teachers, friends, and colleagues. These three pioneers labored hard and with unfailing dedication in the early stages of their careers to come up with better ways to trace neuronal connections; they developed tract-tracing methods and used them with such flair as to change forever the course and character of neuroscientific endeavor.

The recently deceased Alf Brodal improved the Gudden method for studying retrograde changes in cells following interruption of their efferent fibers (Brodal, 1939, 1940). He also became one of the foremost experts in the use of experimental silver methods as witnessed by his many classic investigations of brainstem and cerebellar connections. Walle Nauta was stubbornly convinced of the inherent value of using experimentally induced axonal degeneration in the study of neuronal pathways, and he left no stone unturned in the search for new and better staining solutions. The Nauta silver impregnation method (Nauta, 1950, 1957; Nauta and Gygax, 1951, 1954) and its various modifications breathed new life into neuroanatomy and were fundamental to the subsequent development of the neurosciences in general. János Szentágothai was also a pioneer in the use of experimental silver impregnation techniques (Schimert,* 1938, 1939; Szentágothai-Schimert, 1941); however, he is more often remembered for the finesse with which he combined light and electron microscopic techniques for the defintion of neuronal pathways and is widely acclaimed for his inspiring and imaginative models of neuronal circuitry.

We wish to thank the authors for their contributions and patience during the somewhat lengthy editorial process. Our interactions with Plenum Press, and in particular with Mary Born, have been altogether pleasant. Last, but not least, we would like to acknowledge the continuous encouragement and support of the University of Virginia Medical Center and the generous monetary support provided over many years by the National Institutes of Health.

Lennart Heimer
László Záborszky

Charlottesville

---

*In publications until 1940 Dr. Szentágothai used his original family name, Schimert.

REFERENCES

Brodal, A., 1939, Experimentelle Untersuchungen über retrograde Zellveränderungen in der unteren Olive nach Läsionen des Kleinhirns, *Z. Ges. Neurol. Psychiatr.* **166:**624–704.

Brodal, A., 1940, Modification of Gudden method for study of cerebral localization, *Arch. Neurol. Psychiatr.* **43:**46–58.

Nauta, W. J. H., 1950, Über die sogenannte terminale Degenerations im Zentralnervensystem und ihre Darstellung durch Silberimpregnation, *Arch. Neurol. Psychiatr.* **66:**353–376.

Nauta, W. J. H., 1957, Silver impregnation of degenerating axons, in: *New Research Techniques of Neuroanatomy* (W. F. Windle, ed.), Charles C. Thomas, Springfield, IL, pp. 17–26.

Nauta, W. J. H., and Gygax, P. A., 1951, Silver impregnation of degenerating axon terminals in the central nervous system (1) technic (2) chemical notes, *Stain Technol.* **26:**5–11.

Nauta, W. J. H., and Gygax, P. A., 1954, Silver impregnation of degenerating axons in the central nervous system. A modified technique, *Stain Technol.* **27:**175–179.

Schimert, J., 1938, Die Endigungsweise des Tractus Vestibulospinalis, *Z. Anat. Entwick. Gesch.* **108:**761–767.

Schimert, J., 1939, Das Verhalten der Hinterwurzelkollateralen im Rückenmark, *Z. Anat. Entwick. Gesch.* **109:**665–687.

Szentágothai-Schimert, J., 1941, Die Endigungsweise der absteigenden Rückenmarksbahnen, *Z. Anat. Entwick. Gesch.* **111:**322–330.

Contents

Chapter 4

Combinations of Tracer Techniques, Especially HRP and PHA-L,
with Transmitter Identification for Correlated Light and Electron
Microscopic Studies.. 49
LÁSZLÓ ZÁBORSZKY and LENNART HEIMER

Chapter 7

Intracellular Labeling and Immunocytochemistry.................... 173
STEPHEN T. KITAI, G. RICHARD PENNY, and HOWARD T. CHANG

Chapter 8

Synaptic Relationships of Golgi-Impregnated Neurons as Identified by
Electrophysiological or Immunocytochemical Techniques 201
TAMÁS F. FREUND and PETER SOMOGYI

Chapter 9

Immunocytochemistry and Synaptic Relationships of Physiologically
Characterized HRP-Filled Neurons 239
PETER SOMOGYI and TAMÁS F. FREUND

Chapter 10

In Situ Hybridization Combined with Retrograde Fluorescent Tract
Tracing.. 265
BIBIE M. CHRONWALL, MICHAEL E. LEWIS, JAMES S. SCHWABER,
and THOMAS L. O'DONOHUE

Chapter 13

Processing and Analysis of Neuroanatomical Images 331
MICHAEL T. SHIPLEY, JESUS LUNA, and JOHN H. McLEAN

Tract Tracing for the 1990s

ENRICO MUGNAINI

The development of new techniques can be a straining and sometimes frustrating experience; it is time consuming and not necessarily the kind of activity that can be planned in sufficient detail to attract the attention of grant-awarding agencies. Tinkering with techniques, however, is often instrumental in fostering exciting advancements, because the tinker-and-toil process leads to the development of new experimental procedures that pave the way for enlightened vistas and conceptual breakthroughs. When new protocols have been successfully applied to a variety of experimental subjects and the variable parameters have been critically evaluated, the methods usually become widely applied across laboratories. "How-to-do" handbooks are the catalysts in this process, and it is a tribute to the ingenuity of the investigators when the interval between the publication of successive handbooks shortens and the set of available handbooks thickens.

This volume is, in part, an updated version and, in part, a complement to the book on *Neuroanatomical Tract-Tracing Methods,* edited by Lennart Heimer and Martine T. RoBards and published by Plenum Press in New York, 1981. It also follows in the wake of several other handbooks on neuroanatomical techniques, including *The Use of Axonal Transport for Studies of Neuronal Connectivity* (W. M. Cowan and M. Cuenod, eds., Elsevier, Amsterdam, 1975), *Neuroanatomical Techniques* (N. J. Strausfeld and T. A. Miller, eds., Springer-Verlag, New York, 1980), *Techniques in Neuroanatomical Research* (C. Heym and W.-G. Forssmann, eds., Springer-Verlag, Berlin, 1981), *Neuroanatomical Research Techniques* (R. T. Robertson, ed., Academic Press, New York, 1978), and *Tracing Neural Connections with Horseradish Peroxidase* (M.-M. Mesulam, ed., John Wiley & Sons, New York, 1982). These handbooks, in turn, complemented *New Research Techniques of Neuroanatomy* (W. F. Windle and

ENRICO MUGNAINI • Department of Psychology, University of Connecticut, Storrs, Connecticut 06269–4154.

C. C. Thomas, eds., John Wiley, New York, 1958) and *Contemporary Research Methods in Neuroanatomy* (W. J. H. Nauta and S. O. E. Ebbeson, eds., Springer-Verlag, New York, 1970).

This volume includes substantial refinements in tract tracing and neuronal microcircuit analysis to justify a new edition; for example, the utilization of *Phaseolus vulgaris* leukoagglutinin in anterograde tracing, choleratoxin-conjugated horseradish peroxidase in retrograde tracing, biocytin in intracellular labeling, autoradiography in receptor mapping, *in situ* hybridization for detection of messenger RNAs, and computer-assisted procedures for quantitative analysis. Furthermore, whereas the previously published handbooks were largely dedicated to the exposition of individual procedures, most chapters in this volume contain protocols for the combination of two or more procedures that highlight, even in the same tissue section, complementary aspects of neuronal microcircuits. Many of the following chapters present effective methods affording combined structural and chemical information.

In a sense, this book thus constitutes a guideline for a marriage of neuroanatomy and neurochemistry. Although it is true that chemical neuroanatomy has been in the air since Nissl attempted to relate cell chromatophilic patterns with specific neural functions, it is only recently, and particularly after the advent of immunocytochemistry, that neurochemistry and anatomic brain structure are being precisely and widely integrated. Tract tracing has also been combined with *in situ* hybridization histochemistry, quantitative receptor autoradiography, biochemical assays, and neurophysiology. It is now possible to explore structurally not only static but also dynamic aspects of brain circuitry, such as the transsynaptic regulation of many structure–function relationships.

Exciting possibilities exist to apply many of these new methods to *in vitro* brain-slice preparations for the study of functional neuroanatomy. The successful production of high-titer antibodies to amino acid haptens and enzymes in the chains of second messenger pathways and their substrates, as well as the increasing purity of antisera to receptor proteins and ion channels, is not only increasing the precision of immunolocalization of functionally relevant molecules but is also enlarging the range of questions that one may wish to approach in the study of neural connections. Thus, it is now possible to provide wiring diagrams of distant projections from characterized neurons with wiring diagrams of local circuits, and these diagrams can include information about neurotransmitters, hormones, neuropeptides, growth factors, their respective synthetic enzymes, receptors, and mRNAs as well as cytoplasmic and nuclear messengers and ion carriers. The development of computer-assisted image-analysis systems and postembedding immunoelectron microscopic procedures is opening the way to quantitative approaches that were wishful thinking only a few years ago.

References throughout this volume bear witness to the application of some of the new methods not only to the brain of animals subjected to experimentation in the laboratory but also to human nervous tissues obtained at autopsy, especially if the latter is performed as close as possible to the time of death, or by intraoperative biopsy. The data thus provided, in combination with the realistic pictures of active neural networks generated by the increasingly sophisticated modern imaging techniques, make it possible to extend detailed inquiries into the connections of the human brain, opening fascinating perspectives for neuropsychology, biological psychiatry, neurology, and rehabilitation medicine.

Evidently, the ambitions of tract-tracing neuroanatomists have evolved considerably and encompass molecular, cellular, and system levels. Brain hodology, in its modern expanded sense, contributes enormously to advancements in neuroscience. This trend will undoubtedly continue into the next decade and is likely to bring an even more expanded role for structural approaches. Neuroanatomy will be instrumental in characterizing neuronal phenotypes that determine the functions of neural networks *in vivo* and in exploring the plasticity of the developing, mature, and aging brain, normal or diseased. Although the mushrooming advances in molecular neurobiology and ion channel biophysics will bring about several breakthroughs independently of other neuroscience disciplines, it seems reasonable to suggest that in many other cases and in order to exploit fully the results thus obtained, it will be necessary to integrate the new data at the levels of local microcircuits and neural systems.

The young scientist who aspires to become a first-rate neuroanatomist for the 1990s will quickly realize that neuroanatomy is one of the most exciting and rapidly expanding fields in all of neuroscience, and the possibilities to combine a variety of techniques to probe virgin territory are almost unlimited, as they appear to be determined primarily by the experimenter's own imagination and technical skills. But the dedication must be uncompromising. The myriad successive treatments of brain sections exemplified in this volume, even when performed according to well-proven protocols, are labor intensive and time consuming. The requirements of quantitative approaches and combination of various methods often compound the difficulty of the procedure. The effort and time involved are further magnified when investigations are extended at the electron microscopic level, where well-controlled alteration of native molecules and systems, adequate preservation of ultrastructure, and sufficient sample size require great attention to detail and considerable patience.

The methods described in this volume are becoming well established in many laboratories, although at times they are difficult to employ and exploit in full. Not included are other promising techniques, of which the parameters and mechanisms may not yet have been amply experimented with or resolved (Buhl and Lubke, 1989; Godement *et al.*, 1987; Sagar *et al.*, 1988; Ugolini *et al.*, 1989). These and other newly developed procedures may, in particular cases, hold advantages that cannot be fully appreciated at present. Furthermore, adaptation to tract tracing of new methods designed for other purposes (Lichtman *et al.*, 1985) may help solve specific problems otherwise difficult to approach. In other words, once a good cook, one does not need to always follow established recipes; creative combinations of spices and new flavors are fair game.

The list of contributors to this handbook contains several of the authors whose chapters appeared in the previous volume of *Neuroanatomical Tract-Tracing Methods,* but it also includes many new authors who have contributed to the methodological advances of the present decade. It is to be hoped that this handbook will contribute to the development of novel and progressively more quantitative procedures, and it is a foregone conclusion that its readers will include many new authors of chapters yet to be written. With an increasing role in the generation and consolidation of new knowledge, the emerging neuroanatomists have ample reason to herald the next decade with pride and confidence.

REFERENCES

Buhl, E. H., and Lubke, J., 1989, Intracellular lucifer yellow injection in fixed brain slices combined with retrograde tracing, light and electron microscopy, *Neuroscience* **28:**3–16.

Godement, P., Venselow, J., Thanos, S., and Bonhoeffer, F., 1987, A study in developing visual systems with a new method of staining neurones and their processes in fixed tissue, *Development* **101:**697–713.

Lichtman, J. W., Wilkinson, R. S., and Rich, M. M., 1985, Multiple innervation of tonic endplates revealed by activity-dependent uptake of fluorescent probes, *Nature* **314:**357–360.

Sagar, S. M., Sharp, F. R., and Curran, T., 1988, Expression of *c-fos* protein in brain: Metabolic mapping at the cellular level, *Science* **240:**1328–1331.

Ugolini, G., Kuypers, H. G. J. M., and Strick, P. L., 1989, Transneuronal transfer of Herpes virus from peripheral nerves to cortex and brain stem, *Science* **243:**89–91.

2

Use of Retrograde Fluorescent Tracers in Combination with Immunohistochemical Methods

LANA R. SKIRBOLL, KARL THOR,
CINDA HELKE, TOMAS HÖKFELT,
BRITA ROBERTSON, and R. LONG

I. INTRODUCTION

The use of retrograde markers in combination with methods for visualizing transmitters or related substances dates back to the mid-1970s (Ljungdahl *et al.*, 1975), and since then many different combinations have been successfully applied for the tracing of transmitter specific pathways in the brain. Following the introduction of the fluorescent retrograde markers by Kuypers and his collaborators (Kuypers *et al.*, 1977), several groups have described

LANA R. SKIRBOLL and R. LONG • Clinical Neuroscience Branch, National Institute of Mental Health, Bethesda, Maryland 20205.   KARL THOR and CINDA HELKE • Department of Pharmacology, Uniformed Services University of the Health Sciences, Bethesda, Maryland 20814.   TOMAS HÖKFELT • Department of Histology, Karolinska Institute, Stockholm, Sweden.   BRITA ROBERTSON • Clinical Neuroscience Branch, National Institute of Mental Health, Bethesda, Maryland 20205, and Department of Anatomy, Karolinska Institute, Stockholm, Sweden.

the use of these popular dyes in combination with immuno-histochemistry, formaldehyde-induced fluorescence histochemistry and ace-tylcholinesterase (AChE) staining (Hökfelt *et al.*, 1979, 1980, 1983; Ross *et al.*, 1981; Björklund and Skagerberg, 1979; van der Kooy and Hattori, 1980; Van der Kooy and Stembusch, Van der Kooy *et al.*, 1981a,b; Van der Kooy and Sawchenko, 1982; Albanese and Bentivoglio, 1982; Skirboll and Hök-felt, 1983; Skirboll *et al.*, 1983; Sawchenko and Swanson, 1981, 1982; Saw-chenko *et al.*, 1982; Snyder *et al.*, 1986; Loewy *et al.*, 1986; Thor and Helke, 1987; Charlton and Helke, 1987). The advantage of immunohistochemistry over the latter two techniques lies in its range. In principle, immunostaining permits visualization of any substance against which an antiserum can be raised. Fluorescent immunomarkers, in addition, can be conveniently com-bined with fluorescent immunohistochemistry through the use of multiple filters attached to the fluorescence microscope.

In order to determine if a particular tracer is amenable to combination with immunohistochemistry, several factors must be considered. For ex-ample, is the agent fluorescent in its native state and visible without further histochemical procedures? Is the tracer readily visible in tissue fixed for maximum immunostaining? The main obstacle to combining immunohisto-chemistry and retrograde tracers it the necessity for the dyes to be stable through the water phase when incubation with antisera and rinsing proce-dures are performed. Furthermore, since indirect immunohistochemistry is based mainly on two fluorescent markers, fluorescein isothiocyanate (FITC) and tetramethylrhodamine isothiocyanate (TRITC), it is necessary for the fluorescent dyes to be distinguishable from these secondary immunostains. Finally, the procedure must allow simultaneous evaluation of both types of markers and thus rapid and efficient visualization of colocalization.

In this chapter, we limit the discussion to four fluorescent markers: fast blue, propidium iodide, fluorogold, and rhodamine-filled latex micro-spheres* (rhodamine beads). Additional markers are discussed in a recent review by Skirboll *et al.* (1984). The methodology described in the Appendix has been used in several studies (Skirboll *et al.*, 1983; Skirboll and Hökfelt, 1983; Hökfelt *et al.*, 1979, 1980, 1983; Snyder *et al.*, 1986; Loewy *et al.*, 1986; Charlton and Helke, 1987; Thor and Helke, 1987).

II. METHODOLOGICAL CONSIDERATIONS

A. Choice of Retrograde Fluorescent Marker

Retrograde tracing when combined with immunocytochemistry presents certain problems that may or may not be relevant to the use of either dye or

---

*Fast blue was obtained from Accurate Chemicals, Westbury, NY. Propidium iodide was pur-chased from Sigma Chemical, St. Louis, MO, and rhodamine beads were available from Tracer Technologies, Bardonia, NY. Fluorogold was gift from Fluorochrome, Inc., Engelwood, CO. New and promising fluorescent tracers are continually being developed, one example being the recently introduced green fluorescent microspheres (Katz and Iarovici, 1988).

beads in simple tracing studies. Each tracer has inherent problems with regard to ease of injection, spread from injection site, transport efficiency and time, as well as stability within the labeled cell before and after fixation. In combination with immunocytochemistry, the most important factor when considering the appropriate tracer rests with the stability of the label after several exposures to a water phase. We found that each of the dyes described herein is useful both as a retrograde tracer and in combination with immunohistochemistry. In this regard, each of the four dyes, fast blue, propidum iodide, fluorogold, and rhodamine beads, has advantages and disadvantages depending on its use and the system being traced, and it is not possible to recommend one dye unequivocally over another.

The most important new dyes since our previous review of this approach (Skirboll *et al.*, 1984) are fluorogold and the rhodamine beads. At present, fluorogold does seem to present fewer problems than fast blue and rhodamine beads and seems to be more efficient than propidium iodide. If the experimenter has a preference to the use of one secondary antibody over another, fluorogold or rhodamine beads might be tested first. We have tested the use of retrograde tracers with the avidin–biotin complex (ABC) immunohistochemical method. Although this combination is possible, and one can switch back and forth between light field and fluorescence, the quality of the stain and the viability of the dye are less dependable than that seen when dye is combined with indirect fluorescence.

1. Rhodamine Beads

The primary advantage of rhodamine beads (Katz *et al.*, 1984) as compared to the other fluorescent dyes lies in the ability to make very discrete injections with little spread of the tracer from the site of injection and apparently no uptake into undamaged axons of passage. These properties might well be related to the size of the beads. Rhodamine beads also appear to be particularly efficient with regrade to uptake by terminals and retrograde transport. Preliminary results from experiments that seek to compare the beads directly with other dyes indicate that beads may be more sensitive in the sense that they label a greater number of afferent neurons when compared with other dyes of similar volumes (Liu and Panchura, Department of Anatomy, USUHS, personal communication). In addition, there is no loss of the beads during the immunohistochemical procedure, and there is virtually no fading during examination or photography provided sections are well hydrated. Finally, because of the distinctive nature of the beads, there is little chance of false negative or positive results either with regard to retrograde labeling or in combination with immunostaining.

The primary disadvantage of rhodamine beads is the incomplete morphological profile of the labeled neurons. Since the beads do not diffusely or uniformly fill the cytoplasm, the morphology of a labeled cell cannot usually be appreciated. Furthermore, if two neurons are adjacent and equally labeled, one might count the two cells as one. However, the combination of rhodamine beads with immunostaining resolves some of these problems, since the morphology and the boundaries of an immunostained cell are clear. Another disadvantage that rhodamine beads share with propidium iodide relates to the red fluorescence against a dark background, which reduces the chance of spotting a labeled cell, particularly when scanning a section at low magnification. This necessitates slow and careful examination of slides at high magnification. In combination with immunohistochemistry, rhodamine beads must be used with FITC secondary antibodies.

2. Fast Blue and Fluorogold

Fast blue and fluorogold are equally effective with regard to both transport time and visualization, although fluorogold appears to fill dendrites more readily. Both dyes seem to share many other qualities. Both of them apparently are taken up by damaged fibers of passage but not by intact fibers; they do not seem to be taken up in significant amounts following ventricular administration (Kuypers *et al.*, 1979a,b; Kuypers and Huisman, 1984; Schmued and Fallon, 1986). Fast blue, however, has some disadvantages that fluorogold does not have. Primarily, fast blue washes out of the cells to a greater extent than does fluorogold after being carried through the immunocytochemical cycles. In addition, the intensity of the fluorogold stain is unaffected by exposure to a water phase, whereas fast blue fluorescence appears to become more diffuse in all but the most intensely labeled cells. For this reason, fluorogold does not require the tedious process of photography prior to immunostaining, although when using fast blue this is necessary. Both fast blue and fluorogold allow the use of TRITC and thus will permit visualization of retrograde label and immunostaining by simply switching filter systems.

3. Propidium Iodide

Propidium iodide is more stable in the cells than fast blue. However, it does appear to have a longer transport time, and preliminary studies suggest that it may not be effective in some systems. For example, we found only a few labeled cells in the raphe nuclei after injection of propidium iodide into the spinal cord. In addition, and as with rhodamine beads, faintly labeled cells are difficult to spot at low magnification against a dark background, making initial scans of sections difficult at best.

B. Tracer Injection

It is a prime importance to administer the dyes precisely and with limited spread. Dyes can be administered into the brain using a variety of methods including Hamilton syringe, pressure ejection through a micropipette, iontophoresis, and chronic micropipette implants (for a review see Alheid *et al.*,

1981). Fluorescent tracers are used in solution or suspension in concentrations varying from 1 to 5% (w/v) in water for the dyes and 1 : 1 to 1 : 4 in phosphate-buffered saline (PBS) for the rhodamine beads. Schmued and Fallon (1986) report that mixing fluorogold with PBS rather than with water results in slower uptake and diffusion as a result of suspension formation. In some cases the dyes can be suspended with the aid of an ultrasonic waterbath. Although the solution can be stored in the refrigerator for several weeks, a fresh solution is preferred. The higher concentrations of tracer give a denser neuronal labeling but are more difficult to inject because of greater viscosity. This, in turn, may make it more difficult to control the ejection volume.

In most cases, the injection site consists of a central area of high dye concentration surrounded by a concentric zone of decreasing density. At the periphery of the injection site, individual cell bodies labeled with dye are often observed. The problem of determining the effective injection site is an important one. The uptake site for a particular dye may or may not extend beyond the site of densest tracer deposit. Although we have not studied this issue in detail, it is an important consideration, as is the effect of the dye deposit along the injection track. The problem related to the effective injection site when using HRP was discussed by Warr *et al.* (1981). Injections of 0.2 μl of dye or 50 nl of beads generally produce injection sites with a diameter of 100–150 μm. Ejection of highly concentrated dye solutions (5–10%) using the Hamilton syringe technique sometimes results in a central area of necrosis. Iontophoretic dye injections from glass pipettes reduce the amount of dye deposited and permit a more specific site delineation. Fast blue, propidium iodide, and fluorogold can all be administered successfully using iontophoresis.

C. Tracer Transport

When working with retrograde dyes, it is of primary importance to determine the postinjection survival time that provides optimal neuronal labeling. The optimum time period is that in which the compound may accumulate in the cell in the absence of discernible intracellular breakdown. Different factors determine the optimal survival time for different tracers, and there are no rules that can be applied to all tracers. In practice, the optimal time will vary widely depending on the tracer, the system, and the species being studied as well as the method of tissue processing.

In our experience, fast blue, propidium iodide, and fluorogold are usually adequately transported over a 48-hr to 4-day period, and longer survival times may not lead to markedly brighter fluorescence. On the other hand, with fast blue and propidium iodide some glial labeling was seen after long survival times. In our experience, propidium iodide is transported less effectively over long distances. Rhodamine beads, however, are adequately transported over a 48-hr period in projections from the cerebral cortex to the nucleus of the solitary tract, the longest distance examined in our material. Staining appears to increase slightly with a 5-day survival period, but this increase has not been verified quantitatively. Since none of these agents are metabolized or exocytosed, exceeding calculated transport time is recommended. Finally, in our experience, increasing the concentration of any of the dyes above the optimal levels (fast blue, 3%; propidium iodide, 5%; fluorogold 3%) does not increase either the intensity or the quality of the label.

D. Maintenance of Fluorescent Signal

One of the most serious problems with regard to accurate use of fluorescent dyes comes from fading on exposure to ultraviolet (UV) light. We examined this factor by looking at the effects of exposure times on dye intensity. It was found that fast blue was particularly susceptible to fading, showing discernible differences within 120 sec of exposure. The use of 0.1% *p*-phenylenediamine in the buffered glycerine mounting medium has been reported to retard fading (Johnson and De C Nogueira Araujo, 1981; Platt and Michael, 1983). In comparison, fluorogold and propidium iodide were relatively resistant to UV exposure, showing marked fading only after 20-min exposures. In the case of rhodamine beads, there was no appreciable fading with exposure times as long as 30 min when sections were examined immediately after coverslipping. After 1 day of storage, however, when the sections were dehydrated and the plasticizers in the mounting media had hardened, the beads faded in less than 60 sec. This problem was overcome by (1) removing the coverslip by soaking the slide for 20 min in PBS, (2) rehydrating the tissue sections by briefly dipping the slide in PBS, (3) recoverslipping the slide with Permafluor, and (4) immediately examining the tissue.

E. Visualization of Fluorescent Signal

The emission and activation maxima of each of the retrograde agents result in differences in the color of fluorescence visualized under the microscope. Effective use of these color differences with the appropriate filter combination permits effective separation of the retrogradely transported fluorescent dye from the fluorophores conjugated to the second antibody of the immunocytochemical process. For this purpose, UV excitation was used to visualize fast blue and fluorogold, blue excitation was used for FITC, and green excitation for TRITC, rhodamine beads, and propidium iodide (Fig. 1). Thus, under proper filter combinations (Table I), propidium iodide, rhodamine beads, and TRITC fluoresce red or orange-red, fast blue shows an ice-blue color, fluorogold shows a yellow-gold color, and FITC fluoresces green. If the dye in the case of propidium iodide and fluorogold does not wash out during the immunohistochemical procedure, it is possible to visualize dye

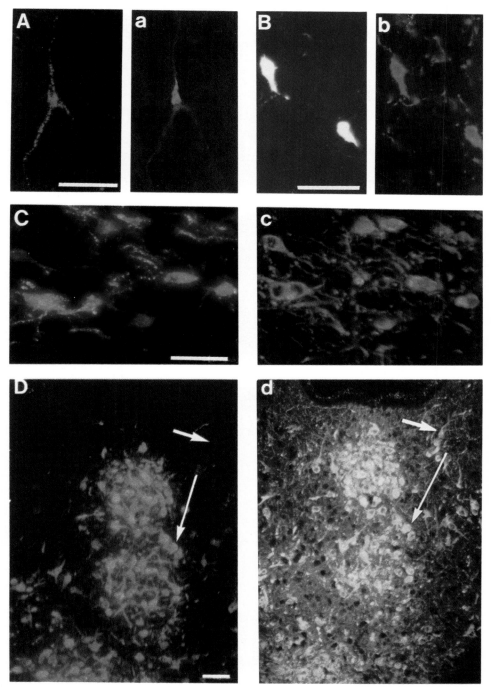

Figure 1. Fluorescence (A,B,C,D) and immunofluorescence (a,b,c,d) micrographs of the medullary raphe (Aa) and dorsal raphe (Dd) nuclei and substantia nigra (Bb,Cc) after injection of retrograde dye into the nucleus tractus solitarius (Aa) or the caudate nucleus (Bb,Cc,Dd). Micrographs show the same area of the same section after processing for immunohistochemistry with antibodies to serotonin (Aa,Dd) or tyrosine hydroxylase (TH) (Bb,Cc). A: Micrograph of cells retrogradely labeled with rhodamine beads. B: Labeled cells filled with fast blue. C: Cells retrogradely labeled with fluorogold. D: Micrograph of cells labeled with propidium iodide. Arrows note the presence of cells labeled by retrograde dye that are (long arrow) and are not (short arrow) immunopositive for serotonin. Bars indicate 50 μm.

and immunostain in the same session by simply switching to the appropriate filter.

More specifically, fast blue gives rise to fluorescence throughout the cytoplasm and in some cases extends into the dendritic processes. Labeled cells show a strongly yellow-gold granular fluorescence. The labeled cells are occasionally surrounded by glial staining. After immunohistochemical staining, the dye can also diffuse into the cell nucleus. The fluorescence of fast blue, which is intense and granular in nature, is routinely viewed through the blue filter system. With the filter combinations described in Table I, minimal fast blue label could be visualized through the FITC filters, and no shinethrough was visible through the rhodamine filters. Thus, when using fast blue as the retrograde dye, it is very important that TRITC-labeled secondary antibodies be used. It should be noted that TRITC-stained cells can be seen through the blue filter system where they appear greenish-brown, a hue that can be clearly distinguished from fast-blue-labeled cells. When the two overlap, there will be a mixed appearance, and the intensity of each will decide the dominant color (Fig. 1C,c).

Fluorogold fills the cytoplasm, and with particularly dense staining it also labels the nucleus. It appears to fill dendritic processes to a greater extent than does fast blue, especially after longer survival times. Its fluorescence has a bright, granular yellow-gold appearance, and it does not appear to migrate into glia or adjacent neurons. This tracer is viewed through the same filter combination as that used for fast blue. Unlike fast blue, however, it does not shine through the rhodamine filters, and it is barely visible through the FITC filters. In very intensely stained cells viewed under the FITC filters, a minimal red stain can be seen in cells that contain the fluorogold. However, since this color is distinct from the green fluorescence of FITC, there is little chance of a false positive result. Thus, when fluorogold is used as the retrograde dye, either rhodamine or FITC secondary labels can be used (Fig. 1B,b).

Propidium iodide is also useful as a retrograde dye. In the microscope under green excitation, it appears red. This dye fills the cytoplasm, and only minimal labeling can be seen in the nucleus of a cell. It fills the dendritic tree to a lesser extent than does fast blue or fluorogold. Some glial labeling can be seen after long survival times. Because of the lesser contrast between

Table I. Filter Combinations with Zeiss and Leitz Microscopes

Signal	Excitation	Dichroic reflector	Barrier filter	Leitz block
True blue	6-365	FT-395	LP-420	System A
FITC	BP 485/20	FT-510	LP-520	System K2 of I2
Rhodamine	BP 546/12	FT-580	LP-590	System N2

red stain and a black background as compared to the blue or gold of the other dyes, this agent is less desirable for scanning of labeled cells at low magnification. A weakly labeled cell is sometimes very hard to distinguish from the background, especially prior to immunostaining. Because of its red appearance under the microscope, an FITC secondary label should be used in combination with this dye. However, under the FITC filters, propidium iodide label can shine through as reddish yellow. Although this is generally clearly distinguishable from FITC immunostaining, the difference can be enhanced by the use of a red elimination filter (Schott KP 560). In addition, since this shinethrough is red in color, there is no risk of a false positive result (Fig. 1D,d).

Rhodamine beads appear in the microscope as red. The number of individual rhodamine beads contained in neurons varies tremendously. Sometimes fewer than five beads may be concentrated in an area appropriate for the size and shape of a neuronal cell body. This makes it difficult to assign labeling to a neuron, especially if some beads are distributed randomly not only in cell bodies but also in axons and dendrites. If more than 100 beads are aggregated in a similar space, the labeling of a neuronal cell body is usually obvious. Generally, we felt confident in describing 20 or more beads in an area of 600 μm^2 or less as being contained in a single neuron, provided the boundaries conform to the morphological shape of a neuron. Subsequent immunostaining then allows a more exact definition of the exact cellular localization of the beads. With regard to the specific location of the beads, it appears that they are limited to the cytoplasm. Rhodamine beads appear red under the appropriate filter system. However when used in combination with FITC immunostaining, they may shine through the FITC filters as yellow dots. The distinctive nature of the rhodamine beads ensures that a cell filled with beads will not be mistaken for an immunostained cell (Fig. 1A,a).

F. Diffusion of Tracer

One of the most important issues with regard to the effective combination of retrograde dye and immunofluorescence is the diffusion of the tracer. This can occur at several stages: *in vivo* prior to sacrifice, during fixation and sectioning, or during the wet immunohistochemical procedure. Diffusion may have several consequences, including a complete or partial loss of the dye, decreased intensity with selective loss of weakly labeled cells, leading to false negative results, or diffusion into surrounding neurons, producing false positive results. This problem is particularly prevalent for fast blue, which appears to change from a more granular to a more soluble form in the cytoplasm, in which case it may invade the nucleus or glia post-mortem during the wet procedure. We reported (Skirboll *et al.*, 1983) a 33% loss of fast-blue-labeled cells during immunostaining, whereas others have reported 5% or 15% loss (Sawchenko and Swanson, 1981; van der Kooy and Sawchenko, 1982).

Although we see little washout with propidium iodide, van der Kooy and Sawchenko (1982) report a 20% loss with this dye. These differences may reflect differences in survival time, fixation, and/or fixation time. In our hands, the retention also varies from system to system. Furthermore, we have found that neither fluorogold nor rhodamine beads appear to diffuse during the water phase of immunohistochemistry. In any one investigator's hands, differences in diffusion may reflect different survival times or fixation procedures or the fact that various neuronal systems are being studied. In any case, diffusion of the tracer during the immunohistochemical procedure is a difficult problem, and it may be worthwhile to photograph labeled cells before submitting the sections to the water phase required in immunohistochemistry. We have found that mounting sections in xylene tends to reduce diffusion of the tracer initiated by mounting media and does not interfere with subsequent immunostaining. It should be noted, however, that xylene is contraindicated for rhodamine beads, since it decreases the fluorescence of the beads. The method of photographing cells before immunostaining is tedious and expensive, since it requires photographing many cells that may subsequently not stain for a particular antigen.

G. Coexistent Antigens and Tracers

Two approaches can be used to combine studies of coexistent antigens with retrograde tracers. One can either stain adjacent sections that have been sectioned thin enough (less than 6 μm) to cut through the same cell twice or make use of the elution technique described by Tramu *et al.* (1978) to visualize two antigens in the same cell. These methods have been described in detail elsewhere (Hökfelt *et al.*, 1980) and are not discussed here. Suffice it to say that since all of the tracers appear to be destroyed by the acidic solution used in Tramu's procedure, the combination of this method with tracing studies requires a specific protocol. Photography of the tracer must be made prior to visualization of the second antigen. For both the adjacent-section method and the elution technique, the primary concern is delineating the dye from the first immunomarker. The choice of methods depends on the antigens being studied; in our hands some antigens do not stain following the acidic elution. Under these conditions, the study of adjacent sections is preferable. It is, however, important to note that other elution methods are available (Vandesande and Dierick, 1975; Nakane, 1969), and it may be possible to employ them in studies on retrograde tracing of multiple-antigen-containing neurons. Alternatively, double-labeling techniques can be used in combination with retrograde tracing (see Wessendorf and Elde, 1986).

III. ADVANTAGES AND LIMITATIONS

A. Advantages

1. The combination of immunohistochemistry with retrograde tracing permits the visualization of neurotransmitters in the same neuron that is labeled for projection to a particular field.
2. Through the use of retrograde dyes and because of their emission characteristics, the research can stimultaneously visualize retrograde dye and immunostaining in the same cell.
3. The primary advantage of rhodamine beads lies in the apparent ability to make very discrete injections. Another advantage is that there is no loss of the intensity of the dye during the immunohistochemical procedure.
4. Fast blue and fluorogold show a strong fluorescence against a dark background, which can successfully be used when scanning of many sections is required.
5. Fluorogold is relatively resistant to both fading and washout during the water phase of immunocytochemistry.

B. Disadvantages

1. The primary disadvantage of the rhodamine beads is the difficulty in evaluating the number of cells that are labeled.
2. Fast blue is susceptible to fading and to some degree of washout.
3. Both fast blue and fluorogold appear to be taken up by fibers of passage, which can lead to false positive results.
4. Propidium iodide is difficult to view against a dark background but is useful in combination with FITC-labeled secondary antibody.
5. It is difficult to make highly discrete injections of fast blue and fluorogold; when neurons with small projection fields are studied, these dyes might not be useful.
6. When fast blue is used, washout is likely to occur, and it may be necessary to photograph the cells prior to immunostaining. This process is both tedious and time consuming.

IV. APPENDIX

In our laboratory injections of dyes are made either by the aid of a Hamilton syringe equipped with a 22-gauge needle or via a glass pipette attached to a Hamilton syringe or small pump. Volumes injected are 0.2–0.3 μl for dyes and 0.02–0.1 μl for the rhodamine beads. Pipettes are pulled and broken back to a tip diameter of 25–100 μm. For iontophoretic administration, the pipettes are attached to constant-current source, and the dye is delivered with 25–30 μA of alternating current.* Finally, the syringe or pipette is held in place for a minimum of 5 min after the injection is complete and then raised slowly (approximately 0.1 mm/min) to reduce tissue damage and reflux movement of the dye up the cannula track. The dorsal surface of the brain and skull is rinsed with saline, and the muscle and skin are closed. Animals should recover from anesthesia before being returned to animal housing. Survival times depend on the fluorescent tracer used and the fiber system studied but usually range from 24 hr to 10 days.

Immunocytochemical visualization of some peptides in cell bodies requires that the animals be treated with colchicine prior to perfusion for immunostaining. Colchicine is used to arrest axonal transport and causes accumulation of antigen in the cell body (Dahlström, 1971). Because this agent has been shown to affect the transport of the dye (Skirboll et al., 1984), colchicine treatment should be performed after optimal survival time and 24 hr prior to perfusion. Colchicine (120 μg in 20 μl) is usually injected into the lateral ventricle ipsilateral to the side of dye injection.

Although all dyes are retained to some degree in unfixed tissue, perfusion is necessary for adequate immunohistochemical staining. After perfusion with cold buffered saline followed by either saturated picric acid in 10% paraformaldehyde made up from 4% paraformaldehyde or 10% paraformaldehyde alone for 10–20 min, brains are removed from the skull and either immersed in the fixative for 90 min or directly rinsed with 0.1 M phosphate-buffered saline (PBS) and immersed in 10–20% sucrose for at least 24 hr prior to sectioning.

Brains are then processed for indirect immunofluorescence according to Coons and collaborators (1958). Briefly, sections are cut on a cryostat at a thickness of 6–14 μm and mounted on chromalum-gelatin-coated glass slides. They are then examined for the presence of retrograde dye or processed immediately for immunocytochemistry. In some cases, prior to primary antiserum, sections are rinsed for 60 min in 10% normal goat serum to reduce background. One of the following three primary antisera was used for the material illustrating this chapter: tyrosine hydroxylase (dilution 1 : 500), 5-hydroxytryptamine (5-HT) (1 : 500), or monoclonal rat substance P (1 : 1000) at 4°C for 24–48 hr. Following rinsing in 0.3–2.0% PBS, the sections were incubated with either FITC-conjugated goat antirabbit or antirat antibodies or tetramethylrhodamine isothiocyanate (TRITC)-labeled goat antirabbit antibodies (1 : 100) for 10–60 min at 37°C. The sections were then rinsed in PBS and mounted in a mixture of glycerol and PBS.† For rhodamine beads, slides mounted with Permafluor and not immediately examined require reimmersion in PBS and recoverslipping prior to visualization.

Sections used for this chapter were examined using either a Zeiss epifluorescence microscope equipped with a ×4 and ×10 Planapo and a ×25 plan

---

*The constant-current source was purchased from Fintronics, Hamden, CT.

†Antisera and reagents were purchased from the following sources: TH, Eugene Tech, Allendale, NJ; 5-HT, Immunonuclear, Stillwater, MN; SP, Pelfreeze, Rogers, AR; TRITC, Boehringer Mannheim, Indianapolis, IN; Permafluor, Immuno, Utica, MI.

neofluar objective or a Leitz Dialux 20 microscope equipped with a Ploempak. Since the emission and activation characteristics of each of the dyes result in clear differences in color, different filter combinations were used to visualize each of the dyes and secondary antibody labels (see Table I).

REFERENCES

Albanese, A., and Bentivoglio, A., 1982, Retrograde fluorescent neuroal tracing combined with acetylcholinesterase histochemistry, *Neurosci. Methods* **6**:121–127.

Alheid, B. F., Edwards, S. B., Kitai, S. T., Park, M. P., and Switzer, R. C., 1981, Methods for delivering tracers, in: *Neuroanatomical Tract-Tracing Methods* (L. Heimer and M. J. Robards, eds.), Plenum Press, New York, pp. 91–113.

Björklund, A., and Skagerberg, G., 1979, Evidence for a major spinal cord projection from the diencephalic A11 dopamine cell group in the rat using transmitter-specific fluorescent retrograde tracing, *Brain Res.* **177**:170–175.

Charlton, C. G., and Helke, C. J., 1987, Substance P containing medullary projections to the intermediolateral cell column: Identification with retrogradely transported rhodamine labeled latex microspheres and immunohistochemistry, *Brain Res.* (in press).

Coons, A. H., 1958, Fluroscent antibody methods, in: *General Cytochemical Methods* (J. F. Danielli, ed.), Academic Press, New York, pp. 394–422.

Dahlström, A., 1971, Effects of vinblastine and colchicine on monoamine containing neurons of the rat with special regard to the axoplasmic transport of amine granules, *Acta Neuropathol. (Berl.)* **5**:226–237.

Hökfelt, T., Terenius, L., Kuypers, H. G. J. M., and Dann, O., 1979, Evidence for enkephalin immunoreactive neurons in the medulla oblongata projecting to the spinal cord, *Neurosci. Lett.* **14**:55–60.

Hökfelt, T., Skirboll, L., Rehfeld, J. F., Goldstein, M., Markey, K., and Dann, O., 1980, A subpopulation of mesencephalic dopamine neurons projecting to limbic areas contains a cholecystokinin-like peptide: Evidence from immunohistochemistry combined with retrograde tracing, *Neuroscience* **5**:2093–2124.

Hökfelt, T., Skagerberg, G., Skirboll, L., and Björklund, A., 1983, Combination of retrograde tracing and neurotransmitter histochemistry, in: *Handbook of Chemical Anatomy. Methods in Chemical Neuroanatomy*, Vol. 1 (A. Björklund and T. Hökfelt, eds.), Elsevier, Amsterdam, pp. 228–285.

Johnson, D. G., and De C Nogueira Araujo, G. M., 1981, A simple method of reducing the fading of immunofluorescence during microscopy, *J. Immunol. Methods* **43**:349.

Katz, L. C., and Iarovici, D. M., 1988, Green fluorescent latex microspheres: a new retrograde tracer, *Neurosci. Abst.* **14**:548.

Katz, L. C., Burkhalter, A., and Dreyer, W. J., 1984, Fluorescent latex microspheres as a retrograde neuronal marker for *in vivo* and *in vitro* studies of visual cortex, *Nature* **310**:498–500.

Kuypers, H. G. J. M., and Huisman, A. M., 1984, Fluorescent tracers, in: *Advances in Cellular Neurobiology*, Vol. 5 (S. Fedoroff, ed.), Academic Press, Orlando, pp. 307–340.

Kuypers, H. G. J. M., Bentivoglio, M., van der Kooy, D., and Catsman-Berrevoets, C. E., 1977, Retrograde transport of bisbenzimide and propidium iodide through axons to their parent cell bodies, *Neurosci. Lett.* **12**:1–7.

Kuypers, H. G. J. M., Bentivoglio, M., van der Kooy, D., and Catsman-Berrevoets, C. E., 1979a, Retrograde axonal transport of fluorescent substances in the rat's forebrain, *Neurosci. Lett.* **6**:127–135.

Kuypers, H. G. J. M., Bentivoglio, M., van der Kooy, D., and Catsman-Berrevoets, C. E., 1979b, Retrograde transport of bisbenzimide and propidium iodide through axons to their parent cell bodies, *Neurosci. Lett.* **12**:1–7.

Ljungdahl, A., Hökfelt, T., Goldstein, M., and Park, D., 1975, Retrograde peroxidase tracing of neurons combined with transmitter histochemistry, *Brain Res.* **84:**313–319.

Loewy, A. D., Marson, L., Parkinson, D., Perry, M. A., and Sawyer, W. B., 1986, Descending noradrenergic pathways involved in the A5 depressor response, *Brain Res.* **386:**313–324.

Nakane, P. K., 1969, Simultaneous localization of multiple tissue antigens using the peroxidase labeled antibody method: A study on pituitary glands of the rat, *J. Histochem. Cytochem.* **16:**557–560.

Platt, J. L., and Michael A. F., 1983, Retardation of fading and enhancement of intensity of immunofluorescence by *p*-phenylenediamine, *J. Histochem. Cytochem.* **31:**840–842.

Ross, C. A., Armstrong, D. M., Ruggiero, D. A., Pickel, V. M., Joh, T. M., and Reis, D. J., 1981, Adrenaline neurons in the rostral ventrolateral medulla innervate thoracic spinal cord: A combined immunocytochemical and retrograde transport demonstration, *Neurosci. Lett.* **25:**257–262.

Sawchenko, P. E., and Swanson, L. W., 1981, A method for tracing biochemically defined pathways in the central nervous system using combined fluorescence retrograde transport and immunohistochemical techniques, *Brain Res.* **210:**31–41.

Sawchenko, P. E., and Swanson, L. W., 1982, Immunohistochemical identification of neurons in the paraventricular nucleus of the hypothalamus that project to the medulla or to the spinal cord in the rat, *J. Comp. Neurol.* **205:**260–272.

Sawchenko, P. E., Swanson, L. W., and Joseph, S. A., 1982, The distribution and cells of origin of ACTH-stained varicosities in the paraventicular and supraoptic nuclei, *Brain Res.* **232:**365–374.

Schmued, L. C., and Fallon, J. H., 1986, Fluoro-gold: A new fluorescent retrograde axonal tracer with numerous unique properties, *Brain Res.* **377:**147–154.

Skirboll, L., and Hökfelt, T., 1983, Transmitter specific mapping of neuronal pathways by immunohistochemistry combined with fluorescent dyes, in: *IBRO Handbook Series: Methods in the Neurosciences. Immunohistochemistry* (A. C. Cuello, ed.), John Wiley & Sons, Chichester.

Skirboll, L., Hökfelt, T., Dockray, G., Rehfeld, J., Brownstein, M., and Cuello, C., 1983, Evidence for periaqueductal cholecystokinin–substance P neurons projecting to the spinal cord, *J. Neurosci.* **3:**1151–1157.

Skirboll, L., Hökfelt, T., Norell, G, Phillipson, D., Kuypers, H. G. J. M., Bentivoglio, M., Catsman-Berrevoets, C. E., Visser, T. J., Steinbusch, H., Verhofstad, A., Cuello, A. C., Goldstein, M., and Brownstein, M., 1984, A method for transmitter identification of retrogradely labeled neurons: Immunofluorescence combined with fluorescence tracing, *Brain Res. Rev.* **8:**99–127.

Snyder, A. M., Zigmond, M. J., and Lund, R. D., 1986, Sprouting of serotonergic afferents into striatum after dopamine-depleting lesions in infant rats: A retrograde transport and immunocytochemical study, *J. Comp. Neurol.* **245:**274–281.

Thor, K. B., and Helke, C., 1987, Central afferents to the nucleus tractus solitarius of the rat: Serotonin and substance P containing neurons in the hindbrain, *J. Comp. Neurol.* (in press).

Tramu, G., Pillez, A., and Leonardelli, J., 1978, An efficient method of antibody elution for the successive or simultaneous location of two antigens by immunocytochemistry, *J. Histochem. Cytochem.* **26:**322–327.

van der Kooy, D., and Hattori, T., 1980, Dorsal raphe cells with collateral projections in the substantia nigra and caudate–putamen. A fluorescent retrograde double labeling study in rat, *Brain Res.* **186:**1–7.

van der Kooy, D., and Sawchenko, P. E., 1982, Characterization of serotonergic neurons using concurrent fluorescent retrograde axonal tracing and immunohistochemistry, *J. Histochem. Cytochem.* **30:**794–798.

van der Kooy, D., and Steinbusch, H. W. M., 1980, Simultaneous fluorescent retrograde axonal tracing and immunofluorescent characterization of neurons, *J. Neurosci. Res.* **5:**479–584.

van der Kooy, D., Coscina, D. V., and Hattori, T., 1981a, Is there a non-dopaminergic nigrostriatal pathway? *Neuroscience* **6:**345–357.

van der Kooy, D., Hunt, S. P., Steinbusch, H. M., and Verhofstad, A., 1981b, Separate populations of cholecystokinin and 5-hydroxtryptamine containing neuronal cells in the rat dorsal raphe, and their contribution to the ascending raphe projections, *J. Neurosci.* **26:**25–30.

Vandesande, F., and Dierick, K., 1975, Identification of the vasopressin producing and of oxytocin producing neurons of the hypothalamic magnocellular neurosecretory system of the cat, *Cell Tissue Res.* **164:**153–162.

Warr, W. B., de Olmos, J. S., and Heimer, L., 1981, Horseradish peroxidase: The basic procedure, in: *Neuroanatomical Tract-Tracing Methods* (L. Heimer and M. J. RoBards, eds.), Plenum Press, New York, 207–256.

Wessendorf, M. W., and Elde, R. P., 1986, Characterization of an immunofluorescence technique for the demonstration of coexisting neurotransmitters within nerve fibers and terminals, *J. Histochem. Cytochem.* **33:**984.

3

The PHA-L Anterograde Axonal Tracing Method

CHARLES R. GERFEN, PAUL E. SAWCHENKO, and JØRN CARLSEN

I. INTRODUCTION

The plant lectin *Phaseolus vulgaris* leukoagglutinin (PHA-L) has unique properties that have made it particularly useful for tracing the axonal projections of neurons (Gerfen and Sawchenko, 1984, 1985). When PHA-L is injected by iontophoresis into the brain and subsequently localized by standard immunohistochemical techniques, neurons at the injection site are labeled in their entirety, revealing the morphology of dendritic arborizations and both local and distant axonal projections. PHA-L appears to label only those neurons that incorporate tracer at the injection site; i.e., there is negligible uptake of the tracer by fibers of passage and negligible retrograde axonal transport of the tracer. In addition, neurons and their axonal projections are labeled with the PHA-L method in a manner that rivals the best Golgi impregnation techniques. With this method the amplification of the signal is generated by the immunohistochemical procedure and both the fluorescent and peroxidase-coupled diaminobenzidine labels provide an accurate visualization of cellular and axonal morphology. Furthermore, because PHA-L is localized with standard immunohistochemical techniques, it may be com-

CHARLES R. GERFEN • Laboratory of Cell Biology, National Institute of Mental Health, Bethesda, Maryland 20892.   PAUL E. SAWCHENKO • Developmental Neurobiology Laboratory, The Salk Institute, San Diego, California 92138.   JØRN CARLSEN • Department of Gastroenterology C, Copenhagen County Hospital, DK-2730 Herlev, Denmark.

bined with other neuroanatomical and neurohistochemical methods. Such combined methods generate information not only concerning the interrelations between separate populations of neurons but also about the neurochemical characteristics of such neurons.

In this chapter the standard procedure for using PHA-L as an anterograde tracer is described, as well as means of combining it with other techniques. Four basic types of combined methods are detailed. First, double anterograde axonal tract tracing to analyze topographic relations of projections of separate populations of neurons (Gerfen, 1985) is accomplished by combining PHA-L with the autoradiographic anterograde axonal tract-tracing method (Cowan *et al.*, 1972). Second, neuroanatomical or neurochemical characterization of the neuronal targets of PHA-L-labeled afferents is accomplished with combinations of the PHA-L method and either retrograde axonal tracing methods or immunohistochemical localization of neurochemical substance in target neurons. Third, the neurochemical characterization of the brain area into which PHA-L-labeled afferents are distributed, either with immunohistochemical techniques (Gerfen, 1984; Heimer *et al.*, 1987) or with autoradiographic localization of receptor binding (Gerfen *et al.*, 1987), provides information that could not be easily determined if the recipient brain area were stained only to show cytoarchitectonic features. Fourth, neurochemical identification of labeled efferent fibers is accomplished by colocalization within PHA-L-labeled fibers of immunohistochemically identifiable substances (Gerfen and Sawchenko, 1985). Such combined methods allow analysis of interrelations between labeled neuronal systems within the same or adjacent sections at the light microscopic level. Electron microscopic localization of PHA-L complements such analysis by demonstrating the ultrastructure of morphological relationships between neurons.

II. PHA-L ANTEROGRADE TRACT TRACING

PHA-L is injected into the brain by iontophoresis through fine-tipped pipettes that are stereotaxically positioned into the brain. During or shortly after injection (within 10 min), the PHA-L is incorporated into a small number of astrocytes and those neurons whose dendrites extend into the vicinity of such astrocytes (Gerfen and Sawchenko, 1984). The number of neurons labeled varies depending on the dendritic topography of the neurons at the injection site and somewhat on the parameters of the iontophoresis. It appears that only neurons labeled at the time of injection incorporate the tracer that is subsequently transported by axons in the anterograde direction. Following this initial period of incorporation, PHA-L diffuses in the neuropil in an area greater than that occupied by labeled astrocytes and neurons. However, because PHA-L does not appear to be incorporated by neurons in those areas to which it diffuses, the effective injection site, which is the area from which PHA-L is incorporated by neurons for anterograde transport, may be definitively determined. The number of neurons labeled does not appear to vary during the survival period, even with long survival periods.

Axonal transport of PHA-L occurs at a relatively slow rate, approximately 4–6 mm per day in the anterograde direction. The optimal survival period is determined by estimating the length of time necessary to label the pathway of interest. Since PHA-L does not appear to be degraded over survival periods of 4–5 weeks, even very long pathways may be traced effectively. Effective and consistent injections have been obtained in virtually all brain areas in a variety of animals, including rats, cats, and primates. Following an appropriate survival period, the animal is sacrificed and the brain processed for immunohistochemical localization of PHA-L.

Figure 1 shows two cases of PHA-L injections that illustrate the typical properties of labeling as seen by an immunofluorescence method. In the first case (Fig. 1A) the injection is centered just to the left of the hippocampal fissure and is marked by the dense labeling of astrocytes (large arrow). The

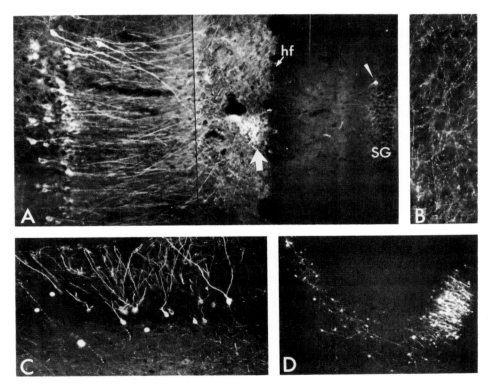

Figure 1. (A) A PHA-L injection to the left of the hippocampal fissure labels a small number of astrocytes (arrow) and CA1 pyramidal neurons whose dendrites extend into the area of the astrocytes. Although tracer diffused into the dentate gyrus outlining the granule cell neurons, only one granule cell is labeled, which extends a dendrite toward the central focus of the injection. (B) Efferents of the CA1 pyramidal neurons in the subiculum are heavily labeled, whereas few mossy fibers, arising from the dentate granule cells, are labeled. (C) In another case an injection of PHA-L into dentate granule cell layer labels many neurons. (D) Many labeled mossy fibers result from the filling of dentate granule cells, in contrast to the small number labeled after the injection shown in A.

great majority of neurons that have incorporated the tracer are located in the CA1 field of the hippocampus. Not every neuron in the CA1 field adjacent to the injection is labeled; rather, it appears that only those neurons are labeled whose dendrites are directed into the area of labeled astrocytes. Spread of the tracer is indicated by the diffuse fluorescence observed in a concentric area on both sides of the hippocampal fissure. On the right side of the fissure, the tracer has spread around the cell bodies of the granule cells of the dentate gyrus. Despite being surrounded by diffuse tracer, only one dentate granule cell has incorporated the tracer, and this cell has a dendrite directed toward the central focus of the injection. Only the axons of neurons that have incorporated the tracer are labeled. In this case the known projections of the CA1 pyramidal cells, e.g., those to the subiculum (Fig. 1B), are densely labeled, and only an occasional mossy fiber from a labeled dentate granule cell is labeled (see also Fig. 2).

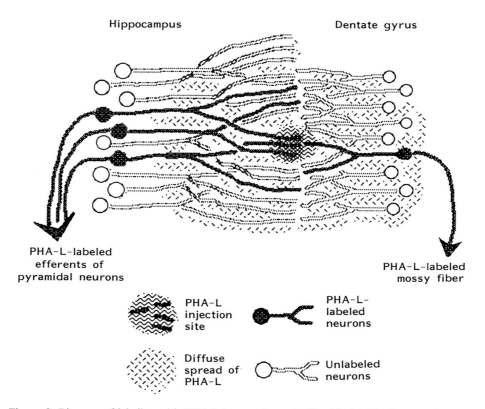

Figure 2. Diagram of labeling with PHA-L in case shown in Fig. 1A. In this diagram the neurons in the hippocampus and the one neuron in the dentate gyrus that are labeled with PHA-L extend dendrites into the center area of the injection. PHA-L diffuses around the central core of the injection but does not label neurons whose dendrites do not extend into the central core of the injection. Only those neurons that are labeled with PHA-L have their efferent axons labeled.

That such specific labeling is due to the location of the injection site, and not to an inability of dentate granule cells to be labeled, is shown by the labeling obtained in another case, in which the injection was located in the dentate gyrus. In this case numerous dentate granule cells are labeled (Fig. 1C; see also Fig. 7A), and so are many of their mossy fiber projections (Fig. 1D).

III. PHA-L INCORPORATION INTO NEURONS

The mechanism of PHA-L incorporation into neurons remains unclear. Differences in the type of labeling obtained with PHA-L and other axonally transported substances suggest different modes of uptake. Tracers commonly used for retrograde transport, including horseradish peroxidase and fluorescent dyes, are most likely incorporated by nonspecific endocytosis into terminals followed by retrograde axonal transport in vesicles with accumulation in perikaryal lysosomes. Such tracers are also incorporated by a similar nonspecific mechanism by dendrites and cell bodies and transported anterogradely in axons. The use of the plant lectin wheat germ agglutinin (WGA), conjugated to peroxidase (Gonatas *et al.*, 1979; Staines *et al.*, 1980), facilitates uptake by the binding of WGA to glycoproteins, which are then endocytosed. Enhanced sensitivity of WGA–HRP as both an anterograde and retrograde tracer over HRP is now commonly recognized (see also Chapter 3).

To compare the uptake and axonal transport properties of PHA-L with WGA we used identical iontophoretic injection parameters and immunohistochemical localization procedures, using diaminobenzindine as a chromogen (Gerfen and Sawchenko, 1984). The advantage of immunohistochemical localization of lectins over TMB histochemical localization of peroxidase is related to the means of signal amplification. Whereas tetramethyl benzidine (TMB) (Mesulam, 1978) histochemistry amplifies the signal by the generation of large reaction crystals, immunohistochemical amplification relies on the layering of immunoglobulins to concentrate more peroxidase (or fluorescent molecules) at the location of each tracer molecule. Figure 3 shows a comparison of the labeling obtained after injections of wheat germ agglutinin (WGA) and PHA-L into the striatum. In the case of PHA-L, the tracer appears to fill a defined population of neurons (Fig. 3A) whose efferent projection fibers to the substantia nigra pars reticulata are labeled (Fig. 3C). On the other hand, after a striatal injection of WGA, the tracer appears diffusely distributed at the injection site (Fig. 3B). With this tracer there is evidence of both retrograde labeling of nigrostriatal neurons in the substantia nigra pars compacta (SNc) and anterograde axonal transport to terminals of the striatonigral afferents in the substantia nigra pars reticulata (Fig. 3D). The labeling is granular in appearance, suggesting a vesicular and/or lysosomal intracellular localization.

The intracellular distribution of PHA-L, as opposed to that of other tracers, may explain its relative longevity; because PHA-L does not enter the lyso-

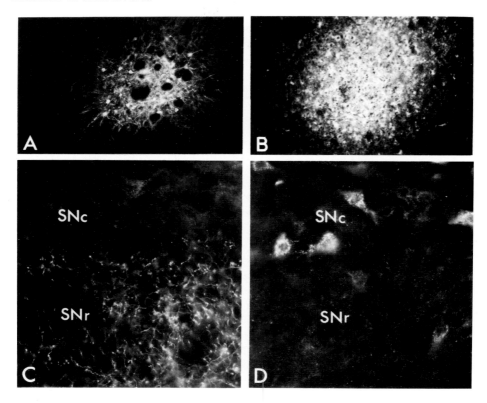

Figure 3. Immunofluorescence localization of two lectins, PHA-L and WGA, after iontophoretic injections into the striatum. (A) Injection of PHA-L into the striatum results in the discrete localization of tracer in medium spiny neurons displaying details of their morphology (see Fig. 4E). (B) An injection of WGA into the striatum appears to spread diffusely, giving nondiscriminate labeling, in contrast to the type of labeling obtained with PHA-L. (C) PHA-L labeling in the substantia nigra after a striatal injection appears specifically to fill the afferent fibers that are distributed in the substantia nigra pars reticulata (SNr). The morphology of the fibers is clearly evident. (D) The WGA labeling in the substantia nigra after a striatal injection takes two forms, retrograde labeling of nigrostriatal neurons in the substantia nigra pars compacta (SNc) and anterograde labeling of striatonigral afferents in the SNr (diffuse and barely detectable). Labeling with WGA appears granular in these fluorescent photomicrographs, as contrasted with the filled appearance of fibers obtained with PHA-L.

somal system, it is not readily degraded. Under some circumstances PHA-L is incorporated in a manner similar to WGA and gives similar labeling. This occurs most often if pressure injections of PHA-L are made or if high currents are used for iontophoresis. It is significant that the granular anterograde and retrograde labeling obtained with WGA, or with PHA-L in some instances, occurs by a fast axonal transport mechanism. The more complete filling of efferent projections obtained with discrete injections of PHA-L occurs by a slow axonal transport mechanism, which has been estimated to be 4–6 mm/day. Figure 4 shows further examples of the type of labeling obtained with PHA-L.

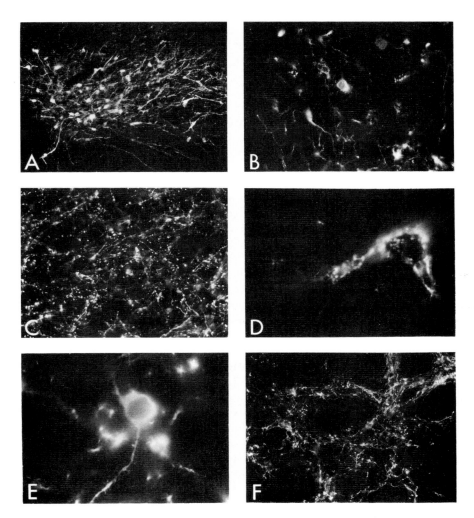

Figure 4. Examples of types of labeling obtained with PHA-L as localized by an indirect immunofluorescence technique. PHA-L-labeled neurons at an injection site in the lateral hypothalamus (A) show the typical morphology of labeled neurons, including their dendritic arbors. Projections of these labeled neurons in the lateral septal area (B, low magnification, and D, high magnification) and in the supramammillary nucleus (C, low magnification) have different morphologies. Labeled hypothalamic afferents in the lateral septal area appear to target the cell bodies and proximal dendrites of neurons (B) that at higher magnification appear to have large boutons making contact with such neurons (D). On the other hand, afferents in the supramammillary nucleus ramify more extensively and appear to be distributed to more distal dendrites of neurons in the area (C, same magnification as B). (E) A high-power photomicrograph of one neuron labeled at an injection site in the striatum shows the detailed morphology obtained with PHA-L labeling. Note the labeling of dendritic spines. (F) PHA-L-labeled afferents in the globus pallidus from a striatal injection. Note the detailed morphology.

The types of labeling obtained with WGA and PHA-L provide some insight as to possible mechanisms of uptake. Wheat germ agglutinin appears to be incorporated by neurons through their dendrites or cell bodies and through axon terminals in the area in which WGA diffuses at the injection site. Incorporated WGA appears to be localized in vesicles and is transported by a fast axonal transport mechanism. PHA-L injected by iontophoresis, on the other hand, appears to be incorporated by a more restricted population of neurons; it is not taken up by all neurons in the area in which it diffuses and is not, in most cases, taken up by axon terminals. Perhaps most significant is the circumstance that PHA-L appears to gain direct access to the cytoplasm and is not restricted to vesicles. This is surmised from the filled appearance of labeled neurons and by the fact that PHA-L moves in the anterograde direction in axons by a slow process. Furthermore, because PHA-L appears to be localized in the cytoplasm and not in vesicles, it is not rapidly degraded by the lysosomal system. Thus, even with very long survival times following the injection, PHA-L remains as an identifiable marker of neurons and their projections.

The difference in the type of labeling obtained with WGA and PHA-L suggests that the latter is not incorporated by endocytosis. Wheat germ agglutinin is thought to bind to membrane glycoproteins that have sialic acid and then to be incorporated by endocytosis (Gonatas *et al.*, 1979). A large number of glycoporoteins contain sialic acid, which presumably accounts for the efficiency of WGA incorporation into neurons. Preliminary evidence suggests that PHA-L binds to a relatively small number of glycoproteins, possibly to a unique glycoprotein (C. R. Gerfen, unpublished observations). Whether the more restricted number of PHA-L binding sites on neurons accounts for the manner of its incorporation remains to be determined.

One possibility is that during the iontophoretic injection of PHA-L the membranes of neurons are temporarily opened, allowing PHA-L to gain direct access to the cell. Such a mechanism may be analogous to the process of electroporation used to transfect cells with viral DNA vectors (Chu *et al.*, 1987). Such a mechanism would not explain why other lectins such as WGA, peanut agglutinin (PNA), or *Phaseolus vulgaris* erthroagglutinin (PHA-E) are not incorporated in a manner similar to PHA-L, unless the specificity of PHA-L labeling results from its binding to an intracellular glycoprotein. Another possibility may be related to the observation that PHA-L labels astrocytes at the center of the injection site. Iontophoretic injections of PHA-L might temporarily disrupt the close association between astrocytes and dendrites, and the site of entry may be related to these contacts. Support for this mechanism comes from the observations of labeling obtained in the developing brain in which PHA-L is incorporated by radial glia but not by neurons at developmental stages when astrocytes have not yet become associated with neurons (C. R. Gerfen, unpublished data). Suffice it to say that at this point the mechanism of PHA-L incorporation is not understood. However, the type of labeling obtained provides an excellent means of tracing efferent axonal projections.

IV. PHA-L COMBINED WITH OTHER TECHNIQUES

Because it is an immunohistochemical technique, the PHA-L method can be combined easily and effectively with other techniques to provide additional data concerning the neuroanatomy of chemically defined circuits within the brain. Although an exhaustive description of such combined methods is not provided, several selected combinations are detailed. Finally, although these methods provide considerable information at the light microscopic level, confirmation of synaptic connections requires the extension of the PHA-L method to the electron microscopic level. These combined methods are diagrammed in Fig. 5.

A. Combined PHA-L and Autoradiographic Axonal Tract Tracing

The PHA-L method shares several advantages with the autoradiographic axonal tract-tracing method. Both methods specifically label the efferent projections of the neurons that incorporate the tracers at the injection sites. Unique to these methods is the relative absence of both retrograde axonal transport from terminals to neuronal cell bodies and the negligible labeling of axons of passage through the injection site. For these reasons the combined use of injections of PHA-L and [^{3}H]-amino acids into separate brain sites provides the most reliable means of comparing the projections from these sites. These methods are easily combined simply by following the procedures for each simultaneously. A brief description of their combined use is provided.

The two tracers are injected according to standard techniques: PHA-L as described in the Appendix and [^{3}H]-amino acids according to the method of Cowan *et al.* (1972). The latter injections are typically made either by pressure injections of a cocktail of [^{3}H]-leucine and [^{3}H]-proline mixed together in equal concentrations of 50 μCi/μl and injected in a volume of 0.1–0.5 μl or, using the same concentrations, iontophoresed with 1–3 μA for 1 min. Although the axonal transport rates of the two tracers are different—PHA-L is transported relatively slowly at rates of 4–6 mm/day, whereas [^{3}H]-amino acids are transported as newly synthesized proteins at rates ranging of 2–100 mm day—it is usually possible to inject both tracers in the same surgical session. If long survival periods are necessary to obtain sufficient labeling with PHA-L, injections of the tracers should be staggered on different days.

The standard procedure for immunoperoxidase localization of PHA-L is then followed. Of particular importance is the step following the DAB reaction in which the sections are immersed in formalin. It is imperative that the DAB–peroxidase reaction be stopped completely, which the formalin step accomplishes. Otherwise low-level residual reaction will also cause chemography of photographic emulsion. Following the DAB–peroxidase reaction and formalin incubation, the sections are then mounted, air dried,

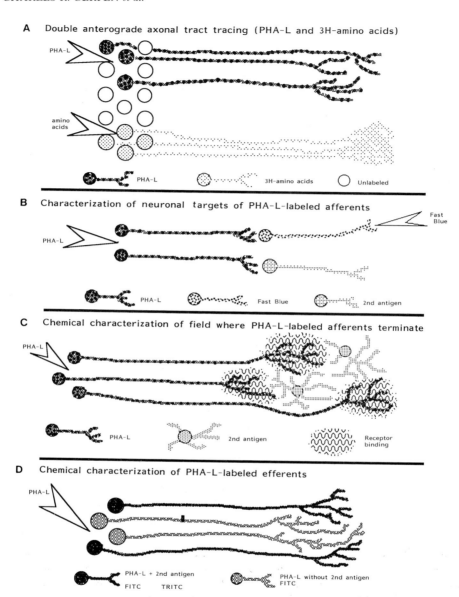

Figure 5. Diagrams of four types of combined neuroanatomical methods using PHA-L.

defatted in chloroform–methanol, and rehydrated. Slide-mounted sections are then dipped in NTB photographic emulsion as is standard for autoradiographic localization of [^{3}H]-amino acids. Following an appropriate exposure time, the slides are then developed by standard procedures, rinsed, dehydrated, and coverslipped out of xylene. This procedure provides both

PHA-L immunoperoxidase and autoradiographic labeling of efferent projections in the same sections. Of course, adjacent sections may also be processed for PHA-L and autoradiographic labeling. However, in this case it may be more difficult to make comparisons between the two projections.

There are a few limitations to this procedure. The first has to do with the relative numbers and distributions of neurons labeled by the two methods. As described above, PHA-L labels neurons determined by the dendritic topographies of the neurons at the site of injection, which in practical terms means that not every neuron in a given volume around the center of the injection is labeled. The autoradiographic method, on the other hand, appears to label nearly every neuron around a given injection site, presumably because neuronal incorporation is accomplished by simple diffusion of the tracer. This prohibits an exact quantitative comparison of the relative projections from the injections. Nonetheless, it is possible to define definitively, especially with the PHA-L method, those neurons that incorporate and transport the tracer. The second limitation has to do with the labeling of projections obtained with the autoradiographic method. Whereas the PHA-L method provides nearly complete labeling of the efferent fibers, labeling with the autoradiographic technique provides no morphological resolution at the light microscopic level. Further, the degree of labeling by the autoradiographic method is dependent to some extent on the metabolic activity of different portions of the fibers themselves. For example, shorter survival periods tend to label terminals more densely than fibers. Thus, the degree of labeling of different portions of the efferent projections is dependent on the survival period, but in an imprecise manner such that it cannot be determined what labeling represents that in fibers versus that in terminals regardless of the survival period used.

The combination of PHA-L and autoradiographic tract-tracing methods may be used to compare the relationships of efferent projections from two distinct areas of the same nucleus, as shown in Fig. 6. For example, by this combined method the striatal projections to globus pallidus and substantia nigra were shown to be arranged in a mediolateral topography (Gerfen, 1985). However, a certain degree of overlap between the projections from different striatal areas was also revealed. Such analysis was facilitated considerably by the ability to label projections of two areas simultaneously, allowing a direct comparison of the distributions of efferents. The combined use of PHA-L and the autoradiographic technique provides the requisite specificity for such analysis since the exact populations of neurons whose efferents are labeled by both methods may be accurately determined. Other anterograde tracers, such as WGA–HRP, do not provide such specificity.

B. Neuroanatomical and Chemical Characterization of Neuronal Targets of PHA-L-Labeled Afferents

The combination of retrograde fluorescent tracers with transmitter immunohistochemistry (Hökfelt et al., 1980; Sawchenko and Swanson, 1981;

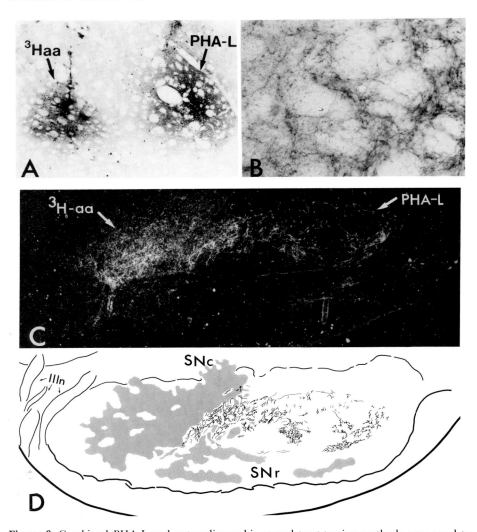

Figure 6. Combined PHA-L and autoradiographic axonal tract-tracing methods were used to examine the topographic organization of striatal projections. (A) Brightfield photomicrograph of the injection sites of [^{3}H]-amino acids (left) and PHA-L (right) into the striatum. Although both tracers diffuse around the central area of the injection, cell bodies that have incorporated each tracer are identified. (B) Brightfield photomicrograph of afferent labeling in the globus pallidus. Autoradiographically generated grains are distributed on the left, and PHA-L labeled fibers and terminals are distributed on the right side, in keeping with a general topography in the labeled striatopallidal projections. (C) Darkfield photomicrograph of afferent labeling in the substantia nigra pars reticulata (SNr). Most autoradiographically labeled afferents from the medial striatal injection are medial to PHA-L-labeled afferents. (D) Camera lucida drawing of the labeling in C shows the general mediolateral topography of labeled striatonigral afferents (autoradiographic labeling indicated with shading). It is apparent that there is a partial overlap of the projections from the two injections and that the projections from each striatal area are discontinuous.

see also Chapter 2) aided considerably in the neurochemical characterization of neuronal circuits. The additional use of the PHA-L method may extend such analysis. The methodology for such combined applications is rather straightforward and depends primarily on the ability to localize the different labels with fluorescent illumination specific for each. Injections of PHA-L and retrogradely transported fluorescent dyes, such as fast blue, may be made during a single surgical procedure. Since both markers are resistant to intracellular degradation, the relatively long survival periods necessary for PHA-L labeling may be used. Although survival periods of over 7 days may provide excessive retrograde labeling with fluorescent dyes, the reduction in dye labeling that occurs because of the subsequent immunohistochemical procedures normally provides adequate correction of this problem.

Since the antigenicity of PHA-L is rather stable, it is advisable to adjust the fixative for optimal labeling of the second neurochemical antigen. Brain sections are processed first by incubating in primary antisera directed against PHA-L and then against the neurochemical antigen. This is the major limiting step of the procedure, and several options are available. First, it is essential that the two primary antisera be raised in different species. For example, if the primary antiserum directed against the neurochemical antigen is raised in rabbits, we typically use a primary antiserum directed against PHA-L that has been raised in guinea pigs (GPαPHA-L, available gratis from C. R. Gerfen, NIMH, Bethesda, MD). Second, the sections may be incubated in a mixture of the primary antisera or sequentially in separate dilutions of the antisera.

Following incubation in the primary antisera, sections are rinsed and incubated in a mixture of fluorescently labeled affinity-purified secondary antisera. Again, it is essential that the secondary antisera not crossreact with the inappropriate primary antiserum. As in the example, rhodamine-labeled goat antiserum directed against guinea pig IgG (GαGP–TRITC, Cappel Labs, diluted 1 : 200) is mixed with fluorescein-labeled goat antiserum directed against rabbit IgG (GαR–FITC, Sigma Chemical, diluted 1 : 200), and the sections are incubated for 45–60 min at room temperature. Sections are then rinsed, mounted, air dried, coverslipped with glycerol buffer (pH 8.5), and viewed with filters to view FITC (excitation filter 460–485 nm, barrier filter 510–545 nm), TRITC (excitation filter 535–550 nm, barrier filter 580 nm), and fast blue (excitation filter 330–380 nm, barrier filter 420 nm).

Examples of these procedures are provided in Fig. 7. In Fig. 7B[1] and B[2] lateral hypothalamic axons labeled with PHA-L seem to contact nigral neurons labeled with fast blue after an injection of the retrograde tracer into the superior colliculus. Figure 7B[4] shows PHA-L-labeled striatonigral afferents distributed amongst fast-blue-labeled nigrotectal neurons. Figure 7B[3] shows PHA-L-labeled striatonigral afferents in relationship to dopaminergic neurons in the pars compacta labeled with rhodamine (rhodamine-labeled secondary antisera to localize TH-containing neurons). These photomicrographs were made by double exposing film first using the appropriate filter

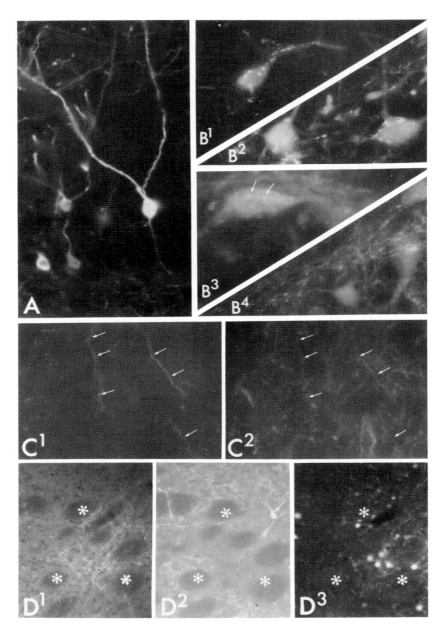

Figure 7. Combined fluorescent techniques and PHA-labeling. (A) Dentate granule cell labeled with PHA-L shows dendritic arborization and the axon labeled with an indirect immunofluorescence method. (B^1 and B^2) PHA-L-labeled afferents (labeled with FITC) with boutons in close apposition to true-blue-labeled substantia nigra neurons that project to the superior colliculus. The afferents, which originate in the contralateral hypothalamus, appear to make contact with the perikarya of nigrotectal neurons. (B^3) PHA-L-labeled striatonigral afferent fiber (labeled with FITC) draped across a TH-positive nigrostriatal neuron (labeled with TRITC). Varicosities of the labeled fiber are in apparent contact with the cell body (arrow). This, however, can be verified only with the electron microscope. (B^4) PHA-L-labeled striatonigral afferents

to view FITC-labeled PHA-L fibers and then using either of the fluorescent
filters to view fast blue or rhodamine.

C. PHA-L-Labeled Afferents in Chemically Defined Brain Areas

With the advent of the immunohistochemical and autoradiographic receptor binding techniques, the characterization of brain areas in terms of their
functional neuroanatomical organization has advanced considerably. Although in some cases cytoarchitectonic features match neurochemical and/
or receptor binding distributions, in other cases new organizational features
have been revealed by these new techniques. A prime example is the striatum, which appears rather homogeneous in terms of its cytoarchitecture but
is observed with immunohistochemical and receptor autoradiographic techniques to be a mosaic of two neurochemically distinct compartments, termed
the patches and matrix. Both types of techniques may be combined with
PHA-L to distinguish labeled afferents into these neurochemically defined
compartments.

To use immunohistochemical markers to define striatal compartments in
relationship to PHA-L-labeled afferents, the same protocol as outlined above
is followed. In the study cited as an example, PHA-L anterograde labeling
and fluorescent retrograde labeling were combined with immunohistochemical localization of markers of striatal compartmentation (Gerfen, 1984) to
examine the input–output organization of the striatum. PHA-L was injected
into the cortex to label corticostriatal inputs (Fig. 7D^1), and fast blue was
injected into the substantia nigra to label striatonigral projection neurons
(Fig. 7D^3). The relationship of these two labels was compared in the same
sections to each other and to the distribution of somatostatin immunoreactivity (to mark the striatal matrix, Fig. 7D^2) or enkephalin immunoreactivity
(to mark the patches).

Figure 8 shows additional photomicrographs from this study. An injection
of PHA-L into the prelimbic cortex (Fig. 8A) labeled striatal afferents (Fig.
8B) that were distributed into patches marked by a paucity of somatostatin

---

(labeled with FITC) distributed among true-blue-containing substantia nigra pars reticulata
neurons labeled by retrograde axonal transport after dye injections into the superior colliculus.
(C^1 and C^2) PHA-L-labeled nigrostriatal fibers (labeled with TRITC in C^1) are shown to be
dopaminergic by colabeling with TH immunoreactivity (labeled with FITC in C^2). (D^1–D^3) PHA-
L-labeled afferents from the prelimbic cortex (labeled with FITC in D^1) distributed to a patch
in the striatum. Somatostatin immunoreactivity (labeled with TRITC in D^2) in the same field as
in D^1, showing the distribution of fibers in the striatal matrix compartment complementary to
the patch into which the prelimbic cortical afferents are distributed. A single somatostatin immunoreactive neuron is located at the boundary between the patch and matrix and extends a
dendrite into the patch, although its local axon collaterals are distributed in the surrounding
matrix. Striatonigral projection neurons (D^3) retrogradely filled from a fast blue injection in the
substantia nigra pars compacta are located in the patch that receives prelimbic inputs. A color
reproduction of this figure appears following p. 352.

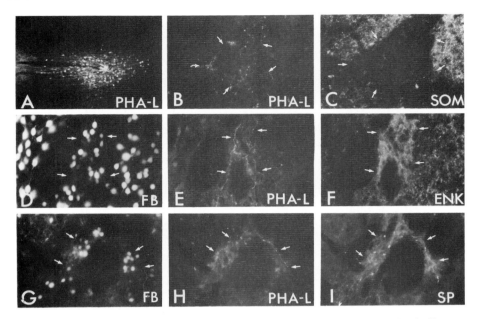

Figure 8. Photomicrographs of combined PHA-L labeling of prelimbic corticostriatal afferents, immunoreactive markers for striatal compartments, and fast blue labeling of striatonigral neurons. (First row) PHA-L injection site in the prelimbic cortex (A). Note the dense astrocytic core of the injection center and labeled cortical neurons with apical dendrites. Distribution of PHA-L-labeled prelimibic corticostriatal afferents in a patch (B, labeled with FITC), which is demarcated as a somatostatin-poor zone (C). (Second row) after a large injection of fast blue into the substantia nigra, both matrix and patch striatonigral neurons are labeled (D). PHA-L-labeled prelimbic corticostriatal afferents (E, labeled with FITC) are distributed in a patch, which overlaps dense enkephalin immunoreactivity (F, labeled with TRITC). (Third row) After a localized injection of fast blue into the substantia nigra pars compacta, patch striatonigral neurons are labeled (G) that are distributed in patches receiving PHA-L-labeled prelimbic corticostriatal afferents (H, labeled with FITC), marked by sense substance P immunoreactivity (I, labeled with TRITC).

fiber labeling (Fig. 8C). Striatonigral projection neurons in both the patch and matrix compartments (Fig. 8D) were labeled by large injections of fast blue into the substantia nigra and are shown in relationship to PHA-L-labeled inputs from the prelimbic cortex (Fig. 8E), which are distributed to patches marked by dense enkephalin immunoreactivity (Fig. 8F). Similar cases revealed that patches project to a particular part of the substantia nigra, the pars compacta (Fig. 8G–I), whereas the matrix neurons project to the substantia nigra pars reticulata. Additionally, other cortical areas, such as the cingulate, sensory, and motor cortical areas were shown to project to the striatal matrix compartment. Thus, by the ability to label corticostriatal and striatonigral systems simultaneously with an immunohistochemical marker of the striatal compartmental organization, the distinct and parallel arrangement of striatal patch and matrix input–output systems was discovered (Gerfen, 1984).

Another means of demarcating striatal compartments is with autoradiographic μ opiate receptor localization, which labels the patches (Herkenham and Pert, 1982). This method allowed the determination of the distribution of the different types of nigrostriatal afferents to either of the "patch" or "matrix" striatal compartments. In sections adjacent to those stained for colabeling of PHA-L and TH fibers, [^{3}H]-naloxone was used to mark dense μ opiate receptor binding in the striatal patches according to the method of Herkenham and Pert (1982) as modified for fixed tissue (Gerfen et al., 1985). With this procedure it was determined that there are two nigrostriatal systems, a dorsal tier of midbrain dopaminergic neurons, which project to the striatal matrix, and a ventral set of dopaminergic neurons in the substantia nigra, which project to the striatal patches. An example of labeling of the patch-directed system is shown in Fig. 9A–A'.

These techniques may also be used in studies of other neural systems, such as afferents to the cortex, in which either neurochemical or receptor binding patterns define subdivisions of areas that are not as readily defined on the basis of cytoarchitectonics. A limitation of such combined methods is that some receptor-binding ligands have altered binding characteristics or do not bind at all in the fixed tissue that is necessary for immunohistochemical localization. Thus, it is essential to determine the compatibility of the receptor ligand to be used with the fixation protocols for PHA-L anterograde tract tracing.

D. Neurochemical Identification of PHA-L-Labeled Efferents

As stated, the immunohistochemical identification of retrogradely labeled neurons promoted the ability to identify neuroanatomical connections chemically. Although this method provides necessary information concerning the neurochemical phenotype of the neurons of origin, it cannot provide detailed information of the axon arborizations of such neurons. This limitation inherent in retrograde tracing of neurochemically defined connections is overcome with a method in which anterogradely transported PHA-L is colocalized with immunohistochemically identifiable neurochemical antigens (Gerfen and Sawchenko, 1985). The basic method is similar to the one described in the previous section except for an absolute requirement to mix the primary antisera during incubations and similarly to mix the secondary antisera. This is essential since it appears that if the antisera are used sequentially, the labeling by the first may block labeling by the second applied antiserum, presumably by steric hindrance within the same structure. When these precautions are taken, the secondary antisera provide reliable labeling of the appropriate antigens without cross activity.

Figures 7C[1], 7C[2], 9B, 9B', and 11 provide examples of the type of information that is obtained with this procedure (see also Gerfen, 1984; Gerfen et al., 1987). Figures 7C[1], 7C[2], 9B, and 9B' show PHA-L-labeled nigrostriatal fibers colocalized with tyrosine hydroxylase (TH) immunoreactivity. The use

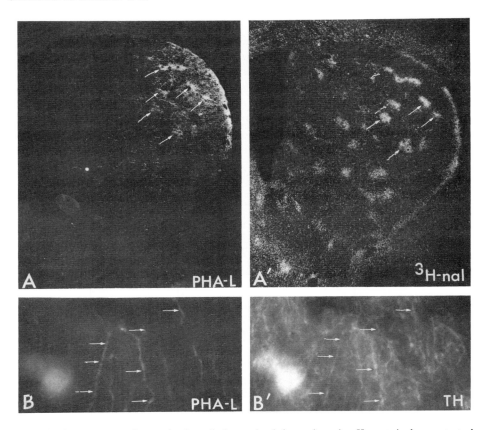

Figure 9. Compartmental organization of nigrostriatal dopaminergic afferents is demonstrated by a comparison of PHA-L-labeled afferents and [³H]-naloxone binding of μ opiate receptors in patches in adjacent coronal sections through the striatum. (A) Darkfield photomicrograph of PHA-L-labeled striatal afferents labeled after an injection into the substantia nigra pars reticulata. Labeled afferents are distributed in patches that overlap the distribution of opiate-receptor-rich patches (A'). That the labeled striatal afferents are dopaminergic was demonstrated by the colabeling of PHA-L-labeled fibers (B) and TH immunoreactivity (B').

of combined fluorescence retrograde tracing and catecholamine histofluorescence technique showed that whereas the majority of neurons in the substantia nigra that project to the striatum are dopaminergic, some 5–10% are nondopaminergic (van der Kooy *et al.*, 1981). PHA-L injections into the substantia nigra labeled both TH-positive dopaminergic and TH-negative nondopaminergic nigrostriatal afferents (not shown). Interestingly, the morphologies of nigrostriatal dopaminergic and nondopaminergic afferents were shown to be distinct. Dopaminergic afferents are relatively thin fibers with small flattened varicosities, whereas labeled nondopaminergic afferents are of much thicker caliber and terminate in large bulbous boutons (Fig. 10).

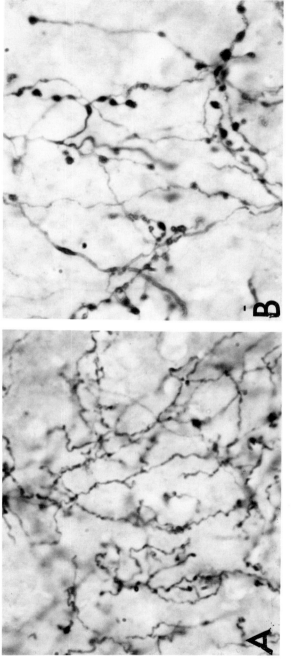

Figure 10. Examples of the morphologically distinct types of PHA-L-labeled nigrostriatal afferents. (A) The most predominant type of labeled nigrostriatal afferent is of relatively thin caliber with slight swellings. This fiber type is colabeled with TH immunoreactivity (see Fig. 7C) and is presumed to be dopaminergic. (B) A distinct morphological nigrostriatal afferent has a large fiber caliber and branches with large bulbous boutons (up to 2.0 μm in diameter). This fiber type is not colabeled with TH immunoreactivity and is presumed to be nondopaminergic.

Another application of the double labeling of PHA-L fibers is shown in Fig. 11 from a study by Cunningham and Sawchenko (1987). In this figure PHA-L-labeled fibers from the nucleus of the solitary tract (NTS) are shown in the supraoptic nucleus in the hypothalamus to express dopamine-β-hydroxylase (DBH), which is the enzyme that converts dopamine to norepinephrine. The fact that the NTS sends a substantial projection to the region just dorsal to the supraoptic nucleus made it impossible to establish the catecholaminergic character of the minor projection that enters the nucleus proper, which had been suggested by combined retrograde transport immunohistochemical studies. In the photomicrographs it is seen that literally every varicosity of the PHA-L-labeled afferent is also stained for DBH (arrows). This established unequivocally the catecholaminergic nature of the NTS input to the supraoptic nucleus.

These examples demonstrate the types of information that may be obtained with the combined use of PHA-L and other neuroanatomical techniques. It is possible to distinguish the morphological and neurochemical determinants of efferent projections arising from a mixed population of neurons that are labeled with PHA-L. Additionally, it is possible to determine the relationship of such labeled afferents to neurochemically and connectionally specified neurons or systems. Because PHA-L is localized with immunohistochemical procedures, the analyses exemplified above can be extended to the electron microscopic level, at which the actual synaptic contacts of the PHA-L labeled fibers can be determined.

E. Electron Microscopic Localization of PHA-L

Although the distinction between fibers and terminals is in general easily made at the light microscopic level, the ultrastructural identification is necessary to confirm the actual synaptic contacts between PHA-L-labeled bulbous end structures and various postsynaptic elements. Wouterlood and Groenewegen (1985) first described the ultrastructural localization of PHA-L, and this technique has since been successfully used by others (e.g., Zahm and Heimer, 1985). Figure 12 shows PHA-L-labeled fibers in the basolateral amygdaloid nucleus (BL) following an injection of PHA-L in the thalamus. Although labeled bulbous end structures were often observed in close contact with the soma of large neurons in the BL (Fig. 12C), electron microscopic analysis invariably showed that synaptic contacts were almost exclusively made with spines and never with the soma of large neurons (Fig. 12D–F).

The PHA-L technique offers exciting possibilities for describing the afferent input to identified postsynaptic cells. For instance, the PHA-L technique can be combined with immunohistochemical identification of transmitter(s) in postsynaptic cells, using different electron-dense markers (Zaborszky and Cullinan, 1989).

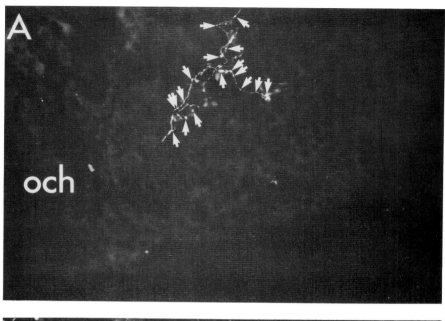

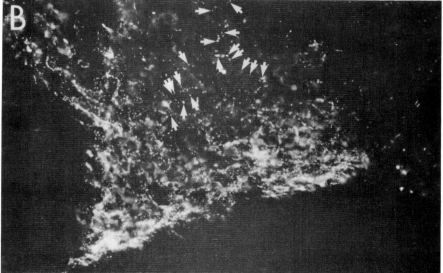

Figure 11. A PHA-L-labeled afferent (A) in the hypothalamic supraoptic nucleus (SON), adjacent to the optic chiasm (och), originating from the nucleus of the solitary tract (NTS) is shown to be colabeled with dopamine-β-hydroxylase (DBH) immunoreactivity. Virtually every PHA-L-labeled varicosity is seen to be DBH-positive (arrows). This demonstrates that NTS inputs to the SON are noradrenergic.

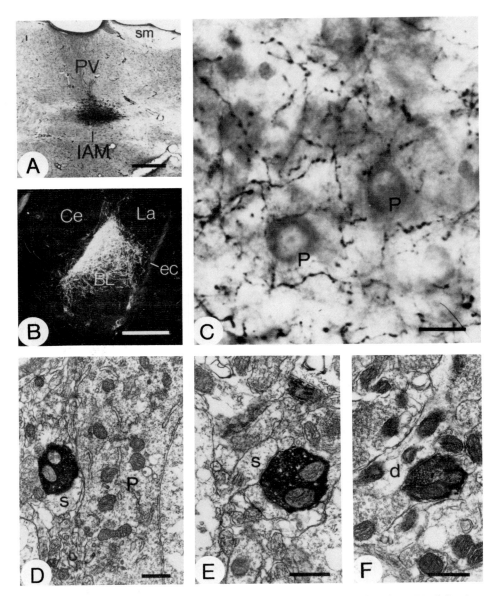

Figure 12. PHA-L-labeled fibers (B and C) in the basolateral amygdaloid nucleus (BL) following an injection in the medial thalamus (A). D–F illustrate PHA-L-labeled terminals in contact with dendritic shaft (d) or spines.

V. APPENDIX

A. The Basic PHA-L Method for Light Microscopy

The protocol originally described for the use of PHA-L as an anterograde axonal tracer remains the basic method for its use (Gerfen and Sawchenko, 1984). With several years of experience there have been slight modifications, primarily as a result of the realization of the stability of the PHA-L itself, which allows a broader latitude in the use of immunohistochemical methods for localization.

1. Injection

Injections of PHA-L are made by iontophoresis. A 2.5% solution of PHA-L (Vector Labs) dissolved in sodium phosphate buffer (0.01 M NaPB, pH 7.4–8.0) is loaded into a glass micropipette with a tip diameter of less than 15 μm. With the animal under anesthesia, the tip is stereotaxically positioned in the brain area of choice, and a 5 to 10-μA positive current is applied for every other 7 sec for 15–20 min using a constant-current source that is capable of generating up to 2000 V (CS-3 current source, Transkinetics Systems, Inc., Canton, MA). To obtain larger injections, which may be necessary in large animals such as primates, currents up to 10 μA are used. It is also possible to make multiple injections to increase the size of the injectioned area.

Although PHA-L may be pressure injected, this method appears to be less effective than iontophoretic application for specific slow anterograde axonal transport. Pressure injections often result in some cellular destruction, presumably because of the toxic effect of PHA-L at high concentrations, and the ability to determine specifically the neurons that incorporate PHA-L at the injection site, one of the best attributes of this method, is considerably compromised by pressure injections.

2. Survival

The estimated axonal transport rate for PHA-L is 4–6 mm per day. The survival period is thus dependent on the length of the pathway to be traced. Typical survival periods are between 7 and 21 days, with up to 3–4 weeks used for injections in primates. There appears to be negligible degradation of neuronally incorporated PHA-L with survival periods up to 5 weeks.

3. Perfusion

The stability of the PHA-L allows a wide range of fixatives. Virtually any paraformaldehyde perfusion fixation method will provide excellent results.

When the PHA-L method is combined with other procedures, such as localization of other antigens with immunohistochemical methods, it is advisable to choose the fixative that is most effective for the other antigen, since that will almost certainly be the limiting factor. Among the many fixatives that have been tried by the authors, the periodate–lysine–paraformaldehyde protocol of McLean and Nakane (1974) is currently the first choice.

The standard perfusion protocol involves deeply anesthetizing the animal before transcardial perfusion with normal physiological saline (0.9% NaCl) to rinse out the blood, followed by the fixative (approximately 500 ml fixative per 300 g rat over 15–30 min). The brain is then removed and postfixed in the fixative plus 20–30% sucrose for 6–72 hr. Because of the stability of the PHA-L, long postfixation periods may be used. Brains that are to be cut with a Vibratome do not need to be postfixed in sucrose.

4. Histochemistry

Brains may be cut either frozen (following sucrose infiltration) or on a Vibratome into 30-μm-thick sections, which are collected in potassium phosphate-buffered saline (KPBS, 0.02 M, pH 7.4). Localization of PHA-L either by indirect immunofluorescence or immunoperoxidase methods provides comparable sensitivity and morphological resolution. The specific application will determine the method to be used. Immunofluorescence provides the simplest method and is used routinely to check quickly the injection site and axonal labeling to determine if the injection was into the desired location and provided adequate labeling. For this procedure, a few test sections through the injection site and from an area in which terminal labeling should be present are reacted using a more concentrated dilution of primary antiserum than is used for more specific labeling.

5. Immunofluorescence Localization

In this protocol goat primary antiserum against PHA-L is used; rabbit antiserum directed against PHA-L may be substituted with the appropriate substitutions of normal goat serum for normal rabbit serum and the use of goat secondary antiserum directed against rabbit IgG. For this procedure free-floating sections are processed in the following manner:

1. *Primary antiserum.* Goat antiserum directed against PHA-L (Vector Labs) diluted 1 : 500 (for rapid processing) or 1 : 1000–1 : 2000 (for longer processing) in KPBS containing 0.5% triton X-100 and 2% normal rabbit serum (NRS) for 2 hr at room temperature (1 : 500 primary antiserum dilution) or for 24–48 hr at 4°C (1 : 1000–1 : 2000 primary antiserum dilution).
2. *Rinse.* Three times for 5 min in KPBS.
3. *Secondary antiserum.* Rabbit antibody directed against goat IgG conju-

gated to fluorescein isothiocyanate (RαG–FITC, affinity purified, Sigma Chemical Co.) diluted 1 : 200 in KPBS containing 0.5% Triton X-100 and 2% normal goat serum (NGS) for 45–60 min at room temperature.

4. *Rinse.* Three times 5 min in KPBS.
5. *Mount sections.* From KPBS onto gelatin coated slides, completely air dry, and coverslip with buffered glycerol containing 0.4% propyl gallate. Sections are then examined with epifluorescence illumination using a filter that specifically excites FITC (excitation filter 460–485 nm, barrier filter 515–545 nm). Labeling is stable for many months if slides are stored at 4°C.

6. Immunoperoxidase Procedure

Virtually any immunoperoxidase method will provide sensitive and specific labeling, including the peroxidase–antiperoxidase (PAP method) or the avidin–biotin–peroxidase method (Hsu *et al.*, 1981). The sensitivity and specificity of the immunofluorescence and immunoperoxidase methods are comparable, so that the initial incubation in primary antisera is the same for the two procedures. The following is the series of solutions in which free floating sections are incubated.

1. *Primary antiserum.* Goat (or rabbit) antiserum directed against PHA-L (Vector Labs), 1 : 1000–1 : 2000 in KPBS plus 0.5% Triton X-100 and 2% normal rabbit serum (or normal goat serum), 24–48 hr at 4°C.
2. *Rinse.* Three times 5 min at KPBS.
3. *Secondary antiserum.* Biotinylated rabbit antigoat (or goat antirabbit) antibody (from the Vectastain kit provided by Vector Labs, Burlingame, CA) diluted 1 : 200 in KPBS plus 2% NGS and 0.5% Triton X-100, 1 hr at room temperature.
4. *Rinse.* Three times 5 min in KPBS.
5. *ABC peroxidase.* Avidin–biotin–peroxidase complex (ABC complex from Vectastain kit), 1 : 100 dilution each of components A and B mixed together in KPBS for 1 hr.
6. *Rinse.* Twice for 5 min in KPBS.
7. *Rinse.* Twice for 2 min in sodium acetate buffer (0.1 M, pH 6.0).
8. *DAB reaction* (modified from Itoh *et al.*, 1979). React for 30–45 min in freshly mixed solution containing (per 10 ml of reaction mixture):

   a. 0.05% 3,3′-diaminobenzidine (DAB, premixed in H_2O).
   b. 0.1 M sodium acetate buffer (pH 6.0).
   c. 20 mM dextrose.
   d. 7.5 mM NH_4Cl.
   e. 5–30 units glucose oxidase.

9. *Stop reaction.* Transfer to 10% formalin (1 : 10 dilution of 33% bottled formaldehyde in 0.9% saline), 5–10 min. This step stops the DAB reaction. This step also bleaches the reaction product, and although

care must be exercised not to overbleach the specific labeling, this step may be used to reduce excessive background labeling.

10. *Rinse.* Three times 5 min in KPBS.
11. *Mount sections.* From the KPBS onto gelatin/chromalum-coated slides, air dry, dehydrate in ascending alcohols, defat in 50/50 chloroform/methanol twice for 30 min, and rehydrate.
12. *Rinse.* 15 min in water, and dehydrate.
13. *Coverslip.* Out of xylene.

B. PHA-L Method for Electron Microscopy

1. Perfusion

Animals under deep anesthesia are perfused transcardially with the following sequence of solutions: first, a brief rinse with 0.1 M sodium phosphate buffer (NaPB, pH 7.4) containing 1% sucrose; second, 350 ml (per 300 g rat) of a fixative solution of 0.12 M PB (pH 7.4) containing 4% formaldehyde (made fresh from paraformaldehyde), 0.1% glutaraldehyde, and 15% saturated picric acid (Somogyi and Takagi, 1982); third, 150 ml (per 300 g rat) of a fixative solution of 0.12 M PB (pH 7.4) containing 4% formaldehyde. The brains are removed immediately and stored in the second fixative for 4 hr at 4°C.

2. Sectioning

Brains are cut into 50-μm-thick sections with a Vibratome. One series of sections is processed with either the immunofluorescence or the immunoperoxidase protocol described above to determine whether the labeling is adequate to proceed with the more involved method for electron microscopic localization.

3. Immunoperoxidase Localization for Electron Microscopy

1. Sections are rinsed for 18–24 hr in several changes of PB.
2. To improve antibody penetration, sections are sunk in 10% sucrose solution and then frozen in liquid nitrogen (Somogyi and Tagaki, 1982).
3. To improve the intensity of the DAB reaction, sections are incubated in 0.5% cobalt chloride for 10 min (Itoh *et al.*, 1979).
4. Antibody incubations. Following the above treatments free-floating sections are incubated in the following series of immunochemical reagents, which are each diluted in Tris-buffered saline (50 mM Tris, pH 7.4, 150 mM NaCl) with 0.25%-carrageenan. Sections are rinsed in three 10-min changes of this buffer before and between each of the following incubations:

a. Primary antisera directed against PHA-L (goat α PHA-L, Vector Labs) diluted 1 : 2000 for 24 hr at 4°C.
b. Secondary antibody (biotinylated rabbit α goat IgG, Vectastain Kit, Vector Labs) diluted 1 : 200 for 2 hr at room temperature.
c. Avidin–biotin–peroxidase complex (mixed ABC complex from Vectastain Kit, Vector Labs) diluted 1 : 400 for 2 hr at room temperature.
d. The peroxidase reaction is carried out by incubating sections according to the protocol of Itoh *et al.* (1979) using a coupled glucose oxidase–DAB mixture. Sections are incubated in a solution containing (per 100 ml 0.1 M NaPB, pH 7.4): 50 mg DAB, 200 mg β-D-glucose, 40 mg ammonium chloride, and 0.4 mg glucose oxidase for 1–2 hr at 37°C.

4. Preparation for Electron Microscopy

The steps for processing sections for dehydration and cutting for electron microscopy are as follows:

1. Postfixation in 2% osmium tetroxide in PB (pH 7.4).
2. Dehydration in an ascending concentration series of the watermiscible resin Quetel 523 M (Ted Pella, Inc.) in distilled water: two 5-min changes each of 35%, 50%, and 70% Quetel; one 10-min change each of 80%, 95%, and 100% Quetel.
3. Sections are treated in mixtures of Quetel 523M and increasing concentrations of Maraglas (Polysciences, Inc.).
4. Sections are then flat embedded in fresh Maraglas using silicone-coated glass slides and coverslips to allow for microscopic examination and photography. Small sections for EM are trimmed from the area of interest and remounted in blank blocks of Maraglas, whereupon serial semi- and ultrathin sections are cut on an ultramicrotome.
5. Sections are collected on Formvar-coated grids and stained with uranyl acetate (10% in 100% methanol for 15–30 min) and lead citrate (0.1% in 0.1 M NaOH for 3–10 min). The sections are then examined and photographed in an electron microscope.

ACKNOWLEDGMENTS. Supported by USPHS grants HL 35137 to P.E.S. and NS 17743 to Lennart Heimer.

REFERENCES

Chu, G., Hayakawa, H., and Berg, P., 1987, Electroporation for the efficient transfection of mammalian cells with DNA, *Nucleic Acids Res.* **15**:1311–1318.
Cowan, W. M., Gottleib, D. L., Hendrickson, A. E., Price, J. L., and Woolsey, T. A., 1972, The autoradiographic demonstration of axonal connections in the central nervous system, *Brain Res.* **37**:21–51.
Cunningham, E. T., Jr., and Sawchenko, P. E., 1987, Anatomical specificity of noradrenergic

inputs to the paraventricular and supraoptic nuclei of the rat hypothalamus, *J. Comp. Neurol.* **274:**60–76.

Gerfen, C. R., 1984, The neostriatal mosaic: Compartmentalization of corticostriatal input and striatonigral output systems, *Nature* **311:**461–464.

Gerfen, C. R., 1985, The neostriatal mosaic: I. Compartmental organization of projections from the striatum to the substantia nigra in the rat, *J. Comp. Neurol.* **236:**454–476.

Gerfen, C. R., and Sawchenko, P. E., 1984, An anterograde neuroanatomical tracing method that shows the detailed morphology of neurons, their axons and terminals: Immunohistochemical localization of an axonally transported plant lectin, *Phaseolus vulgaris*-leucoagglutinin (PHA-L), *Brain Res.* **290:**219–238.

Gerfen, C. R., and Sawchenko, P. E., 1985, A method for anterograde axonal tracing of chemically specified circuits in the central nervous system: Combined *Phaseolus vulgaris*-leucoagglutinin (PHA-L) tract tracing and immunohistochemistry, *Brain Res.* **343:**144–150.

Gerfen, C. R., Baimbridge, K. G., and Miller, J. J., 1985, The neostriatal mosaic: Compartmental distribution of calcium binding protein and parvalbumin in the basal ganglia of the rat and monkey, *Proc. Natl. Acad. Sci. U.S.A.* **82:**8780–8784.

Gerfen, C. R., Herkenham, M., and Thibault, J., 1987, The neostriatal mosaic. II. Compartmental organization of dopaminergic and non-dopaminergic mesostriatal systems, *J. Neurosci.* **7:**3915–3934.

Gonatas, N. K., Haper, C., Mizutani, T., and Gonatas, J. O., 1979, Superior sensitivity of conjugates of horseradish peroxidase with wheat germ agglutinin for studies of retrograde transport, *J. Histochem. Cytochem.* **27:**728–734.

Heimer, L., Zaborsky, L., Zahm, D. S., and Alheid, G. F., 1987, The ventral striatopallidothalamic projection: I. The striatopallidal link originating in the striatal parts of the olfactory tubercle, *J. Comp. Neurol.* **255:**571–591.

Herkenham, M., and Pert, C. B., 1982, Light microscopic localization of brain opiate receptors: A general autoradiographic method which preserves tissue quality, *J. Neurosci.* **2:**1129–1149.

Hökfelt, T., Skirboll, L., Rehfeld, J. F., Goldstein, M., Markey, K., and Dann, O., 1980, A subpopulation of mesencephalic dopamine neurons projecting to limbic areas contains a cholescystokinin-like peptide: evidence from immunohistochemistry combined with retrograde tracing, *Neuroscience* **5:**2093–2124.

Hsu, S. M. L., Raine, L., and Fanger, H., 1981, The use of avidin–biotin peroxidase complex (ABC) in immunoperoxidase techniques: A comparison between ABC and unlabeled antibody (PAP) procedures, *J. Histochem. Cytochem.* **29:**577–580.

Itoh, K., Konishi, A., Nomura, S., Mizuno, N., Nakamura, Y., and Sugimoto, I., 1979, Application of coupled oxidation reaction to electron microscopic demonstration of horseradish peroxidase: Cobalt–glucose oxidase, *Brain Res.* **175:**341–346.

McLean, I. W., and Nakane, P., K., 1974, Periodate–lysine–paraformaldehyde fixative. A new fixative for immunoelectron microscopy, *J. Histochem. Cytochem.* **22:**1077–1083.

Mesulam, M. M., 1978, Tetramethyl benzidine for horseradish peroxidase neurochemistry: A non-carcinogenic blue reaction product with superior sensitivity for visualizing neural afferents and efferents, *J. Histochem. Cytochem.* **26:**106–117.

Sawchenko, P. E., and Swanson, L. W., 1981, A method for tracing biochemically defined pathways in the central nervous system using combined fluorescence retrograde transport and immunohistochemical techniques, *Brain Res.* **210:**31–51.

Somogyi, P., and Takagi, H., 1982, A note on the use of picric acid–paraformaldehyde–glutaraldehyde fixative for light and electron microscopic immunocytochemistry, *Neuroscience* **7:**1779–1783.

Staines, W. A., Kimura, H., Fibiger, H. C., and McGeer, E. G., 1980, Peroxidase-labeled lectin as a neuroanatomical tracer: Evaluation in a CNS pathway, *Brain Res.* **197:**485–490.

van der Kooy, D., Coscina, D. V., and Hattori, T., 1981, Is there a non-dopaminergic nigrostriatal pathway? *Neuroscience* **6:**345–357.

Wouterloud, F. G., and Groenewegen, H. J., 1985, Neuroanatomical tracing by use of *Phaseolus vulgaris*-leucoagglutinin (PHA-L): Electron microscopy of PHA-L-filled neuronal somata, dendrites, and axon terminals, *Brain Res.* **326:**188–191.

Zaborszky, L., and Cullinan, W. E., 1989, Hypothalamic axons terminate on forebrain cholin-ergic neurons: An ultrastructural double-labeling study using PHA-L tracing and ChAT immunocytochemistry, *Brain Res.* **479:**177–184.

Zahm, D. S., and Heimer, L., 1985, Synaptic contacts of ventral striatal cells in the olfactory tubercle of the rat: Correlated light and electron microscopy of anterogradely transported *Phaseolus vulgaris*-leucoagglutinin, *Neurosci. Lett.* **60:**169–175.

Combinations of Tracer Techniques, Especially HRP and PHA-L, with Transmitter Identification for Correlated Light and Electron Microscopic Studies

LÁSZLÓ ZÁBORSZKY and LENNART HEIMER

I. INTRODUCTION

The tracing of neural circuits is greatly facilitated if a neuron's projections and afferent synaptic connections as well as its transmitter content can be identified, and various attempts have been made in recent years to accomplish this goal. Since the analysis of synaptic relations requires the use of the electron microscope, the techniques applied in such investigations must be

LÁSZLÓ ZÁBORSZKY • Department of Otolaryngology, University of Virginia Medical Center, Charlottesville, Virginia 22908.   LENNART HEIMER • Departments of Otolaryngology and Neurosurgery, University of Virginia Medical Center, Charlottesville, Virginia 22908.

compatible with ultrastructural studies. When initial studies by Kristensson and Olsson (1971) and LaVail and LaVail (1972) demonstrated the usefulness of horseradish peroxidase (HRP) as a neuroanatomical tracer, it had already been shown that the end product of the HRP reaction is electron dense if DAB is used as a substrate and the tissue is postfixed in osmium tetroxide (Graham and Karnovsky, 1966; see review by Carson and Mesulam, 1982c). The HRP method, therefore, became increasingly popular in combined light–electron microscopic tracer studies.

Since the late 1970s other macromolecules, e.g., lectins and bacterial toxins, that are more efficiently taken up by neurons have been introduced for tracer studies. Nonetheless, because of the simplicity of HRP techniques, such ligands are often conjugated with HRP. Alone or coupled to HRP, these tracers can also be identified at the EM level and thus can be used for combined light and EM studies. One of the lectins, *Phaseolus vulgaris* leukoagglutinin (PHA-L), has been introduced by Gerfen and Sawchenko (1984) as an anterograde tracer, and since the PHA-L method has already established itself as one of the most effective tracer methods available, it is described separately in Chapter 3. However, its combination with the transmitter identification of the postsynaptic target on the EM level is exemplified in this chapter. Because of their simplicity and easy reproducibility, fluorescent substances have become widely used for tracing connections, either alone or in combination with immunohistochemistry or catecholamine histofluorescence (see Chapter 2). However, since fluorescent dyes are not electron dense, they are generally not useful in ultrastructural analysis, at least not without additional procedures, which may compromise the tissue preservation (Reaves *et al.*, 1982). Recently, fluorescent microspheres have been conjugated to colloidal gold for the purpose of ultrastructural analysis of retrogradely labeled neurons (Quattrochi *et al.*, 1987).

After reviewing the relevant literature on the transport mechanisms of various tracers (Section II), we summarize briefly the developments in HRP histochemistry during the last few years (Section III). We then describe how these tracer techniques can be combined with immunocytochemistry and anterograde degeneration techniques (Section IV) and discuss some general methodological problems (Section V). This is followed by a summary of advantages and limitations (Section VI) and a collection of specific recipes in an Appendix (Section VII).

II. INTRACELLULAR AND INTERCELLULAR TRANSPORT OF VARIOUS TRACERS

Axoplasmic transport (Weiss and Hiscoe, 1948) is in general viewed as a homeostatic mechanism for the maintenance of neural functions. Moreover, there is probably a physiological mechanism by which endogenous macromolecules can be transferred through chains of neurons to subserve trophic functions (Dumas *et al.*, 1979; Lasek, 1980; Grafstein and Forman, 1980;

Schubert and Kreutzberg, 1982; Purves and Lichtman, 1985; Sawchenko and Gerfen, 1985; Weiss, 1986; Ochs, 1987). Macromolecules are taken up by nerve cells through endocytosis, which can be characterized as either receptor-mediated, adsorptive, or bulk- or fluid-phase endocytosis. The most specific of these is the receptor-mediated endocytosis in which the ligands bind to specific cell surface receptors (Pastan and Willingham, 1983; Dautry-Varsat and Lodish, 1984). For example, nerve growth factor (NGF), antibodies to transmitter-related enzymes or synaptic antigens, and radiolabeled transmitters are taken up and transported only in particular systems (Iversen *et al.*, 1975; Stockel *et al.*, 1975; Hendry, 1977; Johnson *et al.*, 1978; Max *et al.*, 1978; Silver and Jacobowitz, 1979; Streit, 1980; Wenthold *et al.*, 1984). In the case of radiolabeled transmitters, specificity of the uptake mechanism depends on the concentration of the tracer delivered. Since these tracers are taken up only by a special class of neurons, their use in combined studies is limited.

One class of ligands binds to cell surface oligosaccharides and enters the cell by adsorptive endocytosis. This type of endocytosis is characteristic of ligands such as wheat germ agglutinin (WGA), ricin II, phytohemagglutinin, concanavalin A.* Bacterial toxins and their nontoxic fragments such as choleragenoid (cholera toxin B subunit) or B or C fragments of tetanus toxin belong to the same class. These probes can be visualized either by using immunohistochemistry (Lechan *et al.*, 1981; Evinger and Erichsen, 1986) or by labeling them with radioligand (Schwab *et al.*, 1979; Büttner-Ennever *et al.*, 1981; Steindler, 1982; Steindler and Bradley, 1983), fluorochromes, ferritin, colloidal gold (Schwab and Thoenen, 1978), or biotin (Shiosaka *et al.*, 1986). The most commonly used technology, however, is to conjugate these probes with HRP (Gonatas *et al.*, 1979; Staines *et al.*, 1980) and subsequently apply HRP enzyme visualization techniques.

Fluid-phase endocytosis allows for the indiscriminate uptake of molecules such as HRP. This endocytotic process reflects the normal turnover of the cell surface membrane and does not involve binding to the plasmalemma. Therefore, all cell types in the peripheral or central nervous system can take up native HRP or lectin-conjugated HRP. The tracer has to be delivered in relatively high amount and concentration, and the degree of uptake depends on the concentration gradient and the neural activity (for references see Warr *et al.*, 1981; Steward, 1981; Mesulam, 1982; Carson and Mesulam, 1982c; Broadwell and Balin, 1985).

Several neurotropic viruses, including rabies, herpes simplex, and poliovirus, can invade the CNS through peripheral nerves (Sabin, 1956; Kristensson *et al.*, 1974, 1978; Kucera *et al.*, 1985; Esiri, 1982; Gillet *et al.*, 1986). Following entry into the target cell and replication in its perikaryon, the virus can be anterogradely, retrogradely, and transneuronally transported. Although the entry of the virus into neurons is probably facilitated by recep-

---

*These substances are termed plant lectins, e.g., carbohydrate-binding proteins that can agglutinate erythrocytes and other cell types.

tor-mediated endocytosis, the cellular mechanisms for the spread of the virus and its transcellular transfer are not fully understood (Vahlne *et al.*, 1980; Tyler *et al.*, 1986). Several reports, however, indicate that viruses may be useful as potential retrograde and transneuronal tracers (Bak *et al.*, 1977, 1978; Kristensson *et al.*, 1974, 1978; 1982; Rouiller *et al.*, 1986; Gillet *et al.*, 1986; Ugolini *et al.*, 1987; Norgren *et al.*, 1988). Futhermore, since the specific visualization of viruses is achieved by immunohistochemical techniques, it is possible to determine the transmitter content of the pathway invaded by the virus by using double immunolabeling protocols (McLean *et al.*, 1988).

A. Uptake of Tracer by Intact Terminals and Retrograde Transport

Electron microscopic studies have shown that at various times after injection of HRP in a terminal field, the tracer appears successively in 40- to 70-nm vesicles, 100- to 125-nm vacuoles, membranous sacs, tubular structures, and multivesicular bodies. After having reached the perikaryon, many of the labeled endocytic organelles concentrate near the Golgi complex in a perinuclear position and fuse with primary and secondary lysosomes, thereby initiating the enzymatic degradation of HRP (Broadwell and Brightman, 1979). Lectins and lectin-conjugated HRP as well as cholera toxin label similar structures. In addition, they consistently label the transmost saccule of the Golgi complex or GERL,* where the lectins are packaged either for intracellular distribution, as primary lysosomes destined to fuse with endosomes (a pre-lysosomal compartment), secondary lysosomes, or plasmalemma, or as exocytic (synaptic) vesicles (Broadwell and Balin, 1985; Balin and Broadwell, 1987). The rate of retrograde transport of native HRP has been estimated as between 48 and 120 mm per day in euthermic animals. The transport rate is slightly faster for lectin–HRP conjugates than for free HRP (Grafstein and Forman, 1980; Mesulam, 1982). The rate of degradation likewise is different for HRP and lectins. For example, HRP is no longer detectable in retrogradely labeled neurons after 4–8 days (Turner and Harris, 1974; Mesulam, 1982), whereas lectins or bacterial toxins have been observed in retrogradely labeled neurons 3 weeks after their administration (Wan *et al.*, 1982; Basbaum and Menetrey, 1987).

---

*Novikoff (1973) has assigned the acronym GERL to an acid-phosphatase-reactive smooth membrane system that lies adjacent to the inner *(trans)* face of the Golgi apparatus, is connected to the rough endoplasmic reticulum, and gives rise to lysosomes. According to studies of Broadwell and colleagues (Broadwell and Cataldo, 1984; Broadwell and Balin, 1985), GERL is considered to be synonymous with the transmost Golgi saccule, involved in the production of secretory granules, but does not appear to be related to ER. Structurally, functionally, and cytochemically, GERL is a distinct entity of the Golgi apparatus.

B. Uptake of Tracer by Perikaryon and Dendrites for Subsequent Anterograde Transport

The perikaryal endocytosis of extracellular HRP is accomplished by 40- to 70-nm coated vesicles (LaVail and LaVail, 1974; Turner and Harris, 1974; Nauta *et al.*, 1975; Broadwell and Brightman, 1979) that fuse with endosomes and later undergo transformation into secondary lysosomes (Broadwell *et al.*, 1980). The HRP does not resist degradation but can undergo an anterograde axonal transport in smooth-surfaced cisterns that are morphologically and enzyme cytochemically distinct from the endoplasmic reticulum (Broadwell and Brightman, 1979; Broadwell and Cataldo, 1984). In contrast, the anterograde axonal transport of WGA–HRP involves Golgi-derived components (vesicles, vacuoles, and dense-core secretory granules) as well as tubules and dense bodies related to perikaryal secondary lysosomes (Broadwell and Balin, 1985).

Although degradation of HRP may take place within the terminal area, especially since proteolytic enzymes and peptide hydrolases are present in the axonal endings (Droz, 1973), it has been suggested that most of the anterogradely transported HRP may eventually be returned to the perikaryon for lysosomal degradation (Mesulam, 1982). There is no unequivocal evidence for exocytosis of native peroxidase at the axon terminal or for transsynaptic transfer to other neurons under normal conditions (Colman *et al.*, 1976; Beattie *et al.*, 1978; Wilczynski and Zakon, 1982; Broadwell and Balin, 1985). In contrast to this, part of the lectins or lectin conjugates are exocytosed from the terminal (Broadwell and Balin, 1985). The clearance of anterogradely transported HRP appears to be a relatively slow process, since reaction product at sites of efferent projections can be demonstrated even at survival times of 7–14 days (Mesulam, 1982). Anterogradely transported lectins can still be detected after survival times of 2–3 weeks.

Dendritic branches also can serve as sites of entry for native HRP and lectin-conjugated peroxidase taken directly from the extracellular space or delivered intracellularly by retgrograde axoplasmic transport. Dendritic lysosomes would sequester the tracer proteins for eventual degradation. Tracer endocytosed by dendrites may undergo anterograde axoplasmic transport. This anterograde transport of tracer would involve secondary lysosomes (e.g., dense and multivesicular bodies and tubular profiles) in the case of native peroxidase and secondary lysosomes, the Golgi complex, Golgi-derived synaptic vesicles, and exocytic vacuoles (e.g., dense-core granules) that would label with lectin-conjugated peroxidase (Broadwell *et al.*, 1979, 1984; Broadwell and Cataldo, 1984; Broadwell and Balin, 1985). Labeling of the Golgi complex with lectin-conjugated peroxidase, but not with native HRP, can explain why the anterograde axonal transport of lectin conjugates is more prominent than that of native HRP followed perikaryal or dendritic uptake.

C. Transport of Tracer into Axon Collaterals

Several investigators (e.g., DeOlmos and Heimer, 1977; Huerta *et al.*, 1983; Hopkins *et al.*, 1984) have shown that an injection of HRP into a terminal field may label not only its cells of origin but also their axon collaterals. The mechanism of transport into axon collaterals is not clear. It may be significant, however, that the phenomenon of collateral labeling was first observed when more sensitive HRP methods became available (DeOlmos and Heimer, 1977). Although a significant amount of the retrogradely transported HRP no doubt reaches the perikaryon and subsequently labels the collateral through anterograde transport, some of it may be rechanneled directly from the main axon into the collateral branch for subsequent anterograde transport to its terminals. The smaller the amount of rechanneled HRP, the more sensitive the HRP method would have to be to detect the collateral labeling. Nonetheless, the phenomenon of collateral labeling can be used to advantage by experienced neuroanatomists, especially to guide and complement studies with double-labeling techniques (e.g., Takeuchi *et al.*, 1985). However, it is probably fair to say that the incidental labeling of collateral pathways has created more problems than it has solved, especially since this potential source of erroneous interpretation may not be generally appreciated.

D. Transganglionic Transport

Horseradish peroxidase and lectin-conjugated HRP applied peripherally are transported not only to the cell bodies in sensory ganglia but also to their projection fields within the CNS (Mesulam and Brushart, 1979; Grant *et al.*, 1979; Carson and Mesulam, 1982b; Nyberg and Blomquist, 1985; Bakker *et al.*, 1984; Nyberg, 1988). If a specific nerve is studied, special care must be taken to avoid spread to other nerves in the surrounding area (Craig and Mense, 1983).

E. Transcellular Transport

Wheat germ agglutinin and its derivatives have been shown to undergo transcellular transfer after both orthograde and retrograde transport (Gerfen *et al.*, 1982; Itaya and van Hoesen, 1982; Ruda and Coulter, 1982; Schnyder and Künzle, 1983; Trojanowski and Schmidt, 1984; Broadwell and Balin, 1985; Peschanski and Ralston, 1985; Baker and Spencer 1986). Jankowska and her colleagues (Harrison *et al.*, 1984; Jankowska, 1985; Jankowska and Skoog, 1986) and Alstermark and Kümmel (1986) have used this phenomenon in a more systematic fashion for functional–anatomic studies of spinal interneurons after peripheral administration of WGA–HRP.

The occurrence and degree of transneuronal labeling are dependent on many variables, including survival time (e.g., Itaya and van Hoesen, 1982;

Takada and Hattori, 1986) and amount of the tracer injected (e.g., Peschanski and Ralston, 1985) and possibly on the type of synapse involved (Porter *et al.*, 1985). Important observations have been made by Takada and Hattori (1986) and Rhodes *et al.* (1987), who found that WGA released from axon terminal can label nearby cellular elements including astrocytes regardless of whether they are related synaptically to the labeled terminals or not. In other words, transneuronal spread of WGA–HRP does not necessarily follow a specific transsynaptic pathway.

Transcellular transfer of tetanus toxin (Schwab *et al.*, 1979) or its C fragment (Evinger and Erichsen, 1986; Fishman and Carrigan, 1987) has also been documented in retrograde tracer studies. In the case of the tetanus toxin, the extracellular space and the synaptic cleft were free of reaction product, which suggests that the transfer of tetanus toxin takes place preferentially in the region of the synapse (Schwab *et al.*, 1977, 1979). Transneuronal transfer of free HRP has apparently been demonstrated in some non-mammalian forms (Nassel, 1981; Wilczynski and Zakon, 1982), but it does not seem to occur in mammals except under exceptional circumstances such as following direct intraneuronal injections (Triller and Korn, 1981; Freund *et al.*, 1985), which invariably cause membrane damage.

Although the mechanism of transneuronal transfer of tracer is not fully understood, Broadwell and Balin (1985) have suggested that the involvement of the transmost Golgi saccule is important for packaging of the tracer and subsequent exocytosis. When lectins or lectin conjugates are used for transneuronal labeling, the signal is usually diminished in the second-order neuron (Ugolini *et al.*, 1987). This problem does not exist in regard to viruses, which typically undergo replication in the cell body, thereby increasing the available tracer in the second-order neuron (e.g., Ugolini *et al.*, 1987). Unfortunately, as in the case of the lectins, the transfer of the viruses is apparently not restricted to areas of synaptic contacts, and glial cells may also be involved (Oppenshaw and Ellis, 1983; Ugolini *et al.*, 1977).

F. Uptake into Fibers of Passage and through Damaged Membrane Surfaces

It appears that free HRP can be taken up by undamaged axons of passage (Herkenham and Nauta, 1977; Aschoff and Schönitzer, 1982; Grob *et al.*, 1982). This is apparently not the case in regard to lectins (e.g., Grob *et al.*, 1982; Steindler, 1982). Damaged neurons, however, can incorporate both types of tracers to a significant degree (Brodal *et al.*, 1983). If the axon is damaged, the label is not membrane bound but rather adheres to the surfaces of intraaxonal organelles including microtubules and filaments, thereby giving the axon a homogeneous appearance at the light microscopic level. Cell bodies and axon terminals of damaged neurons may likewise appear solidly labeled (Fig. 1). On the other hand, it was observed in earlier studies of HRP transport in the peripheral nervous system (Kristensson and Olsson,

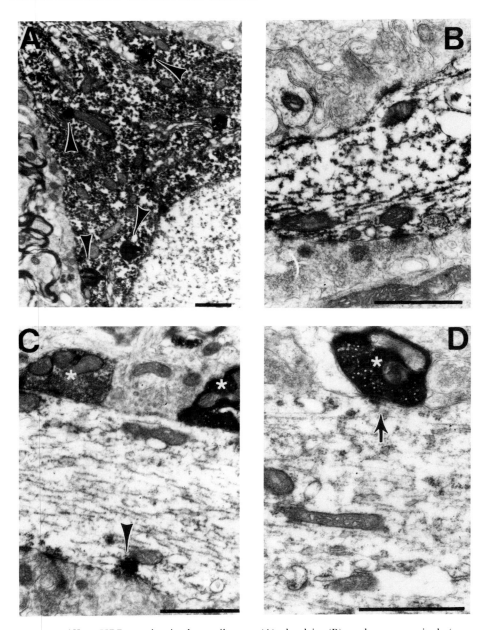

Figure 1. Diffuse HRP reaction in the perikaryon (A), dendrite (B), and axon terminals (stars in C and D) of the ventral pallidum after an HRP injection in the subthalamic nucleus. Sections were processed only for DAB–glucose oxidase reaction. Arrowheads in A and C illustrate transported HRP granules. Arrow in D points to postsynaptic thickening. Bar scale: 1 μm.

1976; Anderson *et al.*, 1979; Malmgren and Olsson, 1979) that in more proximal parts of damaged nerve fibers the HRP may become segregated within vesicles and tubular organelles and be actively transported back to the cell body rather than being diffusely distributed. This would make the labeling in the cell body indistinguishable from retrogradely labeled cell bodies following uptake through intact axon terminal.

G. Summary

Lectins, lectin conjugates, and bacterial toxins used as tracers are consistently more sensitive than free HRP. They are also more suitable for visualizing anterograde and transganglionic transport, and they usually result in more complete dendritic filling of retrogradely labeled neurons. The number of labeled neurons is greater when these tracers are used as compared to free HRP. The use of WGA–HRP in a concentration of 0.5–2%, for instance, results in smaller and better demarcated injection sites than free HRP in 20–30% solutions.

The increased sensitivity achieved by the use of lectins, their conjugates, or bacterial toxins may result from several factors. For instance, lectins and their conjugates remain at the injection site for a considerably longer time than HRP, which is rapidly removed and usually completely eliminated from the injection site after 7 days; WGA–HRP and cholera toxin–HRP, in contrast, can still be identified in the injection site after 13-day survival. Therefore, these tracers may be available for uptake and transport for longer time periods than free HRP. On the other hand, because of their specific uptake sites, lectins or bacterial toxins show little extracellular spread, thereby producing reliable small injections. Other factors that may increase the sensitivity are greater efficiency of the adsorptive endocytosis compared to fluid-phase endocytosis, different transport mechanisms, and differences in the rate of degradation or elimination of the substance.

When results are compared from different studies or decisions are made regarding the tracer to be used in a given experiment, it is important to keep in mind that different regions may show different sensitivity to the same lectin. Different lectin conjugates, e.g., WGA–HRP and choleragenoid–HRP, furthermore, may give rise to markedly different labeling patterns in the same system. These differences can be attributed to several factors such as differences in the distribution of specific binding sites on neuronal membranes or across neuronal populations (Schnyder and Künzle, 1983; Robertson and Grant, 1985). The binding and transport capacities of the lectins may also vary according to the characteristics of the conjugates and the linking reagents used (Trojanowski, 1983; Neal and Cary, 1986).

Although there are indisputable advantages to the use of lectins or bacterial toxins in tract-tracing experiments, one must keep in mind that the increased sensitivity can quickly lead the investigator astray if he or she is not careful. When these tracers are used in the study of less well-known pathways, one should always be alert to the possibility that what may seem like a surprisingly attractive "new discovery" may in fact be a misinterpretation of a labeled collateral system or an insidious case of transneuronal transfer of the label.

III. HORSERADISH PEROXIDASE HISTOCHEMICAL REACTIONS

Three different techniques are available for detecting the transported HRP. One possibility is to label the HRP or its apoenzyme with a radioactive isotope, another is to use immunohistochemistry, and a third and most popular alternative is based on a histochemical reaction. In the last procedure, the sections are incubated in a medium containing hydrogen peroxide and a chromogen, usually a benzidine derivative, that is oxidized to a colored product by the peroxide–peroxidase system. The most commonly used chromogens are diaminobenzidine tetrahydrochloride (DAB), benzidine dihydrochloride (BDHC), tetramethylbenzidine (TMB), o-dianisidine (dimethoxybenzidine dihydrochloride), o-tolidine (dimethylbenzidine), and p-phenylenediamine dihydrochloride pyrocatechol (PPD-PC). There are significant differences in the sensitivity and in the appearance and distribution of reaction product when these different chromogens are used, and there seems to be a general consensus that the TMB method in its various modifications is one of the most sensitive methods (Deschenes *et al.*, 1979; Somogyi *et al.*, 1979; Morell *et al.*, 1981; Warr *et al.*, 1981; Carson and Mesulam, 1982a; Mesulam, 1982; Olsson *et al.*, 1983).

Although the original DAB procedure of Graham and Karnovsky (1966) and its modification by LaVail and LaVail (1974) belong to the least sensitive techniques, the DAB method has so far been the most commonly used technique for electron microscopy. It is simple, easily reproducible, and can be used at neutral pH, although the optimal sensitivity of the enzyme reaction is achieved at a pH of about 5.1 (Malmgren and Olsson, 1977, 1978). The neutral pH, however, facilitates the combination with immunostaining and is compatible with good ultrastructure. The brown reaction product is osmiophilic, thereby making DAB-stained material suited for electron microscopic studies. The traditional DAB procedure is not suitable for the demonstration of anterograde transport at the light microscopic level, but it has been used to identify labeled terminals in the electron microscope (Nauta *et al.*, 1975; Záborszky *et al.*, 1984; see also Fig. 3A).

To potentiate the uptake and transport of HRP, various substances such as dimethyl sulfoxide (DMSO) and adenosine poly-1-ornithine (Warr *et al.*, 1981) have been added to the HRP solution. Efforts have also been made to increase the sensitivity of the DAB procedure by adding 0.01 M imidazole (Malmgren and Olsson, 1977; Strauss, 1982), heavy metals (Adams, 1981), or p-cresol (Streit and Reubi, 1977) to the incubation medium. Itoh *et al.* (1979), furthermore, suggested the use of a coupled oxidation reaction, originally described by Lundquist and Josephson (1971), in which H_2O_2 is continuously supplied in low concentration by the enzymatic reaction of glucose oxidase on glucose. Finally, the lower sensitivity of the DAB procedure can to some extent be counterbalanced by increasing the amount of the tracer injected, but this usually reduces the specificity of the results obtained.

One of the drawbacks with the benzidine derivatives is that they are potentially carcinogenic, and the noncarcinogenic Hanker–Yates substrate (PPD-PC) has therefore received considerable attention (Hanker et al., 1977). Although PPD-PC was considered one of the least sensitive chromogens in the now well-known comparison of different methods published by Mesulam and Rosene (1979), it should be mentioned that investigators with considerable practical experience have a different opinion (e.g., Reiner and Gamlin, 1980; Spreafico et al., 1982; Campbell et al., 1984; Taylor and Lieberman, 1987; Somogyi and Freund, Chapter 9, this volume). The results obtained by these investigators do show that PPD-PC can be used effectively as both a retrograde and an anterograde tracer and furthermore is well suited for ultrastructural studies. It usually takes considerable effort and careful attention to details on the part of the investigator to exploit fully the advantages of a specific method, and unless every method being compared has been granted this kind of affectionate attention, the results of a comparison are likely to be slanted. It should be mentioned in this context that the recently introduced stabilization procedure for the o-tolidine and o-dianisidine (Segade, 1987) techniques may increase the number of alternate HRP histochemical reactions available for ultrastructural studies.

One of the most commonly used chromogens is TMB, which has been claimed to be noncarcinogenic (Holland et al., 1974). However, it is not so much this quality but rather the high sensitivity of the TMB reaction that has made it so popular. Its popularity has so far been restricted mostly to light microscopic tracing experiments, and it is only in the last few years that the TMB reaction has been successfully applied in combined light–EM studies. Some of the problems in using TMB for ultrastructural studies are the relative instability and the excessive crystallization of the product. The TMB reaction, which is optimal at pH 3.3 (Mesulam, 1978), is not osmiophilic, and it is highly soluble in the organic solvents used for preparing tissue for electron microscopy. However, after osmication at higher pH and temperature, the blue TMB product is converted into a dark insoluble product, which can be preserved through dehydration and embedding (Sakumoto et al., 1980; Stürmer et al., 1981; Carson and Mesulam, 1982a; Henry et al., 1985).

Recently, Rye et al. (1984) described a stabilization procedure for TMB histochemistry that involves an additional incubation in a DAB/cobalt/hydrogen peroxide solution. The reaction product obtained with this method is stable in ethanol or aqueous solutions at neutral pH and offers a sensitivity comparable to standard TMB procedures. Tissue reacted with this procedure, is also suited for EM studies (Lehmann et al., 1985; Zahm, 1989). Instead of using sodium nitroferricyanide as stabilizing agent in the TMB procedure, Olucha et al. (1985) introduced ammonium heptamolybdate, which reduces the nonspecific crystallization. Furthermore, a less acidic milieu (pH

6) provides for better ultrastructure (Cunningham and LeVay, 1986; Voigt *et al.*, 1988). Recently Tsai *et al.* (1988) and Chen *et al.* (1989) used a double-label technique by combining the TMB procedure of Olucha *et al.* (1985) with the regular DAB procedure to demonstrate two antigens at the EM level. Hopefully, this protocol may be used also in tract-tracing studies in combination with transmitter identification.

IV. COMBINATION OF TRACER STUDY WITH TRANSMITTER IDENTIFICATION

In order to combine successfully light and EM tract tracing and transmitter identification in the same preparation, one would ideally like to have fulfilled the following conditions: (1) that the tracer be taken up only by undamaged axon terminals or undamaged somatodendritic membranes, (2) that all axon terminals or somatodendritic membranes within the injection site take up the tracer and transport it, independent of the functional state or membrane characteristics of the neuron, (3) that small amounts of injected tracer substance generate large amounts of detectable transported material, (4) that the tracer be transported only in retrograde or anterograde direction, depending on the goal of the investigation, (5) that the transported substance be stable without decomposition for a reasonably long time, (6) that the two (or more) detection systems show the highest sensitivity with the same fixation parameters, (7) that both markers be visible and easily differentiated from each other both on the light and EM level, and, last but not least, (8) that the procedures be compatible with good tissue preservation so that the ultrastructural characteristics of the synaptic profiles can be unequivocally determined.

A double-labeling study of synaptic relations at the EM level is often a natural extension of previous light microscopic studies, in which case the "double-labeling" study at the EM level usually serves the purpose of confirming or rejecting a proposition based on a light microscopic study. Nonetheless, light and EM analyses are often done on the same material in order to facilitate the correlation between the two levels of analysis.

Tables I and II summarize the characteristics of the different tracers and their combinations with methods for transmitter identification. Although some examples of various combinations are mentioned below, it should be emphasized that the possibilities of combining various techniques are limited mostly by the investigator's own imagination.

A. Combining Immunocytochemistry with Ultrastructural Analysis of Anterograde Degeneration

The terminal portion of an axon undergoes degeneration following axon transection or lesioning of the parent cell body. Degenerating synaptic bou-

Table I. Characteristics of Prospective Tracers for Combined Studies

Tracer	Application	Concentration[a] and volume Central	Peripheral	Survival time	References
1. HRP	Anterograde, retrograde Collateral, transganglionic	20–50% 0.05–0.7 µl	20–70% 0.2–10 µl	5 hr–4 days	Warr et al., 1981; Mesulam, 1982; Taylor and Lieberman, 1987
2. WGA	Similar to 1; in addition transcellular	0.1–5% 0.5–2 µl	1% 50 µl	4–5 days	Lechan et al., 1981; Ruda and Coulter, 1982; Porter et al., 1985
3. [^{125}I]-WGA	Same as 2	10–50 µCi/µg 0.7 µl (3.2 µCi/µl)	20 µCi/µg 10 µl (50 pmole)	14 hr–7 days	Dumas et al., 1979; Rhodes et al., 1987
4. N-[acetyl-^{3}H]-WGA	Anterograde Retrograde	0.16–0.88% 0.3–1.9 mCi/mg 0.025–0.6 µl		1–7 days	Steindler and Bradley, 1983
5. WGA–HRP	Same as 2	1–10% 0.01–0.6 µl	0.1–10% 5–50 µl	1–14 days	Gerfen et al., 1982; Itaya and van Hoesen, 1982; Brodal et al., 1983; Trojanowski and Gonatas, 1983; Jankowska, 1985; Lemann et al., 1985; Peschanski and Ralston, 1985; Baker and Spencer, 1986; Rouiller et al., 1986; Takada and Hattori, 1986;
6. Biotin–WGA	Retrograde	2% 1 µl		2 days	Shiosaka et al., 1986

(continued)

Table I. (*continued*)

Tracer	Application	Concentration[a] and volume		Survival time	References
		Central	Peripheral		
7. WGA–apoHRP–Au	Retrograde	2.5–5% 0.2–1 µl		2 days	Basbaum and Menetrey, 1987
8. CGFM	Retrograde	0.5–1 µl		4–7 days	Quattrochi et al., 1987
9. Choleragenoid (CG)	Retrograde	1% 0.2 µl		24 hr	Luppi et al., 1987
10. CG–HRP	Same as 1		0.2% 0.5–1 µl	4 hr–12 days	Robertson and Grant, 1985
11. [^{125}I]-CG	Retrograde		350 pmole 10 µl	14 hr	Dumas et al., 1979
12. [^{125}I]-B-II$_b$[b]	Same as 2		1.3–5 µCi/µl 50 µl (10 µCi/µg)	1–6 days	Büttner-Enever et al., 1981
13. Tetanus C fragment	Transsynaptic		5% 5–20 µl	6 hr–8 days	Evinger and Erichsen, 1986; Fishman and Carrigan, 1987
14. Herpes simplex	Same as 2	10^{4-6} PFU/ml 0.2–1 µl	10^{5-9} PFU/ml 20–100 µl	2–6 days	Bak et al., 1978; Kristensson et al., 1982; Oppenshaw and Ellis, 1983; Ugolini et al., 1987
15. Rabies	Retrograde	10^5 LD$_{50}$ 0.5 µl	4×10^5 PFU/ml 10 µl	1–5 days	Kucera et al., 1985; Gillet et al., 1986
16. [^{125}I]-NGF	Retrograde	88–115 µCi/µg 0.2–0.4 µl	1.5–50 µCi/µg 3–30 µl	4 hr–2 days	Stoeckel et al., 1975; Max et al., 1978; Johnson et al., 1978; Seiler and Schwab, 1984

[a] If radiolabeled substances are used, specific activity is also given.
[b] Tetanus toxin fragment.

Table II. Combinations of Tract Tracing with Transmitter Identification

Tracer	Visualization	Transmitter visualization
Anterograde degeneration	—	DAB
HRP or WGA–HRP	DAB	DAB
HRP or HRP conj.	DAB	BDHC
HRP or HRP conj.[a]	DAB	Immunoautoradiography
HRP or HRP conj.[b]	DAB	Ferritin
Biotin–WGA	Steptavidin–gold	DAB
WGA–apoHRP–gold	Silver intensification	DAB
Gold-microspheres[c]	—	DAB
PHA-L	BDHC	DAB
PHA-L	NiDAB	DAB

[a]See Chapter 5.
[b]See Chapter 6.
[c]This combination apparently has not been attempted.

tons can be easily recognized in the electron microscope (Mugnaini and Friedrich, 1981), but the technique does not provide any information about the chemical nature of the degenerating axons or axon terminals. However, by combining lesion technique with immunocytochemistry at the ultrastructural level (Palkovits *et al.*, 1982), it may be possible to identify the chemical character of the postsynaptic profile contacted by a degenerating bouton (Fig. 2A). It is considerably more difficult to identify the transmitter or peptide content in a degenerating terminal* (Fig. 2B) because the dense axoplasm obscures the immunoprecipitates in dark degenerating systems. On the other hand, in degenerating monoaminergic terminals, where part of the terminal may be free of degenerating material, immunostaining has been observed (e.g., Léránth and Feher, 1983; Léránth *et al.*, 1988). It is also important to remember that different axonal systems may show different types of degeneration and/or different time courses for the degenerating events (Záborszky *et al.*, 1979). These are important considerations that are directly related to the choice of survival time. Degenerating nerve terminals are gradually removed by glial processes, and it is therefore important to choose a reasonably short survival time at which the synaptic contact site is still recognizable. Although a "conglomerate" (Heimer, 1972) engulfed by glia may suggest the presence of a degenerating bouton, the absence of a recognizable synaptic contact prevents an analysis of specific interneural connections. On the other hand, the survival time must be long enough that clear-cut signs of degeneration have had time to develop.

With the use of axon-sparing neurotoxins (ibotenate, kainate), the fibers-of-passage problem can be circumvented, and the application of agents that are toxic only for certain transmitter systems (6-OHDA, 5,7-DHT, AF64A, DSP, etc.) may increase the specificity or selectivity of the lesion.

*At the light microscopic level fields of degenerating terminals can be matched with decline in the immunostaining pattern (Záborszky *et al.*, 1985).

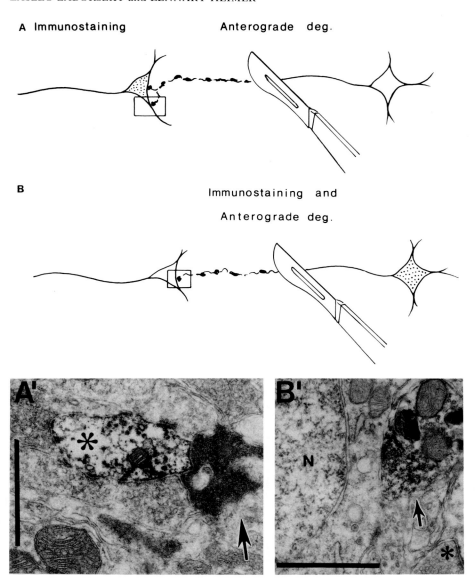

Figure 2. Combination of anterograde degeneration technique with immunocytochemistry. A: The presynaptic profile is identified by anterograde degeneration, and the postsynaptic site by immunocytochemistry. A': Degenerating terminal (arrow) in synaptic contact with a glutamic acid decarboxylase-positive dendrite (asterisk) in the ventral pallidum after lesion of the nucleus accumbens. The animal received a colchicine injection intraventricularly 48 hr before sacrifice, and the lesion was made 30 hr before perfusion. B: The presynaptic site is characterized by both immunocytochemistry and anterograde degeneration. B': Synapse between a degenerated tyrosine hydroxylase-immunoreactive bouton (arrow) and the soma of an immunonegative neuron in the medial preoptic area 48 hr after transection of the ascending noradrenergic bundle. Note the normal bouton in the lower right corner (asterisk). N, nucleus. B' reproduced from Léránth *et al.* (1988) by permission of the editors of *Neuroendocrinology.* Bar scales: 1 μm.

B. Tract Tracing Using HRP or Lectin–HRP Conjugates in Combination with HRP-Based Immunocytochemistry

The procedural steps vary depending on whether both HRP products are visualized by the same chromogen or whether two different chromogens are used.

1. Double Labeling Using the Same Chromogen (DAB–DAB)

Since both the DAB and the DAB–glucose oxidase (Itoh *et al.*, 1979) techniques are simple and characterized by uniform staining products, DAB is an excellent chromogen for ultrastructural studies. The nature of the inquiry determines the experimental design. For instance, one may want to label either the pre- or postsynaptic profile with a tracer and identify the other profile by its transmitter, or it may be useful to label either the pre- or postsynaptic profile with both markers (Figs. 3–5). A neuron, furthermore, can be identified by its target as well as by its transmitter content, and anterograde degeneration can be used for determining one of its afferent inputs.

Oldfield *et al.* (1983) and Záborszky *et al.* (1984) used this type of combination to show HRP-labeled terminals in synaptic contact with immunocytochemically identified postsynaptic neurons (Fig. 3A), whereas Ruda *et al.* (1984) and Záborszky *et al.* (1986) identifed retrogradely labeled neurons in contact with boutons whose transmitter was specified (Fig. 3B). Another combination is shown in Figs. 4 and 5, in which retrogradely labeled basal forebrain neurons are also characterized by their content of choline acetyltransferase, the enzyme that synthesizes acetylcholine (Záborszky and Léránth, 1985).*

In order to preserve the reaction product from both the transported HRP and the peroxidase-labeled tissue antigen, two protocols can be used (Oldfield *et al.*, 1983). One possibility is to sequentially stain the sections, first to localize transported HRP, followed by the immunocytochemical procedure to identify the antigen. The other approach employs a single DAB reaction for simultaneous localization of the two HRP moieties. Oldfield *et al.* (1983) used both approaches in their study of afferents to hypothalamic neurosecretory neurons. In our study of cholinergic amygdalopetal neurons (Záborszky and Léránth, 1985), the simultaneous technique did not retain the retrogradely transported HRP product to a sufficient degree, probably because of the long incubation in the primary antibody. Therefore, it was difficult to distinguish the transported HRP from lysosomes present normally. The sequential technique, on the other hand, allows excellent preservation of the retrogradely transported HRP (Bowker *et al.*, 1981, 1982; Priestley *et al.*, 1981; Wainer and Rye, 1984), and the reactive dense bodies are clearly more electron dense than lysosomes not containing transported peroxidase

---

*A sequential processing for retrograde HRP and AChE was used by Lewis and Henderson (1980) to characterize putative cholinergic projection neurons of the basal forebrain at the EM level.

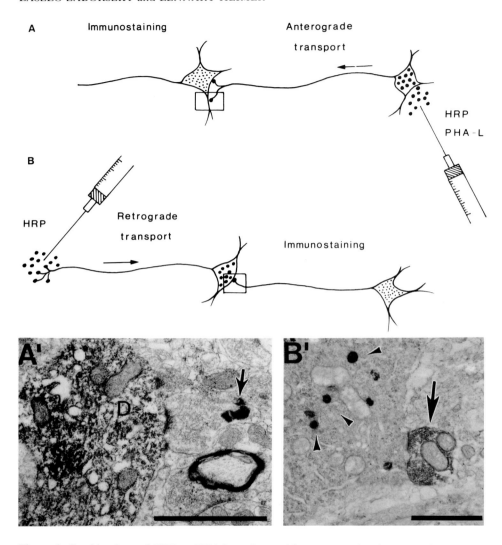

Figure 3. Combinations of HRP or PHA-L tracing and immunocytochemistry. A: The presynaptic terminal is characterized by anterograde transport of HRP, and the postsynaptic site is labeled by immunocytochemistry. A': Electron micrograph showing a choline acetyltransferase (ChAT)-positive dendritic profile (D) in synaptic contact with an axon terminal containing anterogradely transported HRP (arrow) from an injection site in the basolateral amygdaloid nucleus. The section was processed for ChAT immunostaining with DAB. B: The postsynaptic site is characterized by retrograde labeling with HRP, and the presynaptic terminal is stained with immunocytochemistry. B': Retrogradely labeled cell body backfilled from the basolateral amygdaloid nucleus in the ventral pallidum receiving a GAD-containing terminal (arrow). Transported HRP is indicated by arrowheads. The section was first processed with DAB–glucose oxidase reaction and then for GAD immunostaining. Reproduced from Záborszky *et al.* (1984 and 1986) by permission of Elsevier Science Publishers, Inc. (A') and Alan R. Liss, Inc. (B'). Bar scales: 1 μm.

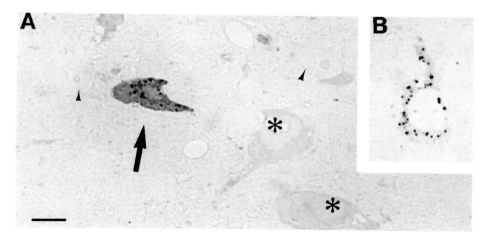

Figure 4. Appearance of unlabeled (arrowhead), retrogradely labeled (B), cholinergic (asterisk) and double-labeled (arrow) cells in a semithin (1-μm) section processed first with the DAB– glucose oxidase reaction and then for choline acetyltransferase immunostaining. Bar scale: 10 μm. Reproduced from Záborszky and Léránth (1985) by permission of Springer Verlag.

(Fig. 5C). In addition, the sequential protocol provides a better correlation between light and electron microscopy, since the retrogradely labeled cells can be identified and photographed in each sequential step of the procedure.

The correlation between LM and EM is very useful since the differences between double-labeled neurons and those exhibiting positive staining either for retrograde HRP or for the transmitter under consideration are not always conclusive at the LM level. For example, the labeling by transported HRP is often quite heavy, especially if HRP has been taken up by damaged axons of passage (Morell *et al.*, 1981; Bowker *et al.*, 1982), in which case retrogradely transported HRP has a tendency to obscure the presence of immunostaining. Immunopositive neurons without retrograde labeling, on the other hand, can occasionally show a granulated rather than diffuse appearance in regular light microscopy, in which case they can be mistakenly identified as retrogradely labeled neurons. Transillumination of the embedded sections or analysis of semithin sections (Fig. 4) usually provides a correct diagnosis. The use of cobalt or nickel salts in the first DAB reaction (Hsu and Soban, 1982) or silver intensification of the DAB end product (Gallyas and Merchenthaler, 1988; Merchenthaler *et al.*, 1989) gives the retrogradely transported HRP a black color, which can be easily separated from the brown DAB product of immunoprecipitates (Bowker *et al.*, 1982).

The immunoperoxidase reaction product is associated with ribosomes, outer membranes of mitochondria, and microtubules of dendrites. This flocculent reaction product is distinct from large dense transported HRP granules related to vesicular, tubular, and lysosomal elements (Fig. 5). By the use of the

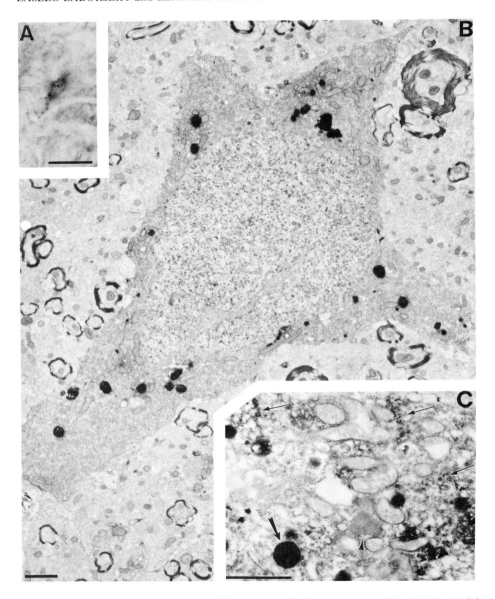

Figure 5. Retrograde tracing of HRP and immunostaining in the same profile. A: Retrogradely labeled neuron prior to immunostaining as seen in the wet section. B: Electron micrograph of the same neuron labeled for ChAT. C: High-power view of a detail of the same neuron in a different plane of section. Thin arrows show the flocculent immunoprecipitates for ChAT, and the thick arrow points to a transported HRP granule. The arrowhead points to a nonreactive lysosome. Note that the electron density of this structure is less than that of dense bodies staining positively for peroxidase. Ultrathin sections were counterstained with lead citrate. Bar scale: 1 μm in B and C, 50 μm in A. Reproduced from Záborszky and Léránth (1985) by permission of Springer Verlag.

DAB–glucose oxidase reaction in the first step (see Appendix, Section VII.A), it is often possible to identify HRP products even in small dendrites.

2. Double Labeling Using Two Different Chromogens (DAB–BDHC)

The two HRP products can be easily distinguished by the use of two different benzidine derivatives. Double-labeling protocols using DAB–BDHC have recently been described both for double antigen localization (Levey *et al.*, 1986) and for transported HRP and antigen determination (Lakos and Basbaum, 1986). Between pH 6 and 7, BDHC generates a crystalline reaction product that is bluish-green as compared to the reddish-brown and homogeneous DAB reaction product. The crystalline BDHC reaction product can easily be differentiated from the flocculent DAB product in the electron microscope. Because the solubility and instability of BDHC increase at higher pH, it is essential to react the tissue first with DAB to identify the transported HRP and then with BDHC for immunocytochemistry.

Although BDHC has many advantages, it also has its difficulties. One is the instability of the reaction product, which, despite several adjustments (see below), still creates some problems. Furthermore, the increased sensitivity and the particle-like nature of the reaction product sometimes makes it difficult to distinguish a positive signal from background. Lakos and Basbaum (1986) have discussed these problems in detail; they also introduced a glutaraldehyde pretreatment to reduce the background, but unfortunately this pretreatment also seems to reduce the sensitivity of the BDHC reaction. Their technique, as well as the one described by Levey *et al.* (1986), are included in the Appendix (Sections VII.B and VII.C).

Best results are usually produced by keeping the pH of the incubation solution in the range of 6.5–6.8. The temperature, time, and H_2O_2 concentration of the incubation solutions are also important. Higher concentrations of H_2O_2, for example, will shorten the incubation time (Lakos and Basbaum, 1986), whereas a lower concentration may reduce the nonspecific staining (Levey *et al.*, 1986). The addition of 0.25% λ-carrageenan (Sigma, Type IV) to the immunocytochemical incubation solution seems to reduce the background (L. Záborszky and W. E. Cullinan, unpublished observation). We also used Triton X-100 (up to 0.1%) to enhance the specific staining without increasing the background deposit, although nuclear staining seemed to be enhanced. To counterbalance the deleterious effect of Triton and the lower pH of the BDHC reaction, we increased slightly the glutaraldehyde concentration of the fixative to 0.2%. Since at higher ionic strength the BDHC crystals are slightly bigger and the nonspecific staining is more pronounced, a lower concentration of buffer, i.e., 0.01–0.02 M, is recommended in the incubation and postrinse solutions (Levey *et al.*, 1986). The type of buffer used also seems to play a role; when acetate buffer is used, the BDHC reaction product appears in both crystalline and diffuse forms, whereas phosphate buffer at the same pH produces only crystalline BDHC deposits (Levey *et al.*, 1986). Since prolonged alcohol dehydration and osmification result in significant loss of BDHC staining, Lakos and Basbaum (1986) suggested the use of *s*-collidine-buffered osmium at 45°C and pH 6.5. We also had good results witth 0.1–0.01 M phosphate-buffered osmium at pH 6.0 at room temperature.

C. Use of Gold-Labeled Tracers in Combination with Peroxidase-Based Immunocytochemistry

The introduction of colloidal gold as an electron-dense label (for references see van den Pol, 1984) has greatly improved our options to use double-labeling procedures for correlated light–EM studies. Several protocols have been published in which the tracer, tagged with colloidal gold, is represented either by lectin conjugates or fluorescent microspheres and in which the identification of the transmitter may be accomplished by the peroxidase–DAB reaction.

1. WGA–apoHRP–Gold

Removal of the heme portion of the HRP molecule eliminates its enzymatic activity but does not interfere with retrograde transport (Hayes and Rustioni, 1979). This observation prompted Basbaum and Menetrey (1987) to prepare a complex containing WGA and enzymatically inactive HRP (apoHRP) and to couple it to colloidal gold. This molecule, i.e., WGA–apoHRP–Au, is visualized with silver intensification and gold toning in retrogradely labeled neurons at the light microscopic level. Mild fixatives compatible with immunohistochemistry can be used according to Basbaum and Menetrey (1987). Since silver intensification does not interfere with fluorescent retrograde tracing or indirect immunofluorescence, sections can be evaluated for the presence of double- or triple-labeled neurons in the light microscope before EM analysis. The colloidal gold is electron dense and can be detected with or without silver intensification at the EM level. Since the appearance of the colloidal gold or its gold-toned product is distinct from HRP-based immunoprecipitation, the technique is also suitable for transmitter identification of retrogradely identified neurons at the electron microscopic level, using HRP-based immunocytochemistry.

Basbaum and Menetrey (1987) did not detect signs of anterograde or transneuronal transport when using the abovementioned protein–gold complex. If this is the case, it may be a valuable feature since labeled cells will never be masked by dense, anterogradely labeled terminals in cases where reciprocal connections are present.* Interpretation of retrograde transport studies, furthermore, which are often complicated by the possibility of trans-neuronal transfer of WGA–HRP (Peschanski and Ralston, 1985), may not be a problem when using the protein–Au complex.

Although the silver intensification and the gold-toning procedure usually reduce the subsequent immunostaining, good results have nevertheless been reported in immunostaining for serotonin, GABA, or tyrosine hydroxylase (Basbaum and Menetrey, 1987). According to our observation, however, no immunostaining was observed after gold toning using a monoclonal antibody against choline acetyltransferase.

2. Colloidal Gold-Labeled Fluorescent Microspheres (CGFM)

Although neurons labeled with retrogradely transported fluorescent tracer tend to show an accumulation of lysosomal structures and myelinated bodies (Schmued *et al.*, 1988), there is no specific sign that characterizes a fluorescently labeled neuron on the ultrastructural level. To bridge the gap between the light and the electron microscope and to make sure that the fluorescently labeled cell is also the one being investigated with the electron microscope may therefore require elaborate reconstructions. The task would be easier if the fluorescent tracer were conjugated with an electron-dense marker, and Quattrochi *et al.* (1987) has recently conjugated rhodamine latex beads with colloidal gold. After the retrogradely labeled neuron is identified in the fluorescence miscroscope, regular EM processing allows the identification of the same cell in the electron microscope because of the electron density of the gold particles.

Gold particles are localized in lysosomes, which suggests that these conjugates are taken up by fluid-phase endocytosis. Since the size and surface properties of latex microspheres are known to affect their uptake and subsequent transport, only microspheres of a certain size (0.02–0.2 μm) can be used for the coupling procedure (Katz *et al.*, 1984; J. J. Quattrochi, personal communication). The conjugation procedure does not seem to compromise the retrograde transport. Since different sizes of colloidal gold can be conjugated to fluorescent beads, collateral projections can also be studied at the EM level. The CGFM tracer represents a promising development, but at the time of this writing it does not seem to have been used in combination with transmitter identification. The protocol of the CGFM coupling technique is presented in the Appendix (Section VII.F).

---

*In cases of reciprocal connections, HRP injections usually result in both anterograde and retrograde label. If the presence of anterogradely labeled terminals interferes with the interpretation of the results, a coinjection of HRP–WGA with a fiber-sparing neurotoxin (e.g., kainic acid or ibotenate) may prevent the appearance of such terminals through lesioning of parent cell bodies at the injection sites.

3. Tracer Labeled with Gold in a Postembedding Protocol

Tohyama and his coworkers (Shiosaka *et al.*, 1986) have applied biotinized WGA as a retrograde tracer and used the streptavidin–Texas red linking for light microscopic visualization. The tracer was identified in the electron microscope by the aid of a postembedding procedure whereby streptavidin-labeled colloidal gold was coupled to the biotinized WGA already present in the thin section. The transmitter was identified with FITC-labeled IgG for light microscopy and with the PAP technique for EM. One of the advantages of this technique is that it uses a lectin rather than free HRP; it also makes use of a visualization technique at the light or EM level that is separate from HRP immunoreaction. The same fixative, furthermore, can be used successfully both for immunocytochemistry and avidin–biotin linking, and it is therefore possible to identify the transmitter of the retrogradely labeled neurons at both the light and EM level with a high degree of sensitivity. The procedure seems to be a useful alternative in the growing number of double-labeling techniques that do not use an HRP-based tracer system. The technique may yet be improved so that the correlation between light and EM can be done in the same section rather than in separate specimens (Shiosaka *et al.*, 1986), which makes the sampling procedure more difficult. Instead of biotinylated WGA, a more sensitive probe, photobiotin (Lacey and Grant, 1987), can be used as the retrograde tracer (M. Tohyama, personal communication, 1988).

D. PHA-L Tracing in Combination with Transmitter Identification of the Postsynaptic Neuron

For demonstrating the transmitter of the target neurons of PHA-L labeled fibers, several procedures have been described for LM application. Basically, such combined studies utilize markers with different colors. Wouterlood *et al.* (1987a) have introduced two basic procedures, a sequential and a "pooled" procedure. According to the sequential protocol peroxidase immunocyto-chemistry is used first to label the transported PHA-L with DAB as substrate. This is followed by alkaline phosphatase immunostaining and Fast Blue as substrate in order to visualize the transmitter in the target neurons. The "pooled" procedure uses coctails of primary and secondary antibodies and subsequent coupling of the PAP complexes. The final demonstration of the PHA-L and the transmitter is achieved by the use of nickel-enhanced DAB (NiDAB) and DAB, respectively. Instead of DAB, aminoethylcarbazole can be used for the transmitter localization. These techniques are discussed in several recent publications (Wouterlood *et al.*, 1987b, Wouterlood, 1988; Luiten *et al.*, 1988).

In order to provide convincing evidence that PHA-L varicosities indeed establish synaptic contact with the chemically identified postsynaptic profile, the above principle has recently been advanced to the EM level (Zaborszky and Cullinan, 1989). The main characteristics of this modified technique are as follows: (1) it employs a sequential protocol which, according to our experience, gives a more consistent staining when compared with the "pooled" protocol. (2) Although it was suggested originally (Hancock, 1984) that NiDAB be used first and then regular DAB, we found that DAB can be used first for transmitter identification with subsequent demonstration of PHA-L with NiDAB. In our experience this protocol does not produce the color mixing referred to by Hancock (1984). The staining sequence is particularly valuable when monoclonal antibodies are used for transmitter localization, since such antibodies may give unsatisfactory staining when used in the second sequence. (3) Instead of using PAP/PAP procedures, we use ABC→PAP or PAP→ABC combinations, since, according to Hsu and Soban (1982), the PAP/PAP procedure results in higher background and color mixing. (4) Instead of using hydrogen peroxide in the DAB solution we use a modification of the glucose oxidase reaction of Itoh *et al.* (1979). (5) In order to preserve the ultrastructure, but at the same time enhance the tissue penetration of the anti-PHA-L antibody, we take advantage of the freeze-thaw technique and low concentration of triton.

This modified double-label protocol allows an excellent preservation of the ultrastructure and satisfactory distinction of the two types of profiles (Fig. 6). The PHA-L labeled profile is strongly electron dense as compared to the more flocculent DAB precipitate in the cholinergic neurons.

A somewhat more elaborate technique uses the DAB–BDHC procedure for such double-label experiments (Fig. 7). In this case we first identify the transmitter with DAB before the PHA-L is visualized with BDHC histochemistry (Záborszky and Cullinan, in preparation).

V. METHODOLOGY

A. Anesthetics

The choice of anesthetic may be important, since some of them have a tendency to affect axonal transport. For instance, Rogers *et al.* (1980) reported that pentobarbital (50 mg/kg) reduced both retrograde and anterograde transport of HRP in rats compared with animals anesthetized with urethane (1.5 g/kg). A much higher dose (400 mg/kg) was required to block axoplasmic transport completely (Mesulam and Mufson, 1980).

B. Delivery

Horseradish peroxidase can be administered in the form of aqueous solutions, crystals, gels, or pastes. Solutions can be injected by pressure or by iontophoresis, and concentration and volume (in the case of pressure injections) depend on the desired size of the HRP deposit and tissue character-

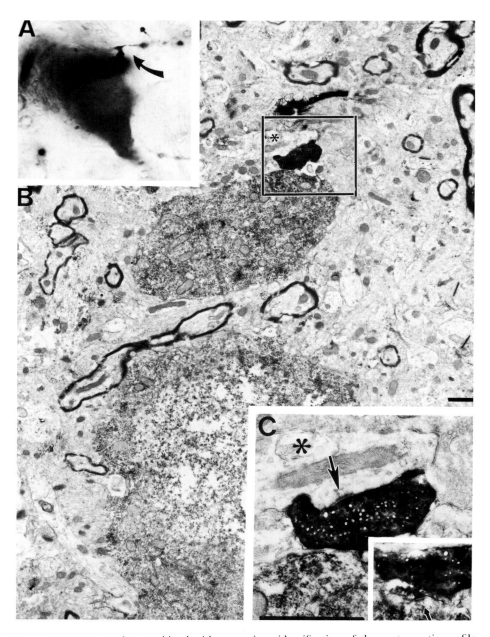

Figure 6. PHA-L tracing combined with transmitter identification of the postsynaptic profile using nickel-enhanced DAB and DAB. A: A cholinergic cell in the basal forebrain (stained for ChAT) is approached by a PHA-L fiber with several varicosities (curved arrow). B: Low-power electron micrograph of the neuron is shown in A. Note that an unlabeled dendrite (asterisk) is located between the two PHA-L profiles, and that the lower PHA-L profile is making an asymmetric synaptic contact with this dendrite as shown in higher magnification in C. An adjacent thin section (inset in C) shows that the same PHA-L bouton also contacts the cholinergic profile. Arrows in C point to the postsynaptic densities. PHA-L was injected into the locus coeruleus. Bar scale: 1 μm. (From Záborszky *et al.*, 1989.)

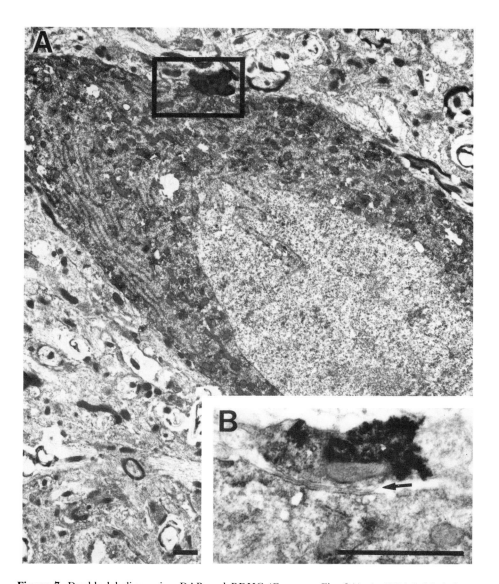

Figure 7. Double labeling using DAB and BDHC (Compare Fig. 3A). A: PHA-L-labeled terminal (boxed area) in close apposition to a cholinergic cell body in the basal forebrain after an iontophoretic injection of PHA-L into the anterior hypothalamic nucleus. ChAT is visualized with the DAB technique, and the PHA-L process is identified with BDHC reaction. B: Higher magnification of the same terminal in an adjacent section. Arrow points to an interposing glial membrane. Note the crystalline BDHC reaction products. Bar scale: 1 μm.

istics (see Table I). With the microiontophoretic delivery technique (Graybiel and Devor, 1974; Alheid *et al.*, 1981), the diameter of the injection can be as small as 100–300 μm. Crystals of HRP can be applied to severed nerve stumps or to exposed surfaces in the CNS to ensure high local concentration of the tracer (Gobel and Falls, 1979). An HRP–polyacrylamide gel has also been applied to superficial CNS structures (Griffin *et al.*, 1979) or through implanted pipettes (Fahrbach *et al.*, 1984), and the improved results probably reflect the fact that this technique provides a sustained slow release of HRP for 24 hr or more as compared to acute injections.

Horseradish peroxidase is usually dissolved in 2% DMSO (Keefer *et al.*, 1976), nonionic detergent solution (5% Nonidet P-40: Lipp and Schwegler, 1980; Escher *et al.*, 1983), or poly-L-ornithine (0.5%: FitzGibbon *et al.*, 1983). These additives have a tendency to enhance the uptake of HRP, thus increasing the amount of HRP available for transport, which in turn may increase the perikaryal and dendritic labeling. The additives, however, may also increase HRP entry into axons of passage, which usually makes the interpretation of the results more difficult.

Wheat germ agglutinin alone or conjugated to HRP can be pressure-injected in lower concentration than free HRP. Slow-release technique (Schwanzel-Fukuda *et al.*, 1983) and iontophoresis have also been used for delivering WGA–HRP (Steindler and Bradely, 1983; Shiosaka *et al.*, 1986). Further details regarding the different tracers can be found in Table I.

Contamination of the tracer alongside the pipette track can create difficulties in interpretation, and this is a problem that does not always get the attention it deserves. The problem is especially pronounced when using pressure injections or tracers with a high diffusion rate, and various efforts have been made to reduce the diffusion of tracer along the pipette track. It seems that most investigators have taken the attitude that a slow withdrawal of the pipette reduces the risk of contamination. To use a pipette with a long thin taper and tip is also an advantage. Unintended labeling through the pipette track can be avoided by injection of HRP through a cannula implanted 1–10 days previously (Wakefield and Shonnard, 1979).

C. Survival Time

The optimal survival time depends on the rate of tracer transport, the length and diameter of the fiber system being studied, and the age of the animal. The survival time is also related to the goal of the investigation, since the rates of anterograde and retrograde transport are different and since degradation of the tracer differs depending on whether it takes place in the cell bodies or in the terminals. A special problem is encountered when HRP tracing is combined with degeneration. Since the rate of the degeneration may differ from the rate of HRP transport, the HRP injection and experimental lesion may have to be done at different times. When HRP tracing is combined with immunocytochemical labeling of the cell bodies, the use of colchicine is often necessary. However, since colchicine arrests the axoplasmic transport, it is advisable first to inject the HRP and then, 24–48 hr later depending on the length of the projection, to administer the colchicine and perform the lesion at the same time. The animal should be perfused after an additional survival time of about 24 hr. Longer survival times (2–3 weeks) are appropriate for lectins, lectin conjugates, or bacterial toxins, and in this case the interval between the tracer and colchicine injection is less crucial (see also Luppi *et al.*, 1987).

D. Fixation

A high concentration of paraformaldehyde in the fixative causes a loss of peroxidase activity, and a high amount of glutaraldehyde, which generally provides for better ultrastructural preservation, reduces the antigenicity and increases nonspecific staining (Malmgren and Olsson, 1978; Mesulam, 1982). A modified Bouin's fixative (Somogyi and Takagi, 1982) provides for a reasonable compromise with adequate preservation of the HRP reaction product as well as good ultrastructure. This perfusion protocol includes a brief rinse (e.g., 50 ml for rat with 200 g body weight) with saline followed by a fixative containing 4% paraformaldehyde, 0.1–0.2% glutaraldehyde, and 15% saturated picric acid in 0.1 M phosphate buffer, pH 7.4 (500 ml).

Following the perfusion of the fixative, a brief rinse with sucrose–saline has been found to be helpful for the purpose of HRP histochemistry (Rosene and Mesulam, 1978). This treatment removes the unbound aldehydes, thereby reducing the effect of the fixative on HRP enzymatic activity throughout the brain (Mesulam, 1982). The rinse also seems to have a positive effect on peptide immunostaining (L. Záborszky and A. Braun, unpublished observation) but may adversely affect the tissue preservation.

Following the removal of the brain from the skull, it is customary to postfix the whole brain for a couple of hours in the same fixative as used for the perfusion but without glutaraldehyde. Although the brain can sometimes be left in the fixative overnight, it is usually not advisable to do so because overly long postfixation reduces the antigenicity and the HRP enzymatic activity.

To improve the preservation of the tissue for ultrastructural study, higher concentrations of glutaraldehyde can be used, provided that sodium borohydride is applied before the immunostaining to remove the excess glutaraldehyde (Kosaka *et al.*, 1986; see also Chapters 5 and 6 for more information about fixation in double-labeling studies).

Sections are cut on a vibratome at 20–40 μm and placed in ice-cold phosphate buffer, pH 7.4.

E. Freeze–Thaw Procedure

The preembedding immunostaining is unfortunately limited to the most superficial parts of the section. Increased penetration can be achieved in different ways, such as using the freeze–thaw procedure (Somogyi and Takagi, 1982), or through the use of improved immunologic binding techniques (e.g., Brandon, 1985; Suresh *et al.*, 1986). The freeze–thaw technique can be applied before or after Vibratome sectioning. In the first case, brains are cut into blocks about $2 \times 2 \times 3$ mm in size. The blocks are then immersed in 0.1 M phosphate-buffered saline containing 10% sucrose (pH 7.4) for 1 hr at 4°C and next in the same buffer containing 20% sucrose for 12 hr at 4°C. The blocks are frozen in liquid nitrogen and immediately thawed in 20% sucrose buffer (Somogyi and Takagi, 1982). When the freeze–thaw technique is used after sectioning, the sections are collected in vials containing 10% sucrose in 0.1 M phosphate buffer. The vials are placed in liquid nitrogen until the fluid is frozen, after which the content is thawed to room temperature (Záborszky and Léránth, 1985).

The specific steps in the double-labeling techniques are described in Section IV of this chapter (see also Appendix, Section VII).

F. Osmication, Dehydration, and Embedding

Unless otherwise stated (see specific recipes for double-labeling studies in the Appendix), sections are postfixed in 1% OsO_4 (pH 7.4) for 30–60 min, dehydrated in a series of alcohols, and stained *en bloc* in 1% uranyl acetate (uranyl acetate is dissolved in 70% ethanol) at the 70% ethanol stage. The sections are then flat embedded in plastic between a glass slide and a coverslip (coated with a mold-releasing compound, EMS) to keeep them flat and allow the light microscopic examination (see also Chapters 6 and 8). The choice of embedding matrix does not seem to be important if preembedding immunostaining is used. We have had good results in most of our preembedding protocols with Spurr-Epon; when BDHC (see Appendix) is used, rapid dehydration and embedding in Durcupan are recommended. Postembedding staining, however, is crucially dependent on the type of embedding medium used (van den Pol, 1985).

Selected sections are then attached to a prepared cylinder of Epon with an adhesive. Ultrathin sections can be collected on single-slot or Formvar-coated mesh grids and examined in the electron microscope with or without additonal uranyl acetate and lead citrate staining. The choice of grids is important if colloidal gold is used; to avoid precipitation, nickel or gold grids should be used.

VI. SUMMARY OF ADVANTAGES AND LIMITATIONS

Each of the procedures discussed in this chapter has its own limitations and advantages, and without some experience in combining various techniques it is not always easy to choose among the various protocols. Nevertheless, considering the nature of the different methods involved, some guiding principles can be identified.

A. Anterograde Degeneration

Experimentally induced axonal degeneration has been widely used in tract tracing, and it offers some distinct advantages in combination with other methods. Degenerating boutons can usually be identifed without much problem in the electron microscope, and the need for good preservation is met with the fixation used for HRP labeling and immunostaining. Since there are no penetration problems to deal with, large tissue samples are available for study. The "fiber-of-passage" problem, however, represents a well-known disadvantage, especially when lesions are made in subcortical structures, but the use of specific neurotoxins may circumvent this problem. Degeneration of an axon may prevent its staining with a peroxidase-based immunohisto-chemical method, and the use of anterograde degeneration, therefore, is most valuable in cases in which the presynaptic element is identifed by degeneration and the postsynaptic structure with HRP retrograde tracing and/or immunostaining technique. Even so, it may still be problematic to distinguish a degenerating bouton from an immuno- or HRP-labeled terminal.

Another problem is that degeneration in itself is usually not visible at the light microscopic level. This makes it difficult to select appropriate areas for EM processing without some type of silver staining on an adjacent semithin section (Heimer, 1970). This type of mapping procedure, however, is less attractive in combination with preembedding immunostaining, since it consumes those parts of the tissue best suited for transmitter identification. However, this method might gain some popularity if postembedding techniques were to become more generally available. Finally, it is important to remember that only a limited number of the affected terminals can be iden-tifed as degenerating terminals at any given time (Dekker and Kuypers, 1976; LeVay and Gilbert, 1976). This problem, however, can to some extent be controlled for by using appropriate mathematical corrections (Lenn *et al.*, 1983).

B. Axonal Transport of HRP or HRP Conjugates

The tracing of HRP or lectin conjugates is as sensitive as autoradiographic fiber tracing (see Chapter 5), and in contrast to the autoradiographic technique, which may take several months, the HRP material can be studied a few days following administration of the tracer. Transcellular transport of WGA–HRP may be a limitation or an advantage depending on the require-ment of the experiment. The experiments, however, can usually be con-ducted in such a way that potential transcellular transport is controlled for. Another limitation of free HRP and HRP conjugates is that intact or dam-aged fibers may take up the tracer. Further characteristics of HRP and HRP conjugated tracers are summarized in Section II of this chapter.

C. The Choice of Chromogen in Double-Labeling Studies

Although DAB is less sensitive than many other chromogens, it is easy to use for both the tracer and the immunoreaction, especially when the tracer DAB and the transmitter DAB are located in different profiles. When tracer- and transmitter-related labels are located in the same profile, it is advisable to use two chromogens that produce distinctly different reaction products, e.g., DAB and BDHC. Although BDHC is more sensitive than DAB, it has some disadvantages, i.e., instability of the reaction product and difficulty controlling for nonspecific precipitates. The fine uniform distribution of the DAB reaction product, as compared to the coarse precipitates of the BDHC reaction, allows for a better identification of fine structural details.

D. Colloidal Gold-Labeled Tracers

Our experience with gold-labeled tracers is limited, but the distinct appearance of colloidal gold on the EM level and the availability of different sizes of gold particles make these techniques appealing in combined studies. Since visualization of colloidal gold is less dependent on fixation, the fixation parameters can be adjusted to suit the immunohistochemical protocol. Unfortunately, the procedures for visualizing the tracers in some cases affect the tissue preservation and eventually the antigenicity for subsequent transmitter identification.

E. Tracing with PHA-L

The introduction of the PHA-L method has presented us with a new option to combine an anterograde tracer with postsynaptic transmitter identification. It is likely that the Ni-DAB-DAB double labeling technique will be most often used, since identification of the two types of markers is easily made on the light-microscopic level, and can be accomplished also on the EM-level at least in the superficial part of the block. In order to obtain convincing discrimination in all places where the two markers occur, other double labeling techniques that are compatible with correlated light–EM methods should be tried, such as the more laborious DAB–BDHC technique.

VII. APPENDIX

A. Double Labeling with DAB–DAB
(Záborszky and Léránth, 1985)

1. *Tracer injection.* Inject 0.05 μl of 20% HRP (Sigma VI, or Boehringer, Grade I) in 2% DMSO.

2. *Perfusion.* According to Somogyi and Takagi (1982).
3. *Tracer visualization.* The sections are reacted with freshly prepared solution of 50 mg DAB, 200 mg β-D-glucose, 40 mg ammonium chloride, and 0.3 mg glucose oxidase (Sigma type VII) per 100 ml of 0.1 M phosphate buffer (PB) for 60–90 min at room temperature (Itoh *et al.*, 1979).
4. *Photography.* After finishing the HRP reaction, the wet sections are mounted from PB on glass slides and coverslipped. The retrogradely labeled cells can be photographed.
5. *Freeze–thaw.* Following several changes in PB, sections are collected in vials containing 10% sucrose in PB. The vials are placed in liquid nitrogen until the fluid is frozen, after which the content is thawed to room temperature.
6. *Immunostaining.* According to the ABC technique of Hsu *et al.* (1981).
7. *Dehydration and embedding.* The immunostained sections are postfixed in 1% OsO_4 for 30 min, dehydrated, stained *en bloc* with 1% uranyl acetate at the 70% ethanol stage, and flat embedded into Spurr–Epon (EMS) between glass slides and coverslips, coated with liquid release agent (EMS) to keep them flat and allow the light microscopic examination and photography.
8. *Reembedding.* Selected plastic embedded sections containing previously photographed cells are mounted on a cylindric Araldite block for electron microscopic examination.

B. Double Labeling with DAB–BDHC
(Levey *et al.*, 1986)

1. *HRP histochemistry with DAB.* Sections should be rinsed in 50 mM Tris-HCl buffer, pH 7.6. They are then preincubated in a solution of DAB (0.05%) in Tris buffer for 10 min before developing in the same solution with hydrogen peroxide added to a final concentration of 0.01%. The reaction is stopped after 5–10 min by rinsing five times in Tris buffer.
2. *Peroxidase histochemistry with BDHC.*
   a. *Rinsing.* Sections should be rinsed two times in Tris buffer and then an additional five times in 0.01 M sodium phosphate buffer, pH 6.8, at room temperature.
   b. *Preincubation.* Sections are then preincubated in a solution of BDHC prepared as follows: for every 100 ml of solution, 10 mg of BDHC (Sigma) is added to 95 ml distilled deionized water and allowed to stir approximately 30 min before filtering. Then 25 mg sodium nitroferricyanide and 5 ml of 0.2 M sodium phosphate buffer (final concentration 0.01 M) are added just before incubation.
   c. *Incubation.* After a 10-min preincubation, the reaction is initiated by adding hydrogen peroxide to a final concentration of 0.005%. Re-

action is terminated after 5–10 min by rinsing extensively in 0.01 M phosphate buffer, pH 6.8.

3. *Dehydration and embedding.* After the incubation, the sections are treated with 1% osmium tetroxide in 0.01 M sodium phosphate buffer (pH 6.8) for 1 hr, rapidly dehydrated in graded alcohols and propylene oxide over 30 min, and embedded in resin (Durcupan, Fluka, Hauppauge, NY) on microscopic slides.

C. Double Labeling with DAB–BDHC
(Lakos and Basbaum, 1986)

1. *DAB procedure to localize transported HRP.* The reaction medium consists of a 0.05% DAB solution in PBS containing 0.01% H_2O_2. An incubation of 5–10 min at room temperature is typical.
2. *BDHC reaction to localize the antigen.*
   a. *Glutaraldehyde pretreatment.* Sections are first rinsed with 0.05% glutaraldehyde in 0.1 M acetate buffer, pH 6.5, for 30–90 sec at room temperature.
   b. *Rinse.* Sections are washed in a 0.1 M acetate buffer, pH 6.5.
   c. *BDHC reaction.* The incubation solution is mixed from freshly made stock solutions A–D:

   A. BDHC 80 mg in 18 ml ethanol (100%) and 40 ml H_2O (warming the solution to 45°C for about 3–10 min will facilitate dissolving the BDHC).
   B. Na nitroprusside (250 mg in 3 ml H_2O).
   C. 0.2 M Na-acetate buffer, pH 6.5.
   D. 3.0% H_2O_2 diluted from 30% stabilized solution (J. T. Baker) and kept in closed jar on ice during the experiment.

   Mix 3.75 ml solution A, 50 μl solution B, and 600 μl solution C. To this mixture add 10–40 μl of solution D.

   d. *Rinse.* To stop the reaction, the sections are washed quickly with cold acetate buffer placed on ice.
3. *Photography.* Color photographs of labeled material can be taken before osmication. Prolonged exposure to light, however, may result in significant loss of the signal. If the tissue is not going to be embedded, the sections should be mounted on gelatin-coated slides. After drying, the sections are rapidly dehydrated through graded alcohols, cleared in xylene, and coverslipped with Permount.
4. *Osmication.* Sections intended for EM are incubated at 45°C in an s-collidine-buffered 1–2% osmium tetroxide solution, pH 6.5. The procedure is done in a rotating water bath for 1 hr. The s-collidine buffer can be prepared ahead of time. For 1 liter of an 0.2 M stock solution, dissolve 26.7 ml s-collidine (trimethylpyridine, EMS), 100 mg $CaCl_2$, 200 mg $MgCl_2$, and 131.7 g sucrose in approximately 750 ml distilled

water. Adjust the pH to 6.5 with 1 N HCl and then bring the final volume to 1000 ml with distilled water.

5. *Dehydration.* After osmication, the tissue is washed in *s*-collidine buffer and dehydrated in graded alcohols: 30% for 5 min; 50% for 5 min; 70% for 10 min; 95% for 15 min; twice 100% for 10 min, followed by propylene oxide twice for 10 min.

D. Double Labeling with Biotin–WGA–Gold and DAB
(Shiosaka *et al.*, 1986; Tohyama, personal communication)

1. *Preparation of the tracer.* Mix 5 μl WGA (200 mM in 0.02 M PBS) with 20 μl photobiotin (1 mg/ml, approx. 200 mM, Bresa, Australia) and illuminated with a mercury vapor lamp (250 W) for 20 min. Solution can be stored in refrigerator.
2. *Staining procedures for light microscopy.* The brains are sectioned in a cryostat (20–30 μm) and rinsed in 0.02 M PBS (pH 7.4). The sections are then incubated in the required primary antibody for the transmitter identification and streptavidin–Texas red (Titus *et al.*, 1982) for the tracer localization. After rinsing with PBS, sections are incubated in PBS with FITC-labeled IgG against the species of the primary antibody. The sections are rinsed with PBS and mounted with PBS–glycerin mixture (1 : 1) or Entellan New (Merck).
3. *Tissue processing for electron microscopy.* After fixation, freeze–thawing, vibratome sectioning, and immunostaining, sections are dehydrated and embedded in plastic. Ultrathin sections are collected on collodion-coated nickel grids.
4. *Postembedding reaction with streptavidin-labeled colloidal gold (SCG).* First, a 15-nm colloidal gold layer is prepared by the method of Frens (1973) and Roth *et al.* (1978). The colloidal gold suspension is adjusted to pH 7.0 with 0.2 M K_2CO_3 and stabilized with a 10% excess of streptavidin (Amersham) by the method of Roth *et al.* (1978). The ultrathin sections on the grids are etched with a 10% H_2O_2–PBS solution for 20 min and incubated in a solution of 2% bovine serum albumin (BSA) and PBS for 30 min at room temperature. They are then incubated in a 1 : 10 mixture of SCG and BSA–PBS for 1 hr at room temperature, washed with doubly distilled water, and stained with aqueous lead citrate.

E. Double Labeling Using WGA–apoHRP–Gold and DAB
(Basbaum and Menetrey, 1987)

1. *Preparation of gold particles.* A volume of 100 ml of chloroauric acid (Sigma; 0.01% w/v in dH_2O) is boiled while being vigorously stirred. Reducing agents (2 ml of trisodium citrate and 100 μl tannic acid, both 1% w/v in

dH$_2$O) are mixed in a separate beaker and rapidly added to the boiling solution. The reaction is complete, usually after 30–50 sec, when the solution quickly turns dark violet and then wine red. Boiling and stirring are continued for 5 min more before the solution is cooled under running water. The solution can be kept at 4°C for several weeks if supplemented with 2% sodium azide (0.2% v/v). If silver intensification is not used, and the preparation of a particular size of gold particles is required, the following guidelines should be used. Gold particles of 6–10 nm are obtained with 2 ml trisodium citrate and 350 μl tannic acid, 12- to 16-nm particles with 2 ml trisodium citrate and 20 μl tannic acid, whereas particles of 20–30 nm require trisodium citrate alone (Menetrey, 1985; Menetrey and Lee, 1985).

2. *Adsorption of Gold to WGA–apoHRP.* The pH range for gold–protein coupling and the amount of protein needed to stabilize gold solution against flocculation by salt are determined according to Geoghegan and Ackerman (1977) and Goodman *et al.* (1981). The pH of the gold solution is raised to 8.4 by adding small quantities (approx. 4 μl/ml solution) of potassium carbonate (0.2 M) and checked on a 1-ml aliquot in the presence of 45 μl of 1% (w/v) polyethylene glycol (PEG, Sigma, mol. wt. 20,000). The gold solution is added to diluted WGA–apoHRP (1 mg protein per milliliter of dH$_2$O) and coupled while being vigorously stirred. After 5 min, filtered PEG is added in a porportion of 1% (v/v) to the complete volume of the solution to prevent aggregation of the complex. The complex is then centrifuged for 120 min at 18,000 rpm. The supernatant is aspirated and discarded, and the soft pellet containing the WGA–apoHRP–gold complex can be injected into the animal without further dilution. Consistent retrograde labeling is obtained when pellets have a final concentration of protein of at least 2.5%. The pellet, if resuspended in destilled water, can be stored at 4°C for 2–3 weeks with no detectable loss of sensitivity. If used after storage, the suspension has to be centrifuged again.

3. *Tissue processing.*
   a. After a brief rinse (5 min) in sodium citrate buffer (0.1 M, pH 3.8), the sections are dipped in physical developer.
   b. Physical developer consists of 60 ml gum arabic (50% solution in dH$_2$O), 10 ml citrate buffer (1 M, pH 3.5), 15 ml hydroquinone (5.6% solution in dH$_2$O), and 15 ml silver lactate solution (Fluka; 0.7% in dH$_2$O). The silver lactate solution should be protected against light and added just before the developer is used. (Menetrey, 1985; Danscher, 1981a, b).
   c. After development, the sections are washed once (5 min) in 0.1 M PO$_4$ (pH 7.4) and transferred into sodium thiosulfate.
   d. Sodium thiosulfate (2.5% solution in 0.1 M phosphate buffer, pH 7.4) for 5 min.
   e. Rinse in 0.1 M PO$_4$.
   f. Gold toning (Fairen *et al.*, 1977).
   g. Immunostaining.

F. Conjugation of Colloidal Gold with Fluorescent Microspheres
(Quattrochi *et al.*, 1987)

1. Activation of Microspheres

1. Suspend 25-mg beads in 5 ml diaminoheptane (Sigma D3266) and buffer (0.01M PO$_4$), pH 6.5, 4°C.
2. Add 10 mg carbodiimide (Sigma C2388).
3. Incubate on shaker 8 hr, 4°C.
4. Dialysis in 0.1 M NaCl/buffer, 24 hr, 4°C.
5. Suspend beads in 0.25 ml glutaraldehyde (1.25% stock) plus 4.75 ml buffer.
6. Incubate 1 hr, 25°C, on shaker.
7. Dialysis in 0.1 M NaCl buffer 25 hr, 4°C.
8. Recover beads (148,000 *g*, 90 min), which are now activated.

2. Covalent Binding of Microspheres with Goat Antimouse IgG

1. Suspend 50 mg activated beads in 5 ml buffer, pH 7.0.
2. Add 2 mg IgG.
3. Incubate on shaker 10 hr, 25°C.
4. Perform 20%/58% sucrose separation with 0.01 M glycine, pH 8, with beads on top of 20%.
5. Centrifuge sucrose separation at 150,000 *g*, 150 min. Collect pellet and centrifuge again.
6. Dialysis 36 hr, 4°C, as in Section VII.F.1, step 4.
7. Centrifuge beads 148,000 *g* for 90 min.
8. Collect pellet, wash in buffer.

3. Incubation of IgG Microsphere with Protein A Colloidal Gold

1. Pellet plus 1 : 10 dilution protein A/AU15 (Jansen) in buffer, 6 hr, 25°C.
2. Incubate 24 hr, 4°C, on shaker.
3. Perform 5%/20% sucrose separation as in Section VII.B.2, step 4.
4. Centrifuge 200,000 *g* 10 min, recover, and repeat.
5. Collect pellet and store in buffer, 4°C.

G. PHA-L Tracing with Transmitter Identification of the Postsynaptic Neuron (NiDAB–DAB)
(Záborszky and Cullinan, 1989)

1. *Injection of PHA-L and perfusion of the animals* as described in Chapter 3 (Gerfen *et al.*) for electron microscopy.
2. *NiDAB reaction to visualize the PHA-L.* Incubation in goat anti-PHA-L (1 : 2000, 36 hr, 4°C) is followed by biotinylated rabbit anti-sheep IgG

(Vector Labs, 1 : 100, 4 hr, 4°C) and the Avidin Biotin Complex (Vector Labs, 1 : 500, 4 hr, 4°C). This is succeeded by the coupled oxidation reaction of Itoh *et al.* (1979) modified as follows:

a. Mix 50 mg DAB and 40 mg NH_4Cl in 100 ml in 0.1 M PB
b. After DAB is dissolved, mix in 0.4 mg glucose oxidase (Sigma)
c. Add 10 ml DAB mixture to the wells in a 6-well dish
d. Add 200 μl from 0.05 M stock nickel–ammonium sulfate solution to each 10-ml well and stir. The final concentration will be 0.001 M.
e. Add tissue sections to the appropriate wells and incubate 5 min
f. After 5 min start the reaction by adding 200 μl 10% β-D-glucose (Sigma)
g. Incubate sections as long as necessary up to approximately 1 hr

3. DAB Procedure to Localize the Transmitter. After the primary and secondary antibodies and the PAP complex, the DAB–glucose-oxidase reaction (Appendix, Section VII.A) is used to visualize the transmitter of the postsynaptic neuron. In the indicated example (Fig. 6) we used rat antiChAT, rabbit antirat IgG and rat PAP. All antibodies are diluted in 0.1 M PB containing 0.04 Triton X-100. Also, in order to further facilitate antibody penetration, the freeze-thaw procedure is used. For dehydration, embedding etc see Appendix (Section VII.A).

ACKNOWLEDGMENTS. The authors extend special thanks to Bruce H. Wainer, Alan I. Basbaum, Steven I. Lakos, James J. Quattrochi, and Masaya Tohyama for use of their material in the Appendix. Regarding the transport mechanisms of HRP and lectins we had several helpful discussion with Richard D. Broadwell. Supported by USPHS-NINCDS grants NS 23945 and 17743.

REFERENCES

Adams, J. C., 1981, Heavy metal intensification of DAB-based HRP reaction product, *J. Histochem. Cytochem.* 29:775.

Alheid, G. F., Edwards, S. B., Kitai, S. T., Park, M. R., and Switzer, R. C. III, 1981, Methods for delivering tracers, in: *Neuroanatomical Tract-Tracing Methods* (L. Heimer and M. J. RoBards, eds.), Plenum Press, New York, pp. 91–116.

Alstermark, B., and Kümmel, H., 1986, Transneuronal labelling of neurones projecting to forelimb motoneurones in cats performing different movements, *Brain Res.* 376:387–391.

Anderson, P. N., Mitchell, J., and Mayor, D., 1979, The uptake of horseradish peroxidase by damaged autonomic nerves *in vitro*, *J. Anat.* 128:401–406.

Aschoff, A., and Schönitzer, K., 1982, Intra-axonal transport of horseradish peroxidase (HRP) and its use in neuroanatomy, in: *Axoplasmic Transport in Physiology and Pathology* (D. G. Weiss, and A. Gorio, eds.) Springer-Verlag, Berlin Heidelberg, New York, pp. 167–176.

Bak, I. J., Markham, C. H., Cook, M. L., and Stevens, J. G., 1977, Intraaxonal transport of herpes simplex virus in the rat central nervous system, *Brain Res.* 136:415–429.

Bak, I. J., Markham, C. H., Cook, M. L., and Stevens, J. G., 1978, Ultrastructural and immunoperoxidase study of striatonigral neurons by means of retrograde axonal transport of herpes simplex virus, *Brain Res.* 143:361–368.

Baker, H., and Spencer, R. F., 1986, Transneuronal transport of peroxidase-conjugated wheat germ agglutinin (WGA–HRP) from the olfactory epithelium to the brain of the adult rat, *Exp. Brain Res.* 63:461–473.

Bakker, D. A., Richmond, F. J. R., and Abrahams, V. C., 1984, Central projections from cat suboccipital muscles: A study using transganglionic transport of horseradish peroxidase, *J. Comp. Neurol.* 228:409–421.

Balin, B. J., and Broadwell, R. D., 1987, Lectin-labelled membrane is transferred to the Golgi complex in mouse pituitary cells *in vivo, J. Histochem. Cytochem.* 35:489–498.

Basbaum, A. I., and Menetrey, D., 1987, Wheat germ agglutinin–apoHRP gold: A new retrograde tracer for light- and electron microscopic single- and double-label studies, *J. Comp. Neurol.* 261:306–318.

Beattie, M. S., Bresnahan, J. C., and King, J. S., 1978, Ultrastructural identification of dorsal root primary afferent terminals after anterograde filling with horseradish peroxidase, *Brain Res.* 153:127–134.

Bowker, R. M., Westlund, K. N., and Coulter, J. D., 1981, Origins of serotonergic projections to spinal cord in rat: An immunocytochemical-retrograde transport study. *Brain Res.* 226:187–199.

Bowker, R. W., Westlund, K. N., Sullivan, M. C., and Coulter, J. D., 1982, A combined retrograde transport and immunocytochemical staining method for demonstrating the origins of serotonergic projections, *J. Histochem. Chytochem* 30:805–810.

Brandon, C., 1985, Improved immunocytochemical staining through the use of fab fragments of primary antibody, fab-specific second antibody, and fab-horseradish peroxidase, *J. Histochem. Cytochem* 33:715–719.

Broadwell, R. D., and Balin, B. J., 1985, Endocytic and exocytic pathways of the neuronal secretory process and transsynaptic transfer of wheat germ agglutinin–horseradish peroxidase *in vivo, J. Comp. Neurol.* 242:632–650.

Broadwell, R. D., and Brightman, M. W., 1979, Cytochemistry of undamaged neurons transporting exogenous protein *in vivo, J. Comp. Neurol.* 185:31–74.

Broadwell, R. D., and Cataldo. A. M., 1984, The neuronal endoplasmic reticulum: Its cytochemistry and contribution to the endomembrane system. II. Axons and terminals, *J. Comp. Neurol.* 230:213–248.

Broadwell, R. D., Oliver, C., and Brightman, M. W., 1979, Localization of neurophysin within organelles associated with protein synthesis and packaging in the hypothalamoneurohypphysial system: An immunocytochemical study, *Proc. Natl. Acad. Sci. U.S.A.* 76:5999–6003.

Broadwell, R. D., Oliver, C., and Brightman, M. W., 1980, Neuronal transport of acid hydrolases and perosidase within the lysosomal system of organelles: Involvement of agranular reticulum like cysterns, *J. Comp. Neurol.* 190:519–532.

Broadwell, R. D., Cataldo, A. M., and Balin, B. J., 1984, Further studies of the secretory process in hypothalamoneurohypophysial neurons. An analysis using immunocytochemistry, wheat germ agglutinin-peroxidase, and native peroxidase, *J. Comp. Neurol.* 228:155–167.

Brodal, P., Dietrichs, E., Bjaalie, J. G., Nordby, T., and Walberg, F., 1983, Is lectin-coupled horseradish peroxidase taken up and transported by undamaged as well as by damaged fibers in the central nervous system? *Brain Res.* 278:1–9.

Büttner-Ennever, J. A., Grob, P., Akert, K., and Bizzini, B., 1981, A transsynaptic autoradiographic study of the pathways controlling the extraocular eye muscles, using [^{125}I]B-II$_b$ tetanus toxin fragment, *Ann. N.Y. Acad. Sci.* 374:157–170.

Campbell, G., So, K.-F., and Lieberman, A. R., 1984, Normal postnatal development of retinogeniculate axons and terminals and identification of inappropriately-located transient synapses: Electron microscope studies of horseradish peroxidase-labelled retinal axons in the hamster, *Neuroscience* 13:743–759.

Carson, K. A., and Mesulam, M.-M., 1982a, Electron microscopic demonstration of neural connections using horseradish peroxidase: A comparison of the tetramethylbenzidine procedure with seven other histochemical methods, *J. Histochem. Cytochem.* 30:425–435.

Carson, K. A., and Mesulam, M.-M., 1982b, Ultrastructural evidence in mice that transganglionically transported horseradish peroxidase–wheat germ agglutinin conjugate reaches the intraspinal terminations of sensory neurons, *Neurosci. Lett.* 29:201–206.

Carson, K. A., and Mesulam, M.-M., 1982c, Electron microscopic tracing of neural connections with horseradish peroxidase, in: *Tracing Neural Connections with Horseradish Peroxidase* (M.-M. Mesulam, ed.), John Wiley, Sons, New York, pp. 153–184.

Chen, W. P., Witkin, J. W., and Silverman, A. J., 1989, Beta-endorphin and gonadotropin releasing hormone neurosecretory cells in the male rat, *J. Comp. Neurol.* (in press).

Colman, D. R., Scalia, F., and Cabrales, E., 1976, Light and electron microscopic observations on the anterograde transport of horseradish peroxidase in the optic pathway in the mouse and rat, *Brain Res.* 102:156–163.

Craig, A. D., and Mense, S., 1983, The distribution of afferent fibers from the gastrocnemius–soleus muscle in the dorsal horn of the cat, as revealed by the transport of horseradish peroxidase, *Neurosci. Lett.* 41:233–238.

Cunningham, E. T., Jr., and LeVay, S., 1986, Laminar and synaptic organization of the projection from the thalamic nucleus centralis to primary visual cortex in the cat, *J. Comp. Neurol.* 254:65–77.

Danscher, G., 1981a, Localization of gold in biological tissue. A photochemical method for light and electronmicroscopy, *Histochemistry* 71:81–88.

Danscher, G., 1981b, Histochemical demonstration of heavy metals, *Histochemistry* 71:1–16.

Dautry-Varsat, A., and Lodish, H. F., 1984, How receptors bring proteins and particles into cells, *Sci. Am.* 250:52–58.

Dekker, J. J., and Kuypers, H. G. J. M., 1976, Quantitative E.M. study of projection terminals in the rat's AV thalamic nucleus. Autoradiographic and degeneration techniques compared, *Brain Res.* 117:399–422.

DeOlmos, J., and Heimer, L., 1977, Mapping of collateral projections with the HRP-method, *Neurosci. Lett.* 6:107–114.

Deschenes, M., Landry P., and Labelle, A., 1979, The comparative effectiveness of the "brown and blue reactions" for tracing neuronal processes of cells injected intracellularly with horseradish peroxidase, *Neurosci. Lett.* 12:9–15.

Droz, B., 1973, Renewal of synaptic proteins, *Brain Res.* 62:383–394.

Dumas, M., Schwab, M. E., Baumann, R., and Thoenen, H., 1979, Retrograde transport of tetaus toxin through a chain of two neurons, *Brain Res.* 145:359–357.

Escher, G., Schönenberger, N., and van der Loos, H., 1983, Detergent-soaked HRP-chips: A new method for precise and effective delivery of small quantities of the tracer to nervous tissue, *J. Neurosci. Methods* 9:87–94.

Esiri, M. M., 1982, Herpes simplex encephalitis: An immunohistological study of the distribution of viral antigen within the brain, *J. Neurol. Sci.* 54:209–226.

Evinger, C., and Erichsen, J. T., 1986, Transsynaptic retrograde transport of fragment C of tetanus toxin demonstrated by immunohistochemical localization, *Brain Res.* 380:383–388.

Fahrbach, S. E., Morrell, J. I., and Pfaff, D. W., 1984, Temporal pattern of HRP spread from an iontophoretic deposit site and description of a new HRP-gel implant method, *J. Comp. Neurol.* 225:605–619.

Fairen, A., Peters, A., and Saldanha, J., 1977, A new procedure for examining Golgi impregnated neurons by light and electron microscopy, *J. Neurocytol.* 6:311–337.

Fishman, P. S., and Carrigan, D. R., 1987, Retrograde transneuronal transfer of the C-fragment of tetanus toxin, *Brain Res.* 406:275–279.

FitzGibbon, T., Kerr, L., and Burke, W., 1983, Uptake of horseradish peroxidase by axons of passage and its modification by poly-L-ornithine and diemethylsulphoxide, *J. Neurosci. Methods* 7:73–88.

Frens, G., 1973, Controlled nucleation for the regulation of the particle size in monodisperse gold solutions, *Nature* 241:20–21.

Freund, T. F., Martin, K. A. C., and Whiteridge, D., 1985, Innervation of cat visual areas 17 and 18 by physiologically identified x- and y-type thalamic afferents. I. Arborization patterns and quantitative distribution of postsynaptic elements, *J. Comp. Neurol.* 242:263–272.

Gallyas, F., and Merchenthaler, I., 1988, Copper–H_2O_2 oxidation strikingly improves silver intensification of the nickel-diaminobenzidine (Ni-DAB) end-product of the peroxidase reaction, *J. Histochem. Cytochem.* 36:808–810.

Geoghegan, W. D., and Ackerman, G. A., 1977, Adsorption of horseradish peroxidase, ovomucoid and anti-immunoglobulin to colloidal gold for the indirect detection of concanavalin A, wheat germ agglutinin and goat antihuman immunoglobulin G on cell surfaces at the electron microscopic level: A new method, theory and application, *J. Histochem. Cytochem.* 25:1187–1200.

Gerfen, Ch. R., and Sawchenko, P. E., 1984, An anterograde neuroanatomical tracing method that shows the detailed morphology of neurons, their axons and terminals: Immunohistochemical localization of an axonally transported plant lectin, *Phaseolus vulgaris* leucoagglutin (PHA-L), *Brain Res.* 290:219–233.

Gerfen, C. R., O'Leary, D. D. M., and Cowan, W. M., 1982, A note on the transneuronal transport of wheat germ agglutinin-conjugated horseradish peroxidose in the avian and rodent visual system, *Exp. Brain Res.* 48:443–448.

Gillet, J. P., Derper, P., and Tsiang, H., 1986, Axonal transport of rabies virus in the central nervous sytem of the rat, *J. Neuropathol. Exp. Neurol.* 45:619–634.

Gobel, S., and Falls, W. M., 1979, Anatomical observations of horseradish peroxidase-filled terminal primary axonal arborizations in layer II of the substantia gelatinosa of Rolando, *Brain Rres.* 175:335–340.

Gonatas, N. K., Harper, C., Mizutani, T., and Gonatas, J., 1979, Superior sensitivity of conjugates of horseradish peroxidase with wheat germ agglutinin for studies of retrograde axonal transport, *J. Histochem. Cytochem.* 27:728–734.

Goodman, S. L., Hodges, G. M., Trejdosiewicz, L. K., and Livingston, D., 1981, Colloidal gold markers and probes for routine application in microscopy, *J. Microsc.* 123:201–213.

Grafstein B., and Forman, D. S., 1980, Intracellular transport in neurons, *Physiol. Rev.* 60:1167–1283.

Graham, R. C., Jr., and Karnovsky, M. J., 1966, The early stages of absorption of injected horseradish peroxidase in the proximal tubules of mouse kidney, ultrastructural cytochemistry by a new technique, *J. Histochem. Cytochem.* 14:291.

Grant, G., Arvidsson, J., Robertson, B., and Ygge, J., 1979, Transganglionic transport of horseradish peroxidase in primary sensory neurons, *Neurosci. Lett.* 12:23–28.

Graybiel, A. M., and Devor, M. A., 1974, A microelectrophoretic delivery technique for use with horseradish peroxidase, *Brain Res.* 68:167–173.

Griffin, G., Watkins, L. R., and Mayer, D. J., 1979, HRP pellets and slow-release gels: Two new techniques for greater localization and sensitivity, *Brain Res.* 168:595–601.

Grob, P., Büttner-Ennever, J., Lang, W., Akert, K., and Fah, A., 1982, A comparison of the retrograde tracer properties of [^{125}I]wheat germ agglutinin (WGA) with HRP after injection into the corpus callosum, *Brain Res.* 236:193–198.

Hancock, M. B., 1984, Visualization of peptide-immunoreactive processes on serotonin immunoreactive cells using two-color immunoperoxidase staining, *J. Histochem. Cytochem.* 32:311–314.

Hanker, J. S., Yates, P. E., Metz, C. B., and Rustioni, A., 1977, A new specific sensitive and non-carcinogenic reagent for the demonstration of horseradish peroxidase, *Histochem. J.* 9:789–792.

Harrison, P. J., Hultborn, H., Jankowska, E., Katz, R., Storai, B., and Zytnicki, D., 1984, Labelling of interneurones by retrograde transsynaptic transport of horseradish peroxidase from motoneurons in rats and cats, *Neurosci. Lett.* 45:15–19.

Hayes, N. L., and Rustioni, A., 1979, Dual projections of single neurons are visualized simultaneously: Use of enzymatically inactive[^{3}H]HRP, *Brain Res.* 165:321–326.

Heimer, L., 1970, Bridging the gap between light and electron microscopy in the experimental tracing of fiber connections, in: *Contemporary Research Methods in Neuroanatomy* (W. J. H. Nauta and S. O. E. Ebbeson, eds.), Springer-Verlag, Berlin, pp. 162–172.

Heimer, L., 1972, The olfactory connections of the diencephalon in the rat, *Brain Behav. Evol.* 6:484–523.

Hendry, I. A., 1977, The effect of the retrograde axonal transport of nerve growth factor on the morphology of adrenergic neurones, *Brain Res.* 134:213–223.

Henry, M. A., Westrum, L. E., and Johnson, L. R., 1985, Enhanced ultrastructural visualization of the horseradish peroxidase–tetramethylbenzidine reaction product, *J. Histochem. Cytochem.* 33:1256–1259.

Herkenhem, M., and Nauta, W. J. H., 1977, Afferent connections of the habenular nuclei in the rat. A horseradish peroxidase study with a note on the fiber-of-passage problem, *J. Comp. Neurol.* 173:123–146.

Holland, V. R., Saunders, B. C., Rose, F. L., and Walpole, A. L., 1974, A safer substitute for benzidine in the detection of blood, *Tetrahedron* 30:3299–3302.

Hopkins, D. A., King, T. R., Morrison, M. A., and Nance, D. M., 1984, Selective effect of kainic acid on axonal transport of anatomical tracers, *Soc. Neurosci. Abstr.* 10:423.

Hsu, S. M., Raine, L., and Fanger, H., 1981, Use of avidin-biotin-peroxidase complex (ABC) in immunoperoxidase techniques, *J. Histochem. Cytochem.* 29:577–580.

Hsu, S. M., and Soban, E., 1982, Color modification of diaminobenzidine (DAB) precipitation by metallic ions and its application for double immunohistochemistry, *J. Histochem. Cytochem.* 30:1079–1082.

Huerta, M., Frankfurter, A., and Harting, J. K., 1983, Studies of the principal sensory and spinal trigeminal nuclei of the rat: Projections of the superior colliculus, inferior olive, and cerebellum, *J. Comp. Neurol.* 220:147–167.

Itaya, S. K., and van Hoesen, G. W., 1982, WGA–HRP as a transneuronal marker in the visual pathways of monkey and rat, *Brain Res.* 236:199–204.

Itoh, K., Konishi, A., Nomura, S., Mizuno, N., Nakamura, Y., and Sugmimoto, T., 1979, Application of coupled oxidation reaction to electron microscopic demonstration of horseradish peroxidase: Cobalt–glucose oxidase method, *Brain Res.* 175:341–346.

Iversen, L. L., Stockel, K., and Thoesen, H., 1975, Autoradiographic studies of the retrograde axonal transport of nerve growth factor in mouse sympathetic neurons, *Brain Res.* 88:37–43.

Jankowska, E., 1985, Further indications for enhancement of retrograde transneuronal transport of WGA–HRP by synaptic activity, *Brain Res.* 341:403–408.

Jankowska, E., and Skoog, B., 1986, Labelling of midlumbar neurones projecting to cat hindlimb motoneurones by transneuronal transport of a horseradish peroxidase conjugate, 1986, *Neurosci. Lett.* 71:163–168.

Johnson, E. M., Jr., Andres, R. Y., and Bradshaw, R. A., 1978, Characterization of the retrograde transport of nerve growth factor (NGF) using high specific activity [^{125}I]NGF, *Brain Res.* 150:319–331.

Katz, L. C., Burkhalter, A., and Dreyer, W. J., 1984, Fluorescent latex microspheres as a retrograde neuronal marker for *in vivo* and *in vitro* studies of visual cortex, *Nature* 310:498–500.

Keefer, D. A., Spatz, W. B., and Misgeld, U., 1976, Golgi-like staining of neocortical neurons using retrogradely transported horseradish peroxidase, *Neurosci. Lett.* 3:233–237.

Kosaka, T., Nagatsu, I., Wu, J.-Y., and Hama, K., 1986, Use of high concentrations of glutaraldehyde for immunocytochemistry of transmitter-synthesizing enzymes in the central nervous system, *Neuroscience* 18:975–990.

Kristensson, L, and Olsson, Y. 1971, Retrograde axonal transport of protein, *Brain Res.* 29:363–365.

Kristensson, K., and Olsson, Y., 1976, Retrograde transport of horseradish peroxidase in transected axons. 3. Entry into injured axons and subsequent localization in perikaryon, *Brain Res.* 115:201–213.

Kristensson, K., Ghetti, B., and Wisniewski, H. M., 1974, Study on the propagation of herpes simplex virus (type 2) into the brain after intraocular injection, *Brain Res.* 69:189–201.

Kristensson, K., Vahlne, A., Persson, L. A., and Lycke, E., 1978, Neural spread of herpes simplex virus types 1 and 2 in mice after corneal or subcutaneous (footpad) inoculation, *J. Neurol. Sci.* 35:331–340.

Kristensson, K., Nennesmo, I., Persson, L. A., and Lycke, E., 1982, Neuron to neuron transmission of herpes simplex virus: Transport of virus from skin to brainstem nuclei, *J. Neurol. Sci.* 54:149–156.

Kucera, P., Dolivo, M., Coulon, P., and Flamand, A., 1985, Pathways of the early propagation of virulent and avirulent rabies strains from the eye to the brain, *J. Virol.* 55:158–162.

Lacey, E., and Grant, W. N., 1987, Photobiotin as a sensitive probe for protein labeling, *Anal. Biochem.* 163:151–158.

Lakos, S., and Basbaum, A. I., 1986, Benzidine dihydrochloride as a chromogen for single- and double-label light and electron microscopic immunocytochemical studies, *J. Histochem. Cytochem.* 34:1047–1056.

Lasek, R. J., 1980, Axonal transport; A dynamic view of neuronal structures, *Trends Neurosci.* 3:87–91.

LaVail, J. H., and LaVail, M. M., 1972, Retrograde axonal transport in the central nervous system, *Science* **176:**1416–1417.

LaVail, J. H., and LaVail, M. M., 1974, The retrograde intraaxonal transport of horseradish peroxidase in the chick visual system: A light and electron microscopic study, *J. Comp. Neurol.* 157:303–358.

Lechan, R. M., Nestler, J. L., and Jacobson, S., 1981, Immunohistochemical localization of retrogradely and anterogradely transported wheat germ agglutinin (WGA) within the central nervous sytem of the rat: Application to immunostaining of a second antigen within the same neuron, *J. Histochem. Cytochem.* 29:1255–1262.

Lemann, W., Saper, C. B., Rye D. B., and Wainer, B. H., 1985, Stabilization of TMB reaction product for electron microscopic retrograde and anterograde fiber tracing, *Brain Res. Bull.* 14:277–281.

Lenn, N. J., Wong, V., and Hamil, G. S., 1983, Left–right pairing at the crest synapses of rat interpeduncular nucleus, *Neuroscience* 9:383–389.

Léránth, C., and Fehér, E., 1983, Synaptology and sources of vasoactive intestinal polypeptide and substance P containing axons of the celiac ganglion. An experimental electron microscopic immunohistochemical study, *Neuroscience* 10:947–958.

Léránth, C., MacLusky, N. J., Shanabrough, M., and Naftolin, F., 1988, Catecholaminergic innervation of LHRH and GAD immunopositive neurons in the rat medial preoptic area: An electron microscopic double immunostaining and degeneration study, *Neuroendocrinology* 48:591–602.

LeVay, S., and Gilbert, C. D., 1976, Laminar patterns of geniculocortical projections in the cat, *Brain Res.* 113:1–19.

Levey, A. I., Bolam, J. P., Rye, D. B., Hallanger, A. E., Demuth, R. M., Mesulam, M.-M., and Wainer, B. H., 1986, A light and electron microscopic procedure for sequential double antigen localization using diaminobenzidine and benzidine dihydrochloride, *J. Histochem. Cytochem.* 34:1449–1457.

Lewis, P. R., and Henderson, Z., 1980, Tracing putative cholinergic pathways by a dual cytochemical technique, *Brain Res.* 196:489–493.

Lipp, H.-P., and Schwegler, H., 1980, Improved transport of horseradish peroxidase after injection with a non-ionic detergent (nonidet P-40) into mouse cortex and observations on the relationship between spread at the injection site and amount of transported label, *Neurosci. Lett.* 20:49–54.

Luiten, P. G. M., Wouterlood, F. G., Matsuyama, T., Strosberg, A. D., Buwalda, B., and Gaykama, R. P. A., 1988, Immunocytochemical applications in neuroanatomy. Demonstration of connections, transmitters and receptors, *Histochemistry* 90:85–97.

Lundquist, I., and Josefsson, J.-O., 1971, Sensitive method for determination of peroxidase activity in tissue by means of coupled oxidation reaction, *Anal. Biochem.* 41:567–577.

Luppi, P.-H., Sakai, K., Salvert, D., Fort, P., and Jouvet M., 1987, Peptidergic hypothalamic afferents to the cat nucleus raphe pallidus as revealed by a double immunostaining techniques using unconjugated cholera toxin as a retrograde tracer, *Brain Res.* 402:339–345.

Malmgren, L., and Olsson, Y., 1977, A sensitive histochemical method for light- and electron microscopic demonstration of horseradish peroxidase, *J. Histochem. Cytochem.* 25:1280–1283.

Malmgren, L., and Olsson, Y., 1978, A sensitive method for histochemical demonstration of horseradish peroxidase in neurons following retrograde axonal transport, *Brain Res.* 148:279–294.

Malmgren, L. T., and Olsson, Y. 1979, Early influx of horseradish peroxidase into axons of the hypoglossal nerve during wallerian degeneration, *Neurosci. Lett.* 13:13–18.

Max, S. R., Schwab, M., Dumas, M., and Thoenen, H., 1978, Retrograde axonal transport of nerve growth factor in the ciliary ganglion of the chick and the rat, *Brain Res.* 159:411–415.

McLean, J. H., Shipley, M. T., and Bernstein, D. J., 1988, Transneuronal transport of herpes simplex virus in the rat brain, *Soc. Neurosci. Abst.* 14:548.

Menetrey, D., 1985, Retrograde tracing of neural pathways with a protein–gold complex. I. Light microscopic detection after silver intensification, *Histochemnistry* 83:391–395.

Menetrey, D., and Lee, C. L., 1985, Retrograde tracing of neural pathways with a protein gold complex, II. Electron microscopic demonstration of projections and collaterals, *Histochemistry* 83:525–530.

Merchenthaler, I., Gallyas, F., and Liposits, Z., 1989, Silver intensification in immunocytochemistry, in: *Techniques in Immunocytochemistry*, Vol. 4, (G. R. Bullock and P. Petrusz, eds.), Academic Press, London (in press).

Mesulam, M.-M., 1978, Tetramethyl benzidine for horseradish peroxidase neurohistochemistry: A non-carcinogenic blue raction-product with superior sensitivity for visualizing neural afferents and efferents, *J. Histochem. Cytochem.* 26:106–117.

Mesulam, M.-M., 1982, Principles of horseradish peroxidase neurohistochemistry and their applications for tracing neural pathways—axonal transport, enzyme histochemistry and light microscopic analysis, in: *Tracing Neural Connections with Horseradish Peroxidase* (M.-M. Mesulam, ed.), John Wiley & Sons, New York, pp. 1–151.

Mesulam, M.-M., and Brushart, T. M., 1979, Transganglionic and anterograde transport of horseradish peroxidase across dorsal root ganglia: A tetramethyl benzidine method for tracing central sensory connections of muscles and peripheral nerves, *Neuroscience* 4:1107–1117.

Mesulam, M.-M., and Mufson, E. J., 1980, The rapid anterograde transport of horseradish peroxidase, *Neuroscience* 5:1277–1286.

Mesulam, M.-M., and Rosene, D. L., 1979, Sensitivity in horseradish peroxidase neurohistochemistry: A comparative and quantitative analysis of nine methods, *J. Histochem. Cytochem.* 27:763–773.

Morrell, J. I., Greenberger, L. M., and Pfaff, D. W., 1981, Comparison of horseradish peroxidase visualization methods: Quantitative results and further technical specifics, *J. Histochem. Cytochem.* 29:903–916.

Mugnaini, E., and Friedrich, V. L., Jr., 1981, Electron microscopy: Identification and study of normal and degenerating neural elements by electron microscopy, in: *Neuroanatomical Tract-Tracing Methods* (L. Heimer and M. J. RoBards, eds.), Plenum Press, New York, pp. 377–406.

Nässel, D. R., 1981, Transneuronal labeling with horseradish peroxidase in the visual system of the house fly, *Brain Res.* 206:431–438.

Nauta, H. J. W., Kaiserman-Abramof, I. R., and Lasek, R. J., 1975, Electron microscopic observations of horseradish peroxidase transported from the caudoputamen to the substantia nigra in the rat: Possible involvement of the agranular reticulum, *Brain Res.* 85:373–384.

Neal, T. L., and Carey, R. C., 1986, Modification of transport specificity of horseradish peroxidase: Anterograde and transneuronal properties, *Soc. Neurosci. Abstr.* 12:1565.

Norgren, R. B., Jr., Lehman, M. N., McLean, J., and Shipley, M. T., 1988, Labeling of hypothalamic neurons after intraocular injection of herpes simplex virus, *Anat. Rec.* 220:70A.

Novikoff, A. B., 1973, Lysosomes: A personal account, in: *Lysosomes and Storage Diseases* (H. G. Hers and F. Van Hoff, eds.), Academic press, New York, pp. 1–41.

Nyberg, G., 1988, Representation of the forepaw in the feline cuneate nucleus: A transganglionic transport study, *J. Comp. Neurol.* 271:143–152.

Nyberg, G., and Blomqvist, A., 1985, The somatotopic organization of forelimb cutaneous nerves in the brachial dorsal horn: An anatomical study in the cat, *J. Comp. Neurol.* 242:28–39.

Ochs, S., 1987, Axoplasmic transport, in: *Encyclopedia of Neuroscience* (G. Adelman, ed.), Birkauser, Boston, pp. 105–108.

Oldfield, B. J., Hou-Yu A., and Silverman, A.-J., 1983, Technique for the simultaneous ultrastructural demonstration of anterogradely transported horseradish peroxidase and an immunocytochemically identified neuropeptide, *J. Histochem. Cytochem.* 31:1145–1150.

Olsson, Y., Arvidson, B., Hartman, M., Pettersson, A., and Tengvar, C., 1983, Horseradish peroxidase histochemistry. A comparison between various methods used for identifying neurons labeled by retrograde axonal transport, *J. Neurosci. Methods* 7:49–59.

Olucha, F., Martinez-Garcia, F., and Lopez-Garcia, C., 1985, A new stabilizing agent for the tétramethyl benzidine (TMB) reaction product in the histochemical detection of horseradish peroxidase (HRP), *J. Neurosci. Methods* 13:131–138.

Openshaw, H., and Ellis, W. G., 1983, Herpes simplex virus infection of motor neurons: Hypoglassal model, *Infect. Immun.* 42:409–413.

Palkovits, M., Leranth, C., Jew, J. Y., and Williams, T. H., 1982, Simultaneous characterization of pre- and postsynaptic neuron contact sites in brain, *Proc. Natl. Acad. Sci. U.S.A.* 79:2705–2708.

Pastan, I., and Willingham, M. C., 1983, Receptor-mediated endocytosis: Coated pits, receptosomes and the golgi, *Trends Biochem. Sci.* 8:250–254.

Peschanski, M., and Ralston, H. III, 1985, Light and electron microscopic evidence of transneuronal labeling with WGA–HRP to trace somatosensory pathways to the thalamus, *J. Comp. Neurol.* 236:29–41.

Porter, J. D., Guthrie, B. L., and Sparks, D. L., 1985, Selective retrograde transneuronal transport of wheat germ agglutinin-conjugated horseradish peroxidase in the oculomotor system, *Exp. Brain Res.* 57:411–416.

Priestley, J. W., Somogyi, P., and Cuello, A. C., 1981, Neurotransmitter-specific projection neurons revealed by combining PAP immunohistochemistry with retrograde transport of HRP, *Brain Res.* 220:231–240.

Purves, D., and Lichtman, J. W., 1985, *Principles of Neural Development*, Sinauer Associates, Boston.

Quattrochi, J. J., Madison, R., Sidman, R. L., and Kljavin, I., 1987, Colloidal gold fluorescent microspheres: A new retrograde marker visualized by light and electron microscopy, *Exp. Neurol.* 96:219–224.

Reaves, T. A., Jr., Cumming, R., Libber, M. T., and Hayward, J. N., 1982, A technique combining intracellular dye-marking, immunocytochemical identification and ultrastructural analysis of physiologically identified single neurons, *Neurosci. Lett.* 29:195–199.

Reiner, A., and Gamlin, P., 1980, On noncarcinogenic chromogens for horseradish peroxidase histochemistry, *J. Histochem. Cytochem.* 28:187–193.

Rhodes, C. H., Stieber, A., and Gonatas, N. K., 1987, Transneuronally transported wheat germ agglutinin labels glia as well as neurons in the rat visual system, *J. Comp. Neurol.* 261:460–465.

Robertson, B., and Grant, G., 1985, A comparison between wheat germ agglutinin– and choleragenoid–horseradish peroxidase as anterogradely transported markers in central branches of primary sensory neurones in the rat with some observations in the cat, *Neuroscience* 14:895–905.

Rogers, R. C., Butcher, L. L., and Novin, D., 1980, Effects of urethane and pentobarbital anesthesia on the demonstration of retrograde and anterograde transport of horseradish peroxidase, *Brain Res.* 187:197–200.

Rosene, D. L., and Mesulam, M.-M., 1978, Fixation variables in horseradish peroxidase neurohistochemistry. I. The effects of fixation time and perfusion procedures upon enzyme activity, *J. Histochem. Cytochem.* 26:28–39.

Roth, J., Bendayan, M., and Orci. L., 1978, Ultrastructural localization of intracellular antigens by the use of protein A–gold complex, *J. Histochem. Cytochem.* 26:1074–1081.

Rouiller, E. M., Capt, M., Dolivo, M., and De Ribaupierre, F., 1986, Tensor tympani reflex pathways studied with retrograde horseradish peroxidase and transneuronal viral tracing techniques, *Neurosci. Lett.* 72:247–252.

Ruda, M., and Coulter, J. D., 1982, Axonal and transneuronal transport of wheat germ agglutinin demonstrated by immunocytochemistry, *Brain Res.* 249:237–246.

Ruda, M. A., Coffield, J., and Dubner, R., 1984, Demonstration of postsynaptic opioid modulation of thalamic projection neurons by the combined techniques of retrograde horseradish peroxidase and enkephalin immunocytochemistry, *J. Neurosci.* 4:2117–2132.

Rye, D. B., Saper, C. B., and Wainer, B. H., 1984, Stabilization of the tetramethylbenzidine (TMB) reaction product: Application for retrograde and anterograde tracing, and combination with immunohistochemistry, *J. Histochem. Cytochem.* 32:1145–1153.

Sabin, A. B., 1956, Pathogenesis of poliomyelitis: Reappraisal in the light of new data, *Science* 123:1151–1157.

Sakumoto, T., Nagai. T., Kimura, H., and Maeda, T., 1980, Electron microscopic visualization of tetramethyl benzidine reaction product on horseradish peroxidase neurohistochemistry, *Cell. Mol. Biol.* 26:211–216.

Sawchenko, P. E., and Gerfen, C. R., 1985, Plant lectins and bacterial toxins as tools for tracing neuronal connections, *Trends Neurosci.* 5:378–384.

Schmued, L. C., Kyriakidis, K., Fallon, J. H., and Ribak, C. E., 1989, Neurons containing retrogradely-transported fluorogold exhibit a variety of lysosomal profiles: A combined brightfield, fluorescent, and electron microscopic study, *J. Neurocytol.* (in press).

Schnyder, H., and Künzle, H., 1983, Differential labeling in neuronal tracing with wheat germ agglutinin, *Neurosci. Lett.* 35:115–120.

Schubert, P., and Kreutzberg, G. W., 1982, Transneuronal transport: A way for the neuron to communicate with its environment, in: *Axoplasmic Transport in Physiology and Pathology* (D. G. Weiss and A. Gorio, eds.), Springer-Verlag, Berlin, Heidelberg, New York, pp. 32–43.

Schwab. M. E., and Thoenen, H., 1978, Selective binding, uptake and retrograde transport of tetanus toxin by nerve terminals in the rat iris. An electron microscope study using colloidal gold as a tracer, *J. Cell Biol.* 77:1–13.

Schwab, M., Agid, Y., Glowinski, J., and Thoenen, H., 1977, Retrograde axonal transport of ^{125}I-tetanus toxin as a tool for tracing fiber connections of the rostral part of the rat neostriatum, *Brain Res.* 126:211–224.

Schwab. M. E., Suda, K., and Thoenen, H., 1979, Selective retrograde transsynaptic transfer of a protein, tetanus toxin, subsequently to its retrograde axonal transport, *J. Cell Biol.* 82:798–810.

Schwanzel-Fukuda, M., Morrell, J. I., and Pfaff, D. W., 1983, Polyacrylamide gel provides slow release delivery of wheat germ agglutinin (WGA) for retrograde neuroanatomical tracing, *J. Histochem. Cytochem.* 31:831–836.

Segade, L. A. G., 1987, Pyrocatechol as a stabilizing agent for *o*-tolidine and *o*-dianisidene: A sensitive new method for HRP neurochistochemistry, *J. Hirnforsch.* 28:331–340.

Seiler, M., and Schwab, M., 1984, Specific retrograde transport of nerve growth factor (NGF) from neocortex to nucleus basalis in the rat, *Brain Res.* 300:33–39.

Shiosaka, S., Shimada, S., and Tohyama, M., 1986, Sensitive double-labeling technique of retrograde biotinized tracer (biotin–WGA) and immunocytochemistry: Light and electron microscopic analysis, *J. Neurosci. Methods* 16:9–18.

Silver, M. A., and Jacobowitz, D. M., 1979, Specific uptake and retrograde flow of antibody to dopamine-β-hydroxylase by central nervous system noradrenergic neurons *in vivo*, *Brain Res.* 167:65–75.

Somogyi, P., and Takagi, H., 1982, A note on the use of picric acid–paraformaldehyde–glutaraldehyde fixative for correlated light and electron microscopic immunocytochemistry, *Neuroscience* 7:1779–1784.

Somogyi, P., Hodgson, A. J., and Smith, A. D., 1979, An approach to tracing neuron networks in the cerebral cortex and basal ganglia. Combination of Golgi staining, retrograde transport of horseradish peroxidase and anterograde degeneration of synaptic boutons in the same material, *Neuroscience* 4:1805–1852.

Spreafico, R., Cheema, S., Ellis, L. C., Jr., and Rustioni, A., 1982, On comparison of horseradish peroxidase visualization methods, *J. Histochem. Cytochem.* 30:487–488.

Staines, W. A., Kimura, H., Fibiger, H. C., and McGeer, E. G., 1980, Peroxidase-labeled lectin as a neuroanatomical tracer: Evaluation in a CNS pathway, *Brain Res.* 197:485–490.

Steindler, D. A., 1982, Differences in the labeling of axons of passage by wheat germ agglutinin after uptake by cut peripheral nerve versus injections within the central nervous system, *Brain Res.* 250:159–167.

Steindler, D. A., and Bradley, R. H., 1983, N-[Acetyl-^{3}H]wheat germ agglutinin: Anatomical and biochemical studies of a sensitive bidirectionally transported axonal tracer, *Neuroscience* 10:219–241.

Steward, O., 1981, Horseradish peroxidase and fluorescent substances and their combination with other techniques, in: *Neuroanatomical Tract-Tracing Methods* (L. Heimer and M. J. RoBards, eds.), Plenum Press, New York, pp. 279–310.

Stoeckel, K., Schwab, M., and Thoenen, H., 1975, Specificity of retrograde transport of nerve growth factor (NGF) in sensory neurons: A biochemical and morphological study, *Brain Res.* 89:1–14.

Strauss, W., 1982, Imidazole increases the sensitivity of the cytochemical reaction for peroxidase with diaminobenzidine at a neutral pH, *J. Histochem. Cytochem.* 30:491–493.

Streit, P., 1980, Selective retrograde labeling indicating the transmitter of neuronal pathways, *J. Comp. Neurol.* 191:429–463.

Streit, P., and Reubi, J. C., 1977, A new and sensitive staining method for axonally transported horseradish peroxidase (HRP) in the pigeon visual system, *Brain Res.* 126:530–537.

Stürmer, C., Bielenberg, K., and Spatz, W. B., 1981, Electron microscopical identification of 3,3′, 5,5′–tetramethylbenzidine-reacted horseradish peroxidase after retrograde axoplasmic transport, *Neurosci. Lett.* 23:1–5.

Suresh, M. R., Cuello, A. C., and Milstein, C., 1986, Advantages of bispecific hybridomas in one-step immunocytochemistry and immunoassays, *Proc. Natl. Acad. Sci. U.S.A.* 83:7989–7993.

Takada, M., and Hattori, T., 1986, Transneuronal transport of WGA–HRP from the ipsi- to contralateral medial habenular nucleus through the interpeduncular nucleus in the rat, *Brain Res.* 384:77–83.

Takeuchi, Y., Allen, G. V., and Hopkins, D. A., 1985, Transnuclear transport and axon collateral projections of the mamillary nuclei in the rat, *Brain Res. Bull.* 14:453–468.

Taylor, A. M., and Lieberman, A. R., 1987, Ultrastructural organisation of the projection from the superior colliculus to the ventral lateral geniculate nucleus of the rat, *J. Comp. Neurol.* 256:454–462.

Titus, J. A., Haugland, R., Sharrow, S. O., and Segal, D. M., 1982, Texas red, a hydrophilic, red-emitting fluorophore for use with fluorescein in dual parameter flow microfluorochrometric and fluorescence microscopic studies, *J. Immunol. Methods* 50:193–204.

Triller, A., and Korn, H., 1981, Interneuronal transfer of horseradish peroxidase associated with exo/endocytic activity on adjacent membranes, *Exp. Brain Res.* 43:233–236.

Trojanowski, J. Q., 1983, Native and derivatized lectins for *in vivo* studies of neuronal connectivity and neuronal cell biology, *J. Neurosci. Methods* 9:185–204.

Trojanowski, J. Q., and Gonatas, N. K., 1983, A morphometric study of the endocytosis of wheat germ agglutinin–horseradish peroxidase conjugates by retinal ganglion cells in the rat, *Brain Res.* 272:201–210.

Trojanowski, J. Q., and Schmidt, M. L., 1984, Interneuronal transfer of axonally transported proteins: Studies with HRP and HRP conjugates of wheat germ agglutinin, cholera toxin and the B subunit of cholera toxin, *Brain Res.* 311:366–369.

Trojanowski, J. Q., Gonatas, J. O., and Gonatas, N. K., 1982, Horseradish peroxidase (HRP) conjugates of cholera toxin and lectins are more sensitive retrogradely transported markers than free HRP, *Brain Res.* 231:33–50.

Tsai, Y., Norgren, R. B., and Lehman, M. N., 1988, Double-label electron microscopic immunocytochemistry using tetramethylbenzidine (TMB) as a chromagen, *Soc. Neurosci. Abst.* 14:546.

Turner, P. T., and Harris, A. B., 1974, Ultrastructure of exogenous peroxidase in cerebral cortex, *Brain Res.* 74:305–326.

Tyler, K. L., McPhee, D. A., and Fields, B. N., 1986, Distinct pathways of viral spread in the host determined by reovirus S1 gene segment, *Science* 233:770–774.

Ugolini, G., Kuypers, H. G. J. M., and Simmons, A., 1987, Retrograde transneuronal transfer of herpes simplex virus type 1 (HSV 1) from motoneurons, *Brain Res.* 422:242–256.

Vahlne, A., Svennerholm, B., Sandberg, M., Hamberger, A., and Lycke, E., 1980, Differences in attachment between herpes simplex type 1 and type 2 viruses to neurons and glial cells, *Infect. Immun.* 28:675–680.

van den Pol, A. N., 1984, Colloidal gold and biotin–avidin conjugates as ultrastructural markers for neural antigens, *Q. J. Exp. Physiol.* 69:1–33.

van den Pol, A., 1985, Dual ultrastructural localization of two neurotransmitter-related antigens: Colloidal gold-labeled neurophysin-immunoreactive supraoptic neurons receive peroxidase-labeled glutamate decarboxylase- or gold-labeled GABA-immunoreactive synapses, *J. Neurosci.* 5:2940–2954.

Voigt, T., LeVay, S., and Stamnes, M. A., 1988, Morphological and immunocytochemical observations on the visual callosal projections in the cat, *J. Comp. Neurol.* 272:450–460.

Wainer, B. H., and Rye, D. B., 1984, Retrograde horseradish tracing combined with localization of choline acetyltransferase immunoreactivity, *J. Histochem. Cytochem.* 32:439–443.

Wakefield, C., and Shonnard, N., 1979, Observations of HRP labeling following injection through a chronically implanted cannula—a method to avoid diffusion of HRP into injured fibers, *Brain Res.* 168:221–226.

Wan, X.-C. S., Trojanowski, J. Q., and Gonatas, J. O., 1982, Cholera toxin and wheat germ agglutinin conjugates as neuroanatomical probes: Their uptake and clearance, transganglionic and retrograde transport and sensitivity, *Brain Res.* 243:215–224.

Warr, W. B., de Olmos, J. S., and Heimer, L., 1981, Horseradish peroxidase: The basic procedure, in: *Neuroanatomical Tract-Tracing Methods* (L. Heimer and M. J. RoBards, eds.), Plenum Press, New York, pp. 207–262.

Weiss, D. G., 1986, The mechanism of axoplasmic transport, in: *Axoplasmic Transport* (Z. Igbal, ed.), CRC Press, Boca Raton, FL, pp. 275–307.

Weiss, P., and Hiscoe, H. B., 1948, Experiments on the mechanism of nerve growth, *J. Exp. Zool.* 107:315–395.

Wenthold, R. J., Skaggs, K. K., and Reale, R. R., 1984, Retrograde axonal transport of antibodies to synaptic membrane components, *Brain Res.* 304:162–165.

Wilczynski, W., and Zakon, H., 1982, Transcellular transfer of HRP in the amphibian visual system, *Brain Res.* 239:29–40.

Wouterlood, F. G., 1988, Anterograde neuroanatomical tracing with *Phaseolus vulgaris*-leucoagglutinin combined with immunocytochemistry of gamma-amino butyric acid, choline acetyltransferase or serotonin, *Histochemistry* 89:421–428.

Wouterlood, F. G., Bol. J. G. J. M., and Steinbusch, H. W. M., 1987a, Double-label immunocytochemistry: Combination of anterograde neuroanatomical tracing with *Phaseolus vulgaris* leucoagglutinin and enzyme histochemistry of target neurons, *J. Histochem. Cytochem.* 35:817–823.

Wouterlood, F. G., Steinbusch, H. W. M., Luiten, P. G. M., and Bol, J. G. J. M., 1987b, Projection from the prefrontal cortex to histaminergic cell groups in the posterior hypothalamic region of the rat. Anterograde tracing with *Phaseolus vulgaris* leucoagglutinin combined with immunocytochemistry of histidine decarboxylase, *Brain Res.* 406:330–336.

Záborszky, L., and Cullinan, W. E., 1989, Hypothalamic axons terminate on forebrain cholinergic neurons: An ultrastructural double-labelng study using PHA-L tracing and ChAT immunocytochemistry, *Brain Res.* 479:177–184.

Záborszky, L., and Léránth, C., 1985, Simultaneous ultrastructural demonstration of retrogradely transported horseradish peroxidase and choline acetyltransferase immunoreactivity, *Histochemistry* 82:529–537.

Záborszky, L., Léránth, C., and Palkovits, M., 1979, Theoretical review: Light and electron microscopic identification of monoaminergic terminals in the central nervous system, *Brain Res. Bull.* 4:99–117.

Záborszky, L., Léránth, C., and Heimer, L, 1984, Ultrastructural evidence of amygdalofugal axons terminating on cholinergic cells of the rostral forebrain, *Neurosci. Lett.* 52:219–225.

Záborszky, L., Alheid, G. F., and Heimer, L., 1985, Mapping of transmitter-specific connections: Simultaneous demonstration of anterograde degeneration and changes in the immunostaining pattern induced by lesions, *J. Neurosci. Methods* 14:255–266.

Záborszky, L., Heimer, L., Eckenstein, F., and Léránth, C., 1986, GABAergic input to cholinergic forebrain neurons: An ultrastructural study using retrograde tracing of HRP and double immunolabeling, *J. Comp. Neurol.* 250:282–295.

Zahm, D. S., 1989, The ventral striatopallidal parts of the basal ganglia in the rat: II. Compartmentation of ventral pallidal efferents, *Neuroscience* (in press).

5

Interchangeable Uses of Autoradiographic and Peroxidase Markers for Electron Microscopic Detection of Neuronal Pathways and Transmitter-Related Antigens in Single Sections

VIRGINIA M. PICKEL and TERESA A. MILNER

I. INTRODUCTION

In the past several years, there has been a rapid expansion in use of immunocytochemical methods for identifying neuronal molecules. These include

VIRGINIA M. PICKEL and TERESA A. MILNER • Department of Neurology and Neuroscience, Division of Neurobiology, Cornell University Medical College, New York, New York 10021.

neurotransmitter-synthesizing enzymes, several transmitters such as norepinephrine (NE), dopamine (DA), 5-hydroxytryptamine (5-HT), and γ-aminobutyric acid (GABA), and a variety of neuropeptides (Cuello, 1983; Heym and Lang, 1986; Pickel, 1985; Polak and Van Noorden, 1983; Steinbush *et al.*, 1978; Storm-Mathisen *et al.*, 1983). The increasing use of immunocytochemistry is largely attributable to both commercial and individual production of a large number of mono- and polyclonal antibodies (MacMillan and Cuello, 1986; M. E. Ross *et al.*, 1981; Sofroniew *et al.*, 1978). Many of the available antibodies have a high titer and can be specifically localized by several different immunocytochemical methods. The most common methods employ secondary immunoglobulins (IgGs) produced against serum from the same species as the primary antibody. The secondary IgG is conjugated with either fluorescence, peroxidase, gold, or radiolabeled markers (i.e., tritium or iodine) for localization of the antibodies in sections of tissue (DeMey, 1983; Glazer *et al.*, 1984; Hunt and Mantyh, 1984; Pickel *et al.*, 1986). Alternatively, the secondary IgG can be immunologically bound to a peroxidase–antiperoxidase (PAP) complex with the antiperoxidase being produced in the same species as the primary antibody (Sternberger, 1979). In our laboratory, the PAP method is used routinely for localization of single antigens in light and electron microscopic preparations (Pickel, 1981; Pickel, 1985).

The localization of single neuronal antigens has broadened our knowledge of the regional distributions and ultrastructural localization of a large number of transmitters and related substances in the central nervous system (CNS). However, these studies give limited information on the relationship of the neurotransmitter-specific neurons and neuroanatomically defined pathways. Information regarding the existence of a specific immunocytochemical marker in an identified pathway can be achieved by dual light microscopic labels (Sawchenko and Swanson, 1981; 1982; Milner *et al.*, 1984; Milner and Pickel, 1986a,b; Priestly *et al.*, 1981; Rye *et al.*, 1984; Sakumoto et al., 1978). Many of these dual-labeling studies employ peroxidase markers whose reaction product can be detected by electron microscopy. The differential labeling seen with two combined peroxidase methods for electron microscopy depends largely on the distinction between the granularity of anterogradely or retrogradely transported horseradish peroxidase (HRP) and the immunocytochemical reaction that is more diffuse (Isaacson and Tanaka, 1988; Oldfield *et al.*, 1983; Priestly *et al.*, 1981; Zaborszky and Leranth, 1985). However, the difference between the two peroxidase products is most readily apparent when the transport and immunocytochemical markers are in separate cells and processes.

Alternative approaches described in this chapter take advantage of the clear distinction between autoradiographic silver grains and the peroxidase reaction product for dual labeling of transport and neuronal antigens. In the first approach, the autoradiographic demonstration of neuronal pathways labeled by anterograde transport of tritiated amino acids (see Cowan and Cuenod, 1975, for a detailed review of the autoradiographic technique) is combined with the immunocytochemical localization of neuronal markers by the PAP technique. In the second approach, the autoradiographic localization of radioiodinated secondary IgG (McLean *et al.,* 1983; Pickel *et al.,* 1986) is combined with transport of HRP or wheat germ agglutinin-conjugated horseradish peroxidase (WGA–HRP). Retrograde transport has been shown to be enhanced by use of WGA–HRP, which specifically binds to the plasma membranes and is more readily internalized by neurons (Brushart and Mesulam, 1980; Gonatas *et al.,* 1979; Mesulam, 1982).

The interchangeable use of autoradiographic and peroxidase markers provides two reliable methods for the demonstration (1) that afferents from a peripheral ganglion or specific nucleus in brain contain a specific transmitter or form synapses with neurons having identifiable transmitters, and (2) that central perikarya that project to peripheral targets or to another brain region either contain or receive afferents having identifiable transmitters. The specific questions that can be answered by combining anterograde transport of [^{3}H]-amino acids with PAP labeling of antibodies are shown schematically in Fig. 1, whereas the synaptic associations revealed by combining retrograde and anterograde transport of WGA–HRP and immunoautoradiography are illustrated in Fig. 2. As can be seen in these figures, the necessity for two contrasting electron-dense markers is most evident when the transport and immunocytochemical labels are in the same neurons. However, one often cannot predict prior to experimentation whether the transmitter under investigation will be in the same or separate populations of neurons. Thus, although the contrasting markers are not absolutely essential for demonstrating synaptic junctions between anatomically and chemically distinct neurons, they do provide more versatility and avoid unnecessary ambiguity regarding input from afferents containing the same transmitter.

II. AUTORADIOGRAPHIC LOCALIZATION OF ANTEROGRADELY TRANSPORTED AMINO ACIDS COMBINED WITH IMMUNOPEROXIDASE LABELING

Technical aspects and examples of the combined use of autoradiography for localization of anterogradely transported [^{3}H]-amino acids and PAP immunocytochemistry for labeling of putative transmitter systems are described. The examples include immunocytochemical identification of catecholaminergic and peptidergic neurons in relation to afferents from sensory ganglia and intrinsic pathways of the brain.

A. Methodology

The methods described are based primarily on the procedures currently used within our laboratory. The sequence of events includes injection of the labeled amino acids, fixation, processing of the tissue for immunocytochemistry, autoradiography, and data analysis.

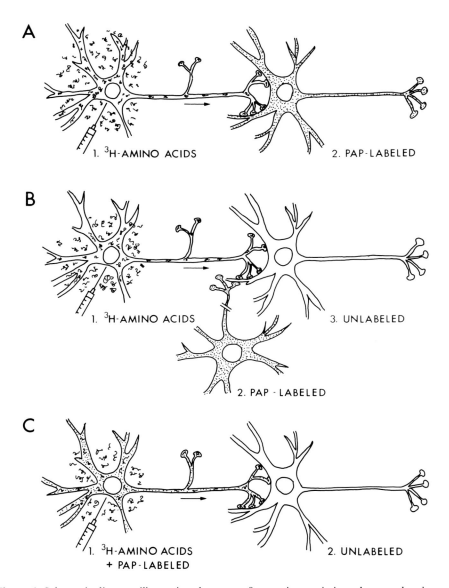

Figure 1. Schematic diagram illustrating the types of synaptic associations that may be observed by combining anterograde transport of [³H]-amino acids and PAP immunocytochemistry. A: Anterograde autoradiographic labeling (squiggled lines) in terminals which form direct synaptic contacts with neurons containing PAP (dots) reaction product. B: Convergence of the anterogradely labeled terminals and other PAP-immunoreactive (dots) terminals on a common unlabeled target. C: Colocalization of the autoradiographic and PAP labels within the same neuron, which forms synapses with a second, unlabeled cell.

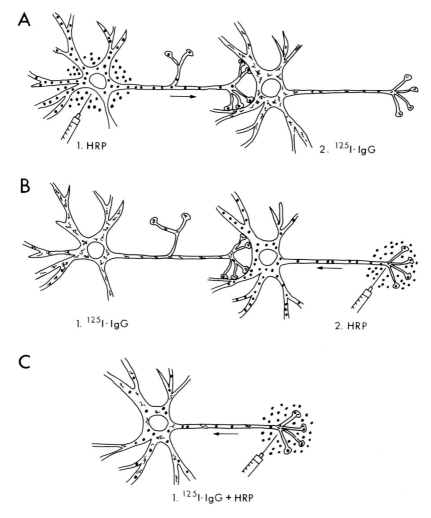

Figure 2. Schematic diagram illustrating the types of associations that may be observed by combining anterograde or retrograde transport of HRP and immunoautoradiography. A: Anterograde labeling of HRP (large dots) in terminals forming direct synaptic contacts with a second neuron containing the immunoautoradiographic (squiggled lines) labeling. B: Immunoautoradiographic labeling in a neuron which directly synapses with a second neuron showing retrograde transport of HRP. C: Colocalization of the retrogradely transported HRP (large dots) and immunoautoradiographic (squiggled lines) label.

1. Injection of Labeled Amino Acids

Details of the methodology for the use of anterograde axonal transport for tracing neuronal pathways are given by Cowan *et al.* (1972) and Cowan and Cuenod (1975). In brief, a small quantity, e.g., 1 mCi [2-³H]-L-proline in 1 ml of 0.1 N HC1 (specific activity 30–50 Ci/nmole; New England Nuclear Corporation) is concentrated in a vacuum centrifuge and then reconstituted with the appropriate volume of sterile Ringer's solution to yield a final dilution of 100 μCi/μl (Milner et al., 1984). The [^{3}H]-proline also can be combined with a similarly prepared solution of [^{3}H]-leucine to improve the observed transport through uptake of more than one amino acid. The labeled solution is delivered to selective loci of halothane (2% in 100% O$_2$) anesthetized animals using a glass micropipette with an outer tip diameter of 10–50 μm. The micropipette is first attached to an air pressure delivery system (Amaral and Price, 1983), then visually placed in peripheral ganglia or stereotaxically placed in selected brain regions using standard atlas coordinates (Paxinos and Watson, 1986). In peripheral ganglia, quantities ranging from 0.5 to 1.0 μl of the reconstituted solution are injected over a 30-min interval. To confine the injection sites within the anatomical boundaries of small central nuclei, the volume of radioactive solution delivered is necessarily much smaller (30–60 nl) than that used in the peripheral ganglia (Milner et al., 1984). Following either peripheral or central injections, the animals are allowed to survive for an experimentally determined interval (usually 24–48 hr) to allow transport to areas of terminal innervation.

2. Tissue Preparation

a. Fixation. At the time of sacrifice, these animals are anesthetized with pentobarbital (50 mg/kg), and the brains are fixed by vascular perfusion. Since amino acids that have been incorporated into proteins are maintained in tissues after most aldehyde fixation procedures, the fixation method is optimized for immunocytochemistry. Immunocytochemical labeling is best achieved by minimal fixation. Reduced interactions between antigen and antibody and/or inadequate penetration of immunoreagents may account for diminished detection of immunoreaction product when tissues are exposed to high concentrations of aldehydes. Fixation by perfusion with 200 ml of 4% paraformaldehyde in 0.1 M phosphate buffer (pH 7.3) usually is suitable for light microscopy of brains from 200- to 250-g rats. Additional fixation by immersion in the same solution for 30–60 min does not diminish immunoreactivity. Aortic arch perfusion with either (1) 200 ml of 4% paraformaldehyde and 0.2% glutaraldehyde, or (2) 50 ml of 3.75% acrolein and 2% paraformaldehyde in 0.1 M phosphate buffer are used routinely for electron microscopy of brain tissues from 200- to 250-g rats, (Milner and Pickel, 1986 a,b). Perfusions with aldehydes or acrolein are preceded by a rapid delivery of 10 ml of heparin saline (1000 units) to prevent fixation of blood cells to the walls of the vessels. The acrolein fixation is also followed by perfusion with 200 ml of 2% paraformaldehyde in 0.1 M phosphate buffer. After removal, the fixed tissue (brain or spinal cord) is cut into 2–5 mm slices, then postfixed for an additional 30 min either in the glutaraldehyde–paraformaldehyde mixture (perfusion 1) or in 2% paraformaldehyde (perfusion 2). The rapid perfusion with a small volume of 3.75% acrolein results in considerably less fixation than originally proposed by King *et al.* (1983). This quantity was experimentally determined to give optimal preservation of ultrastructure without loss of immunocytochemical labeling for all antibodies that have been tested except for monoclonal antibodies against choline acetyltransferase (CAT) and 5-HT. Whenever applicable, the improved morphology seen after acrolein fixation at least partially offsets the inconvenience of having to use extreme caution to avoid the toxic effects of the compound. Preparation of the acrolein solutions as well as the perfusions must be carried out under a well-ventilated hood. The use of reducing agents such as sodium borohydride, as described below (Abdel-Akhner *et al.*, 1952), also is virtually essential for immunocytochemical labeling following fixation with acrolein (see Chapter 6).

b. Sectioning. For both light and electron microscopy, the fixed brain slices are sectioned routinely at 30–40 μm on a vibrating microtome (Vibratome). However, 10-μm cryostat sections can be used for light microscopy whenever it is necessary to obtain numerous consecutive sections or when sections of a more consistent thickness and/or greater penetration are necessary. In brain, the sections through the injection site are processed by light microscopic autoradiography to establish the size and location of the diffused isotope. The regions expected to contain terminal autoradiographic labeling are processed by the immunoperoxidase method for the identification of transmitter-specific antigens.

c. Sodium Borohydride Treatment. Prior to initiation of immunocytochemical labeling, the sections from acrolein-fixed brains are incubated for 30 min in a 1% solution of sodium borohydride (NaBH$_4$) in 0.1 M phosphate buffer and then washed through successive changes of the same buffer until gas bubbles disappear. Improved immunocytochemical labeling may be attributed (1) to reduction of dialdehydes to their corresponding alcohols (Abdel-Akher *et al.*, 1952; Schachner *et al.*, 1977) and (2) to greater penetration of immunoreagents to intracellular storage compartments due to damage to cellular membranes by the gas bubbles.

3. Immunoperoxidase Labeling

a. Antibodies. Specific rabbit polyclonal antibodies against catecholamine-synthesizing enzymes, particularly tyrosine hydroxylase (TH) and phenylethanolamine N-methyltransferase (PNMT) used in the examples of this chapter, were produced and generously supplied by Dr. Tong H. Joh, Department of Neurology and Neuroscience, Division of Molecular Neurobiology, Cornell University Medical College. Antibodies prepared by his protocol are available from Eugene Tech, Allentown, NJ. The antibodies against TH and PNMT are shown to be specific by immunoelectrophoresis and selective inhibition of the activity of the respective enzymes (Joh *et al.*, 1973;

M. E. Ross *et al.*, 1981). A monoclonal antibody to CAT (Eckenstein and Thoenen, 1982), the acetylcholine-synthesizing enzyme, also is commercially available from Boeringer Mannheim. There are a number of excellent sources of commercial antisera to 5-HT, and neuropeptides including enkephalin (ENK), substance P (SP), neurotensin (NT), and somatostatin. A number of the companies that produce antibodies and other immunoreagents are listed in a directory from Linscott Inc., Glen Mill Valley, CA 94941. All antibodies should be tested for specificity by published methods (Cuello, 1983; Larsson, 1981; Milner *et al.*, 1984; Pickel, 1981).

b. Labeling Procedure. The detailed PAP-labeling method, as used for the localization of antibodies in free-floating Vibratome sections, has been described in a number of reports (Leranth and Pickel, Chapter 6, this volume; Milner and Pickel, 1986a,b; Pickel, 1981; Pickel *et al.*, 1986). Thus, the method is described only with regard to details that pertain to combined use with autoradiographic localization of transported [^{3}H]-amino acids. The sections through the regions expected to contain autoradiographic labeling in axon terminals are transferred to a Tris-saline solution (9.0 g NaCl in 1 liter of 0.1 M Tris at pH 7.6). The sections to be labeled with rabbit antibodies are then incubated in the following solutions: (1) a 1 : 30 dilution of normal goat serum in Tris-saline for 30 min; (2) an empirically derived optimal dilution of primary antibodies or control serum for 18–24 hr at room temperature; (3) a 1 : 50 dilution of goat antirabbit IgG (Sternberger–Meyer) in Tris-saline for 30 min; and finally (4) a solution of 1 : 100 diluted rabbit PAP in Tris-saline for 30 min. Each incubation is separated by at least 2×10-min. washes. The diluent and washes are prepared with 1% goat serum Tris-saline. The serum is omitted in the final wash after step 4. To localize the antibodies produced in sheep or goat, the secondary IgG is produced in another species, for example, rabbit, and the antiperoxidase in sheep or goat (Dako, Inc.) and the goat serum is substituted with 0.1% bovine serum albumin. Similarly, rat antibodies can be localized by immunocytochemical reactions with rabbit or goat antirat IgG and rat PAP (Dako, Inc.) The bound peroxidase is visualized by reaction for 4–6 min in a solution containing 44 mg 3,3'-diaminobenzidine (DAB) and 20 μl of 30% hydrogen peroxide in 200 ml of 0.1 M Tris-saline, pH 7.6 (Sternberger, 1979). A few of these sections are examined by light microscopy to verify the immunocytochemical labeling; the remainder are processed for light or electron microscopic autoradiography.

4. Autoradiography

For light microscopy, the immunolabeled sections are mounted on acid-cleaned slides previously coated with 0.25% gelatin. The sections are air dried on the slides, then defatted by processing through two 15-min changes of chloroform–100% ethanol (1 : 1) followed by a graded ethanol series to deionized water. The slides are air dried for a second time and dipped in Ilford L4 emulsion (at 50°C) diluted 1 : 1 with distilled water. These are then allowed to dry in a dark room at >60% humidity to prevent cracking of the emulsion. The autoradiographic preparations are then exposed in light-proof boxes with desiccant at 4°C for periods of 15–30 days. At the end of the exposure period, the slides are developed for 2 min at 16–17°C using Kodak D-19 developer, rinsed in water, and then placed in Kodak Ektaflo fixer for 8 min, washed in running water for 1 hr, dehydrated, cleared in xylene, and mounted with resin under a coverslip. All the chemicals for autoradiography are prepared on the day of use. The final autoradiographic preparations are examined and photographed with brightfield, darkfield, or differential interference contrast optics on a light microscope.

For electron microscopy, the immunolabeled sections are postfixed for 2 hr in 2% OsO_4, in 0.1 M phosphate buffer then washed in phosphate buffer, dehydrated through a graded series of ethanols followed by propylene oxide, and flat embedded in Epon 812 (Pickel, 1981). For flat embedding the sections are placed in Epon between two sheets of Aclar plastic (Masurovsky and Bunge, 1968). Lead weights are placed on top of the plastic sheets to maintain flatness of the section; and the Epon is hardened at 60°C for 18–24 hr. Plastic is peeled from one surface that is to be placed in direct contact with Epon to insure adhesion. The desired area of the tissue is chosen using a light microscope. This region is cut from the larger section then placed in the flat base of a Beam capsule that is subsequently filled with Epon and hardened in the oven at 60°C.

The autoradiographic procedure is the same as that described in detail by Beaudet (1982), Bosler *et al.* (1986), Descarries and Beaudet (1983), and Pickel and Beaudet (1984). In brief, ultrathin sections are collected from the extreme outer (about 1 μm) surface of the flat embedded Vibratome sections and deposited on slides with a wire loop containing water. These slides were previously acid cleaned and coated with 2% parlodion in amyl acetate. After drying, on the parlodion-coated slides, the sections are counterstained for 20 min with 2.5% uranyl acetate in 50% ethanol and washed through several quick changes of 50% ethanol; stained for 5 min with Reynold's lead citrate diluted 1 : 1 with 0.1 N NaOH and washed in distilled water. After drying, the slides and sections then are coated with a silver-gray layer of carbon (Varian Vacuum Evaporator). Care should be taken not to produce either an excessively thick or thin layer of carbon. The stained and carbon-coated slides are then dipped in Ilford L4 emulsion (50°C) diluted 1 : 4 with distilled water and air dried in a dark room at >60% humidity. These are exposed in light-proof boxes with desiccant at 4°C for 3–12 months. Longer exposure periods may enhance the incidence of randomly scattered silver grains. The autoradiographs are developed 1–2 min at 16–17°C with Kodak Microdol X developer which has been freshly prepared with deionized water and filtered. The size of the grains reflects the duration of incubation, the temperature of the developing solution, and the type of developer (Salpeter *et al.*, 1969, 1977).

Following the developing procedure, the slides are rinsed in water and fixed for 4 min in 30% fresh, filtered sodium thiosulfate followed by four 5-min washes in deionized water. Prior to drying, the slides are rinsed individually with distilled water using a squirt bottle. The entire counterstaining and development procedure is done with minimal agitation to insure that the parlodion coating is not dissociated from the slides. The parlodion coating with autoradiographic thin sections is floated onto the surface of double-distilled water in a glass container. The position of the thin sections on the parlodion film can be seen by reflections from an appropriately positioned lamp from above. Two-hundred-mesh or slotted slim-bar grids are placed directly on top of the ribbons of sections. These are then picked up on filter paper by approaching from above the water–parlodion surface. After drying, the grids on the parlodion coating and sections are removed from the filter paper with forceps and immersed for 3 min in fresh EM-grade amyl acetate under a well-ventilated hood. These are allowed to dry in an oven (45°C) prior to electron microscopic examination.

5. Data Analysis

The localization of reduced silver grains to specific neuronal profiles in electron microscopic autoradiographs is determined by the method described by Salpeter et al. (1969). Briefly, the micrographs are enlarged to a final magnification appropriate for profiles under investigation, and the grain densities (grains per unit area) are tabulated as density distribution around the axon terminal or suspected source of the radiation. The presence of silver grains over the same axon terminal in consecutive or even near adjacent sections is also considered evidence for specific labeling of the identified terminal. The number of grains is frequently so small that they may be detected only in one of two or three sections. Thus, ribbons of four or more thin sections are needed to confirm the reproducibility of autoradiographic labeling. Isolated grains or series of three or more grains in a straight line (α tracks) usually can not be followed in adjacent sections.

B. Applications

The described method of combining autoradiographic localization of anterogradely transported [^{3}H]-amino acids and immunoperoxidase labeling can be applied to any central or peripheral neural pathway. The examples chosen are from previous or ongoing studies in our laboratory that have shown autoradiographically labeled terminals in synaptic contact with PAP-labeled dendrites (Fig. 1A) or the convergence of these terminals on unlabeled dendrites also receiving input from other PAP-labeled afferents (Fig. 1B). In all studies numerous autoradiographically labeled terminals also formed synapses with unlabeled neurons that were not contacted by other afferents showing detectable levels of the antigen under investigation.

1. Transmitter-Specific Neurons in Relation to Afferents from Peripheral Ganglia

The autoradiographic localization of anterogradely transported [³H]-amino acids has been combined with immunoperoxidase labeling for TH to demonstrate the synaptic input of vagal afferents on catecholaminergic neurons in the rat medulla (Sumal *et al.*, 1983). Catecholaminergic neurons of the A2 group (Dahlström and Fuxe, 1964) are located in the medial and commissural nuclei of the solitary tract (NTS) in the medulla oblongata (Howe *et al.*, 1980; Palkovits and Jacobowitz, 1974). The catecholaminergic neurons within the NTS have been implicated in several autonomic functions including regulation of arterial blood pressure (Chalmers *et al.*, 1978; DeJong, 1974). In addition, the baroreceptor afferents from the inferior (nodose) ganglion of the vagus nerve terminate in portions of the NTS that contain the catecholaminergic neurons (Kalia and Mesulam, 1980; Katz and Karten, 1979). In the simultaneous autoradiographic tracing of [³H]-amino acids and PAP immunocytochemistry of TH, the brown peroxidase labeling for TH in neuronal perikarya in the NTS can be easily differentiated from overlying silver grains using either darkfield (Fig. 3A) or brightfield optics. Darkfield provides better resolutions of the silver grains and more details of the underlying myelinated bundles of axons, which can be used in mapping studies. However, the brown peroxidase reaction product is more easily identified with brightfield optics as can be seen in the examples in Fig. 3B–D.

After usual exposure periods of 3–8 months, electron microscopic autoradiographic preparations show accumulations of silver grains over selective axon terminals. The autoradiographic labeling of transported [³H]-amino acids is readily differentiated from the immunoperoxidase reaction product as shown in Fig. 4 for enkephalin in the NTS. The electron density produced by interaction of osmium tetroxide with the peroxidase reaction for enkephalin is seen as a faint precipitate surrounding vesicles, mitochondria, and other organelles in the enkephalin-labeled terminal. The peroxidase labeling in this terminal can be appreciated most readily by comparing the overall density with that seen in the autoradiographically labeled terminal that does not contain immunoreactivity (Fig. 4). In this example, the terminal labeled by anterograde transport and the enkephalin-containing terminal converge on a common unlabeled dendrite. The low intensity of immunocytochemical labeling probably reflects both the depth from the surface (greater depths have less density) and the presence of the overlying emulsion. In this specific preparation, the density of immunoreactivity for enkephalin in the axon terminal and the quality of the ultrastructural morphology were reduced by prior treatment of the animal with colchicine (see Section III.A).

2. Transmitter-Specific Central Neurons in Relation to Central Afferents

The combined use of autoradiography for identifying the location of anterogradely transported [³H]-amino acids and immunoperoxidase labeling

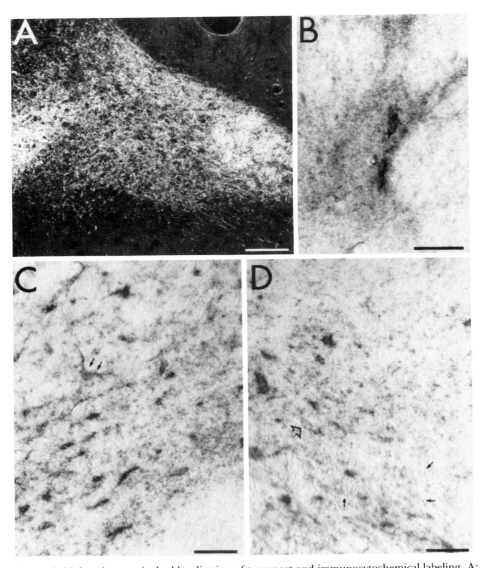

Figure 3. Light microscopic dual localization of transport and immunocytochemical labeling. A: Darkfield photomicrograph showing the autoradiographic labeling for anterogradely transported [^{3}H]-amino acids in the medial nucleus of the solitary tract combined with PAP labeling for tyrosine hydroxylase. Amino acids were injected in the nodose ganglion 24 hr prior to sacrifice. B: Brightfield photomicrograph showing retrograde transport of HRP in neuronal perikarya of the intermediolateral column of the thoracic spinal cord combined with immunoautoradiographic labeling for substance P. Cervical sympathetic nerve was dipped in HRP 24 hr prior to sacrifice. C: Brightfield photomicrograph showing the retrograde transport of WGA–HRP (brown) and immunoautoradiographic labeling for TH (black) in the ventral tegmental area 24 hr after injection of the tracer in the nucleus accumbens. Perikarya with only TH (single arrow) and both TH and HRP (double arrows) are evident. D: Brightfield photomicrograph showing the anterograde transport of WGA–HRP in the medial substantia nigra 23 hr following injection of the tracer in the nucleus accumbens. The anterogradely labeled processes (small arrows) are easily distinguished from the retrogradely labeled perikarya (open arrow) and from the black silver grains indicating immunoautoradiographic labeling for TH. The autoradiographic exposure period for A was 1 month; for B–D, it was 1 week. Bar in A, 100 μm; in B–D, 50 μm. A color reproduction of this figure appears following p. 352.

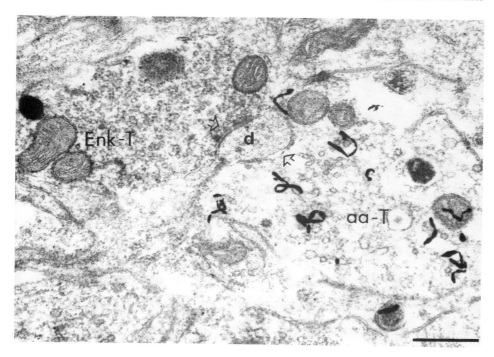

Figure 4. Electron micrograph showing autoradiographic labeling of [³H]-amino acids in axon terminal (aa-T) in the commissural nucleus of the solitary tract. The tracer was injected in the nodose ganglion 48 hr prior to colchicine treatment and followed 24 hr later with fixation by perfusion with 4% paraformaldehyde and 0.1% glutaraldehyde. The aa-T and a terminal showing light peroxidase labeling for enkephalin (Enk-T) form synapses (open arrows) with a small unlabeled dendrite (d). Autradiographic exposure period was 6 months. Bar, 0.5 μm.

of neurotransmitters in central pathways is illustrated by our studies of efferents from the NTS in relation to neuropeptides in the parabrachial nuclei of rat brain (Milner *et al.*, 1984). The medial NTS is known to project to the parabrachial region (Loewy and Burton, 1978; Norgren, 1978; Sawchenko and Swanson, 1982). Following a circumscribed, small (30-nl) injection of [³H]-amino acids (see Section II.A.1) in the medial NTS at the level of the area postrema, anterograde labeling is seen in the parabrachial region. Autoradiographic exposures range from 4–8 weeks for light microscopy and 8–14 months for electron microscopy depending in part on the specific activity and concentration of the isotope. In electron micrographs clusters of silver grains can be observed over axon terminals in the lateral parabrachial region (Fig. 5). Three or more labeled terminals are often found within the same field, whereas other areas are completely devoid of labeling. A few randomly scattered silver grains located over structures other than axons or axon terminals are probably attributed to background labeling or α tracks. In these cases, the labeled profiles can not be traced in serial sections. Several neuropeptides are found in cell bodies in the NTS and in terminals of the parabrachial region (Cuello and Kanazawa, 1978; Elde *et al.*, 1976;

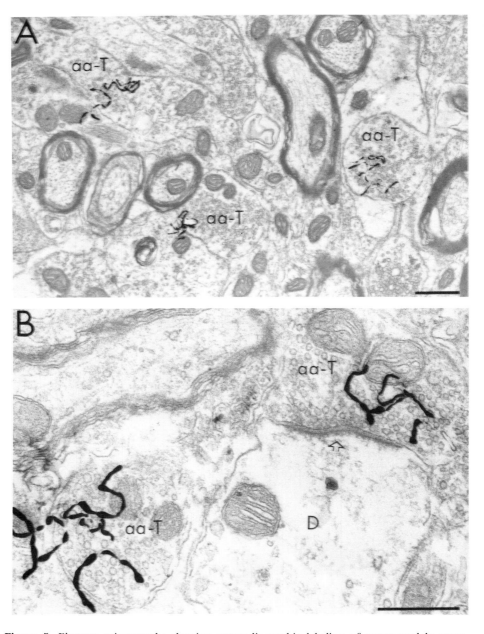

Figure 5. Electron micrographs showing autoradiographic labeling of anterogradely transported tritiated amino acids in terminals (aa-T) in the parabrachial region of a rat that received injections of the isotope in the solitary nucei 24 hr prior to sacrifice. The aa-T in micrograph B forms an asymmetric synapse (open arrow) with an unlabeled dendrite (D). The autoradiographic exposure period was 12 months. Bar, 0.5 μm.

Khachaturian and Watson, 1982; Ljungdahl *et al.*, 1978; Maley and Elde, 1982; Uhl *et al.*, 1979a,b).

Combined autoradiographic labeling of afferents from the NTS and immunoperoxidase-labeling of SP was analyzed in the parabrachial region. The peroxidase product for SP was easily differentiated from clusters of silver grains. The axons or terminals labeled with SP were sometimes in direct apposition to terminals or axons containing anterograde autoradiographic labeling. However, quantitative evaluation (Salpeter *et al.*, 1969) of the distribution of silver grains in serial sections indicated that the autoradiographic and peroxidase labels were always in separate processes. In sections taken more than 5 μm away from the surface of the tissue, the PAP reaction product was faint and difficult to distinguish from background even with light counterstaining. The fact that silver grains were not superimposed on the peroxidase reaction product indicates the absence of chemographic interactions with the overlying emulsion and also demonstrates that the solitary efferents to the parabrachial region do not contain detectable levels of SP.

C. Limitations

One of the major limitations of combining anterograde transport of [^{3}H]-amino acids with immunoperoxidase labeling is the difficulty in selecting the appropriate area for maximal detection of terminal labeling in thin sections prepared for electron microscopy. The area must be chosen either on the basis of previous knowledge regarding the transmitter under investigation or by a comparative analysis with light microscopic autoradiographs. Since these light microscopic autoradiographs require exposure periods of approximately 1 month, there is a delay in processing the tissue for electron microscopy. However, tritium has a long half-life, thus the delay in processing should not significantly diminish the observed labeling.

A second limitation is the long exposure periods of 6–14 months that may be required to reach detectable levels of autoradiographic labeling in axon terminals. Although the shorter periods may be useful in studies of transport from peripheral ganglia or larger central nuclei where larger volumes of isotope are used. However, studies of efferents from small nuclei such as those of the solitary tracts invariably require reduced volumes of tracer to achieve selective labeling. As a consequence, longer autoradiographic exposure periods usually are necessary even with maximal concentrations of the radioisotope.

III. ANTEROGRADE OR RETROGRADE TRANSPORT OF HORSERADISH PEROXIDASE COMBINED WITH IMMUNOAUTORADIOGRAPHIC LABELING

Anterograde and retrograde transport of HRP and WGA-HRP following microinjections into selective brain areas have been used extensively for light microscopic tracing of neuronal pathways. These methods also are compatible with electron microscopy (LaVail and LaVail, 1974; Falls, 1988; Mesulam and Mufson, 1980). Moreover, HRP is taken up from the cut end of centrally projecting portions of either preganglionic (Chan *et al.*, 1988; Milner *et al.*, 1988) or postganglionic nerves (Higgins *et al.*, 1984). The transport may be anterograde and/or retrograde depending on placement of the peroxidase (see Fig. 6 for example of HRP applied to the cervical vagus nerve).

The protocol used for combining peroxidase transport histochemistry with immunoautoradiographic demonstration of antibodies is described with respect to reagents and sequence of each labeling procedure. Examples are given from ongoing studies in the rat spinal cord and brain that serve to illustrate (1) anterograde transport of HRP in terminals forming synapses with immunoautoradiographically labeled dendrites (Fig. 2A) and (2) immunoautoradiographic labeling in neurons that either form synaptic contacts with a second cell retrogradely labeled with HRP (Fig. 2B) or are themselves retrogradely labeled (Fig. 2C). Some of the specific questions that can be addressed with the nerve dip preparation are illustrated for enkephalin and vagal sensory and motor neurons in Fig. 6.

A. Methodology

The primary methods include application of the tracers, tissue preparation, peroxidase histochemistry, and immunoautoradiography.

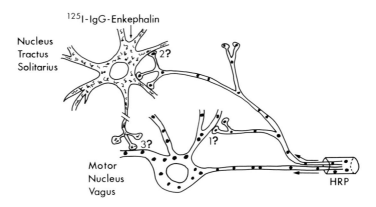

Figure 6. Schematic drawing illustrating the use of horseradish peroxidase (HRP) applied in a glass cuff around the cut end of the cervical vagus nerve. Anterogradely labeled sensory vagal afferents are depicted in relation to dendrites that are retrogradely labeled in the dorsal motor nucleus of the vagus and to enkephalin-labeled neurons in the nuclei of the solitary tracts in the rat medulla. The questions that can be addressed by use of this method in the model system include: (1) do vagal sensory neurons terminate on vagal motor neurons; (2) do the vagal afferents terminate on enkephalin-labeled neurons; and (3) do the enkephalin-labeled terminals form synapses with dendrites of vagal motor neurons.

1. Application of Peroxidase Tracers

The animals are anesthetized with halothane (2% in 100% O_2) or chloral hydrate (420 mg/kg i.p.) prior to and during the application of HRP or WGA–HRP (Schwab *et al.*, 1978). For studies of transport from peripheral nerves, the central end of the cut nerve trunk is placed in the open end of a piece of capillary tubing (1.6 mm × 15 mm) previously sealed at the other end and filled with 1 µl of 30% HRP (Boehringer-Mannheim) as described by Higgins *et al.* (1984) and shown in Fig. 6. For transport between sites within the CNS, small quantities (10–40 nl) of 10% WGA–HRP (Sigma) in saline are used (Mesulam, 1978). A small volume of highly concentrated tracer helps to insure a relatively small effective injection site, particularly when the conjugate is administered by iontophoresis or a controlled pressure system (Amaral and Price, 1983). Leaving the micropipette in position for 10–20 min after delivery also helps to prevent seepage of the WGA–HRP along the pipette tip. The method of injection is essentially the same as that described for injections of radioactive amino acids in the previous section. The optimal time for transport is usually 18–24 hr depending on the size of the injections and/or length of the neuronal pathways (Vanegas *et al.*, 1978). After an appropriate survival period, the animals can be reanesthetized and given intraventricular injections of colchicine (100 µg in 7.5 µl saline) to enhance perikaryal and dendritic labeling of neuropeptides and other rapidly transported proteins (Ljungdahl *et al.*, 1978). These animals are then allowed to survive for another 18–24 hr prior to sacrifice. The colchicine-treated animals show some reduced levels of transport as compared with untreated controls (Karlsson and Sjostrand, 1969). Moreover, use of colchicine is often associated with relatively poor perfusions and poor preservation of morphology, presumably because of disruption of cytoskeletal proteins.

2. Tissue Preparation

a. Fixation. Fixation is a critical step for both immunocytochemistry and peroxidase transport methods. The detected labeling of both markers is greatly reduced by high concentrations or long exposure to aldehydes (Courville and Saint-Cyr, 1978; Pickel, 1981; Rosene and Mesulam, 1978). Modifications of double aldehyde fixation methods employing buffered glutaraldehyde and paraformaldehyde (Graham and Karnovsky, 1966) have been most widely used. The best combination of aldehydes for dual labeling largely reflects a balance between the optimal conditions for each method. High concentrations (1–2%) of glutaraldehyde greatly diminish immunocytochemical labeling but improve the detection of transported WGA–HRP. In contrast, higher concentrations (up to 4%) and long exposure (1–2 hr) to buffered paraformaldehyde usually does not markedly reduce immunoreactivity but severely depresses the detection of transported peroxidase (Kim and Strick, 1976). Using 4% paraformaldehyde and 0.1 to 0.2% glutaraldehyde or 2% paraformaldehyde and 3.75% acrolein preserves both peroxidase and immunoautoradiographic labels reasonably well. Prior to perfusion with either fixative, the peroxidase-injected animals are first anesthetized with pentobarbital (50 mg/kg, i.p.). Following perfusion, the tissues are removed and postfixed in 4% or 2% paraformaldehyde for 30 min and then transferred through several changes of 0.1 M phosphate buffer.

For light microscopy, the brain or spinal cord is stored overnight at 4°C in 10% sucrose in 0.1 M phosphate buffer prior to sectioning at 30 μm on a sliding microtome. The ice-crystal artifacts produced by freeze–thawing generally render the tissue unusable for electron microscopy unless precautions are taken to cyroprotect (e.g., infiltrate with 20% sucrose) and rapidly freeze relatively small pieces of tissue. Frozen sections are useful for light microscopy both because they can be collected rapidly and because the damage induced by freeze–thawing facilitates penetration of the reagents. However, vibratome sections also can be used for light microscopy and provide better morphology for electron microscopy. For initial determination of the specificity of injection, sections through the injection site are processed for HRP histochemistry alone (see Section III.A.3), and examined by light microscopy to determine the size and location of the diffusion sphere for the HRP or WGA–HRP. The volume, survival time, type of fixation, and sensitivity of the histochemical reaction are important factors in determining the apparent size of the injection (Mesulam, 1982). If the injection is restricted to the area of interest, the regions of afferent and efferent connections are processed for immunoautoradiography. The transport to sites of interest is also evaluated by light microscopy of a few test sections prior to processing the remaining sections for immunocytochemisty.

b. Sodium Borohydride. In addition to the previously described advantages of sodium borohydride for immunocytochemistry on aldehyde-fixed tissues, use of this compound appears to improve the sensitivity of the detection of transported HRP and WGA–HRP. The mechanism is likely due to removal of the aldehyde double bonds, which react with HRP to form Schiff bases that interfere with HRPs enzymatic activity (Molin *et al.*, 1978; Rosene and Mesulam, 1978). Thus, the previously collected sections from acrolein-fixed tissues are always treated with sodium borohydride as described in the previous section.

3. Peroxidase Histochemistry

Several chromogens have been advocated for the detection of transported WGA-HRP. One of the most sensitive is tetramethylbenzidine (TMB) as used by DeOlmos *et al.* (1978); Mesulam (1978); Mesulam and Rosen (1979); and Mesulam *et al.* (1980). This method provides excellent light microscopic demonstration of both anterogradely and retrogradely transported WGA-HRP (Mesulam, 1982). However, for electron microscopy it is limited by its relative lack of stability, the large crystallike product which obscures cytolog-ical details, and the low pH of the incubation medium which damages the ultrastructural morphology (Carson and Mesulam, 1982). By several modi-fications in the incubation conditions and stabilization with osmium tetrox-ide, Sakumoto *et al.* (1980) and Sturmer *et al.* (1981) were able to use TMB for electron microscopic localization of transported WGA-HRP in small den-drites and axon terminals. More recently, Rye *et al.* (1984) have demon-strated that the TMB reaction product can be stabilized by incubation with diaminobenzidine (DAB). Use of DAB as the only chromogen as described by LaVail and LaVail (1974) improves the morphology, but usually is not adequately sensitive for detecting anterogradely transported WGA-HRP in terminals or retrogradely transported WGA-HRP in small dendrites and spines. Thus the DAB-stabilized TMB reaction seems to be one of the better methods presently available for the light and electron microscopic detection of transported HRP and is the method currently in use in our laboratory for dual labeling studies. This procedure is a modification of that described by Mesulam (1976, 1978). Sections are incubated at room temperature using the following protocol:

Presoak (20 min; in the dark)

1–0.1% sodium nitroferricyanide, 2% ethanol, and 0.005% 3,3′,5,5′ tetramethylbenzidine in 0.01 M sodium acetate buffer (pH 4.8)

↓

Reaction solutions (a) or (b) (in the dark)

(a) To 100 ml presoak mixture add: 1 ml 0.3% H_2O_2; 1 × 20 min incubation   (b) To 100 ml presoak mixture add: 0.3 ml 0.3% H_2O_2; approximately 4 × 15 min

↓

Rinse (2 × 1 min)
0.01 M sodium acetate buffer (pH 4.8)

↓

Stabilization (4 min)
0.05% diaminobenzidine and 0.01% H_2O_2 in 0.1 M phosphate buffer pH 7.4

All incubations are carried out with constant agitation. Choice of reaction mixture (a) or (b) depends upon the quantity of transported HRP. Usually solution (a) is used for microinjections (i.e., small quantities of HRP); whereas solution (b) is used for nerve dips (i.e., large quantities of HRP). In the latter case, the solution is changed upon appearance of precipitate in the reaction solution. Addition of 0.02% colbalt acetate to the stabilization solution im-proves the visualization of the DAB-reaction product (Rye *et al.,* 1984), but may be omitted in dual light microscopic labeling studies to enhance the contrast between the black silver grains and brown peroxidase reaction product (which turns black with cobalt). At the end of the DAB-reaction, the sections are either: (1) postfixed for 10 min in 1% glutaraldehyde in 0.1 M phos-phate buffer, rinsed through several changes of phosphate buffer, and processed for autoradiography as described in Section II.A.4; or (2) processed for immunocytochemistry as described for protocol II in the next section and then prepared for autoradiography.

4. Immunoautoradiographic Labeling

Several radiolabeling methods are compatible with peroxidase reactions for axonal transport at the light and electron microscopic levels of analysis. These include ^{3}H-secondary IgG (Glazer *et al.*, 1984), ^{125}I-secondary IgG (Pickel *et al.*, 1986), and ^{3}H-biotin for avidin–biotin labeling (Hunt and Mantyh, 1984). However, the high sensitivity of labeling with radioiodine makes this compound somewhat preferable for electron microscopy (Fertuck and Salpeter, 1974). For dual peroxidase and immunoautoradiographic labeling using ^{125}I-IgG, the previously prepared sections are processed sequentially using protocol I or II diagrammed below.

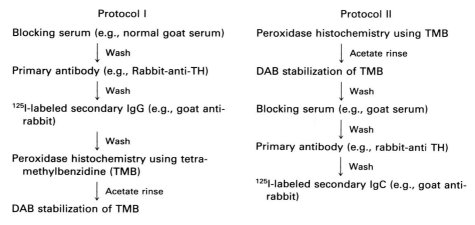

The blocking serum is used at a 1 : 30 dilution and a 30-min incubation; whereas the primary antibody is diluted according to an experimentally determined values and an 18- to 24-min incubation (Leranth and Pickel, Chapter 6, this volume). The dilution of the ^{125}I-IgG and duration of the secondary incubation depend on the specific activity of the isotope. For example, a 2-hr incubation is used with a 1 : 50 dilution (about 100 μCi/μl) of ^{125}I-labeled IgG (Amersham, Arlington Heights, IL) (Pickel *et al.*, 1986). Three 15-min washes precede the incubation with radiolabeled secondary IgG. The incubations are carried out at room temperature with continuous agitation and using a lead shield to protect the investigator. All dilutions and washes are prepared in 0.1 M Tris-saline (pH 7.6). For rabbit antibodies using goat antirabbit secondary IgG, 1% goat serum is added to the diluent of the primary antibody and to the wash before and after incubation with the primary antibody. In protocol II, 0.05% Triton-X 100 is also included in the diluent of the primary antibody. In protocol I, the washes (approximately 10) following incubation with the radioisotope are continued for a total of 2–3 hr or until negligible radioactivity is detected in the wash solution. This extensive washing diminishes background autoradiographic labeling in the section, but also may remove part of the TMB reaction product when using protocol II. Thus the most optimal washing time for specific detection of both labels in protocol II must be experimentally determined and is usually less than 2 hr with frequent changes of wash solution.

5. Sequence of Reactions: Choice of Protocol I versus II

Protocol I and II differ in the sequence of reactions and in the use of detergent in the primary antibody solution. In protocol I, sections are first incubated with immunoreagents then processed for peroxidase histochemistry. This protocol avoids nonspecific attachments of IgG to broken membranes or to the TMB-reaction product. These attachments can give a false positive with respect to colocalization of the two markers. A few sections should be examined following incubation with each label separately as well as using protocol II to evaluate possible nonspecific interactions and/or loss of markers during subsequent incubations in the dual labeling procedure. Use of low concentrations of 0.05% Triton-X 100 with the primary antibody diminishes nonspecific attachments using protocol II. Moreover, this concentration of Triton does not seriously compromise the morphology in acrolein-fixed tissue. Under these conditions, protocol II appears to give more intense immunolabeling, possibly due either (1) to enhanced penetration of immunoreagents when using Triton X-100 or (2) to loss of bound primary or secondary antibodies during the TMB reaction in protocol I. The second protocol was developed in the studies by Chan *et al.* (1988) and Velley *et al.* (1989).

B. Applications

1. Transmitters in Central Neurons in Relation to Peripherally Projecting Neurons and Sensory Afferents

Immunoautoradiography for PNMT has been combined with retrograde transport of HRP following application of the tracer to cut cervical sympathetic nerves in rat (Milner *et al.*, 1988). The method is similar to that used for transport from the cut cervical vagus nerve in Fig. 6. However, only efferents are contained in the central sympathetic nerves. Thus, only retrograde labeling is seen in the spinal cord. Light microscopy of coronal sections through the intermediolateral (IML) column of the spinal cord showed immunoautoradiographic silver grains distributed over and around perikarya containing retrogradely transported reaction product for HRP similar to that shown for SP in Fig 3B. Electron microscopy established that terminals containing PNMT formed direct synapses with the preganglionic sympathetic neurons in the IML. The osmicated HRP-reaction product is recognized as irregular electron-dense clumps in the cytoplasm of perikarya and dendrites while the immunoautoradiographic silver grains appear as black squiggles (Fig. 7A). The tissue shown in Fig. 7A was processed using protocol I with cobalt intensification of the HRP reaction product. For comparison, Fig. 7B showing antetrograde transport of HRP from the cut cervical vagus (see methods in Fig. 6) was processed using protocol II and without cobalt intensification.

2. Transmitters in Central Neurons in Relation to Afferent and Efferent Pathways

Studies of the dopaminergic (TH-containing) neurons of the A10 cell group (Dahlström and Fuxe, 1964) in the ventral tegmental area and their afferent and efferent connections with the nucleus accumbens (Mogensen *et al.*, 1980; Nauta *et all.*, 1978) illustrate the combined use of immunoautoradiography and transport of WGA–HRP within pathways in the CNS. These studies were carried out in collaboration with V. Bayer, Cornell University Medical College. Coronal sections through the ventral tegmental area of animals receiving injections of WGA-HRP in the nucleus accumbens were processed for peroxidase histochemistry and TH immunoautoradiography by protocol I as described above. Figure 2c depicts the dual labeling approach used in this study. By light microscopy, numerous perikarya contain the brown granular peroxidase reaction product alone; other perikarya contain only black silver grains indicating immunoreactivity for TH (single arrow in Fig. 3c); and a few cells exhibit both peroxidase and autoradiographic labeling (double arrow in Fig. 3c). In electron micrographs from the same preparation, perikarya and dendrites also show only retrograde transport, only autoradiographic labeling for TH or both markers (Fig. 8). The perikarya with retrograde transport of WGA–HRP show dense clumps of reactive material throughout their cytoplasm. In the micrographs of Fig. 8, the density of the reaction product was enhanced by cobalt. Cobalt intensification appears to be most useful for better visualization of anterograde transport but leads to some compromise in the ultrastructural morphology of retrogradely labeled cells. Thus, our more recent studies have not used cobalt intensification (see Fig. 7B from studies by Velley *et al.*, 1989).

As anticipated from previous anatomical studies (Groenewegen and Russchen, 1984; Nauta *et al.*, 1978), the anterogradely labeled terminals in the ventral tegmental area were sparse in comparison to those seen in the medial portions of the adjacent substantia nigra. In light micrographs through the medial substantia nigra, punctate brown varicosities anterogradely labeled with WGA–HRP are distinguishable from retrogradely labeled perikarya and from perikarya and dendrites containing immunoautoradi-

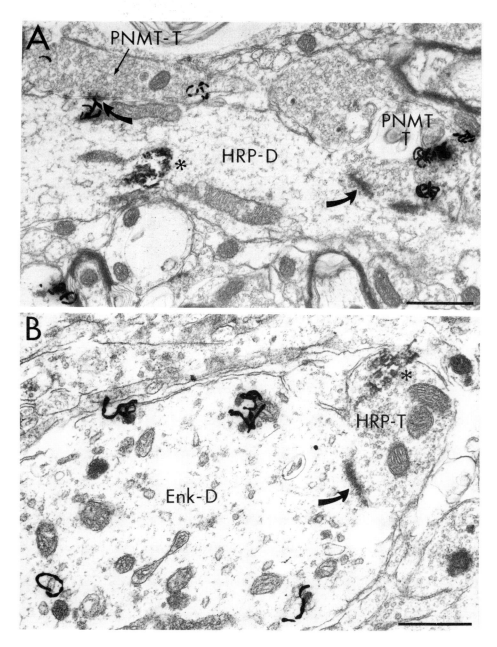

Figure 7. Ultrastructural demonstration of retrogradely transported HRP in a dendrite and immunoautoradiographic localization of substance P in a terminal of the intermediolateral column of the thoracic spinal cord. Serial micrographs in A and B show the labeled dendrite (HRP-D) and a continuous (solid arrow) spiny process that receives an asymmetric contact from the substance-P-immunoreactive terminal. A junction between the HRP dendrite and another unlabeled dendrite is shown by the open arrow in A, and a junction with the SP-T is shown by the open arrow in B. The single silver grain within the HRP-labeled dendrite of the section in B is background labeling or spread of radioactivity from the adjacent terminal. Autoradiographic exposure period was 3 months. Bar, 0.5 μm.

ographic labeling for TH (Fig. 3D). Electron microscopy confirms that the anterograde label is in axon terminals (Fig. 9A). The cobalt-intensified and diaminobenzidine-stablized TMB reaction product for anterogradely transported WGA–HRP is seen as dense aggregates clustered within selective axon terminals. The dual-labeling method is shown schematically in Fig. 2A. In the micrograph of Fig. 8A, the anterogradely labeled terminal forms a symmetrical synapse with a transversely sectioned dendrite that contains sparse immunoautoradiographic labeling for TH (the labeling was confirmed in adjacent sections). In longitudinal sections of dendrites within the same thin section (Fig. 8B), the autoradiographic labeling for TH is far more obvious, even though in both examples the exposure period was 2 months. The distribution of grains in the longitudinally sectioned dendrite illustrates that numerous coronal sections are necessary to achieve the same level of confidence with regard to the specificity of the immunoautoradiographic labeling. Slightly longer exposure periods of 6–8 months will increase the number of silver grains in both transverse and longitudinally sectioned dendrites. However, excessively long exposure periods (usually greater than 8 months) also may increase the background labeling. Optimal autoradiographic exposure periods thus must be experimentally determined by developing test sections at monthly intervals.

C. Limitations

The combined transport of WGA–HRP or HRP with immunoautoradiography has three known limitations. First, the ultrastructural morphology and cytological details can be compromised by (1) the size and electron density of peroxidase reaction product, particularly in retrogradely labeled cells; (2) the short duration of fixation and low concentration of aldehydes in fixatives needed for immunocytochemistry and transport of WGA-HRP to be compatible; and (3) the low pH necessary for the histochemical reaction. Second, false localization of an antigen within an identified pathway may be attributed to (1) chemographic interactions between the peroxidase product and overlying emulsion, or (2) attachments of immunoreagents to the histochemical reaction product. Third, the numbers of synaptic interactions are likely to be underestimated, since (1) less than optimal conditions are used for combining immunocytochemistry and transport; (2) the number of silver grains in individual thin sections of transversely sectioned dendrites or small terminals is relatively small; (3) the distribution of peroxidase reaction product within processes can vary depending upon the plane of section; and (4) differential penetration of immuno- versus histochemical reagents. These limitations can be partially overcome by careful execution of the described protocols and judicious use of appropriate control experiments.

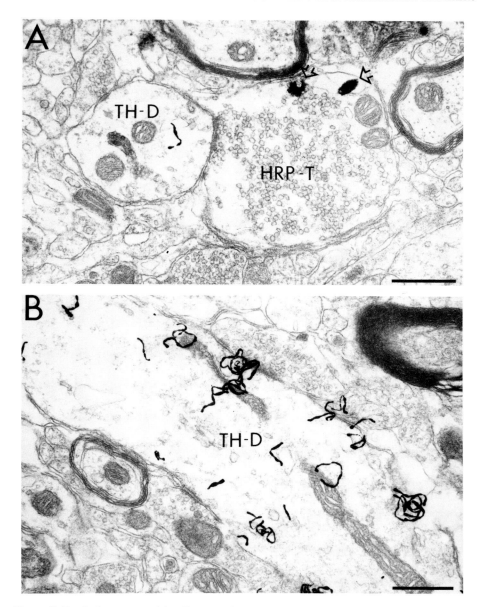

Figure 8. Dual ultrastructural localization of anterogradely transported WGA–HRP and tyrosine hydroxylase in the medial substantia nigra. A: Electron micrograph showing two electron-dense agregates (open arrows) of anterogradely transported WGA–HRP in an axon terminal (HRP-T) that forms a synapse with a coronally sectioned dendrite containing a silver grain, which may represent immunoautoradiographic labeling for TH (TH-D). B: Electron micrograph of a longitudinally sectioned dendrite with more evident immunoautoradiographic labeling for TH. In both A and B the autoradiographic exposure period was 2 months, and the fixation was by perfusion with 2% paraformaldehyde and 3.75% acrolein. Bar, 0.5 μm.

IV. SUMMARY OF ADVANTAGES AND LIMITATIONS

Two general methods have been described for combined analysis of transport and immunocytochemistry using autoradiographic and peroxidase markers. Awareness of some of the overall advantages and limitations of the described techniques is important for deciding whether these methods are the most appropriate for addressing specific problems.

A. Advantages

1. Differences in color as seen by light microscopy or shape as seen by electron microscopy provide a means for recognizing the two markers in the same or separate neurons.
2. The markers are sufficiently large to permit their identification by electron microscopy at magnifications as low as ×10,000. Thus, serial sections can be scanned rapidly to detect associations.
3. The markers are stable for long-term storage and examination.
4. The peroxidase and autoradiographic markers are morphologically distinguishable from colloidal gold, which is a third widely used electron-dense marker. Thus, these two markers may be combined with colloidal gold for identification of two antigens in relation to specific neuronal pathways.
5. The markers offer reliable means to confirm ultrastructurally the presence of antigens in common or synaptically linked neurons.

B. Limitations

In addition to the specifically outlined limitations for each method, the following limitations are generally applicable to autoradiography.

1. The autoradiographic exposure periods are relatively long. This limitation is more important for the methods employing [^{3}H]-amino acids because of the low emission spectra of the isotope, particularly when restricted sizes of injections are required.
2. Demonstration of differential light microscopic labeling in photomicrographs of combined autoradiography and immunocytochemistry is most optimal at relatively low magnification, which enables greater depth of focus. In studies in which sections are to be used exclusively for light microscopy, this limitation can be minimized by using thinner sections.
3. The overlying emulsion partially masks the peroxidase product. This problem is most evident in electron microscopic autoradiographs of sections that are collected away from the surface of the tissue where the peroxidase product is less evident.

4. Serial sections are required for confirmation of autoradiographic labeling.

ACKNOWLEDGMENTS. The authors gratefully acknowledge the support provided by grants from NIH (HL18974), NIMH (MH00078, MH42834, and MH40342), NIDA (DA 04600), and NSF (BNS 8320120) as well as technical support from June Chan.

REFERENCES

Abdel-Akher, M., Hamilton, J. K., Montgomery, R., and Smith, F., 1952, A new procedure for the demonstration of the fine structure of polysaccharide, *J. Am. Chem. Soc.* **74:**4970–4971.

Amaral, D. G., and Price, J. L., 1983, An air pressure system for the injection of tracer substances into the brain, *J. Neurosci. Methods* **9:**35–44.

Beaudet, A., 1982, High resolution radioautography of central 5-hydroxytryptamine (5-HT) neurons, *J. Histochem. Cytochem.* **9:**765–768.

Bosler, O., Beaudet, A., and Pickel, V. M., 1986, Characterization of chemically defined neurons and their cellular relationships by combined immunocytochemistry and radioautographic localization of transmitter uptake sites, *J. Electron Microsc. Tech.* **4:**21–39.

Brushart, T. M., and Mesulam, M. M., 1980, Transganglionic demonstration of central sensory projections from skin and muscle with HRP–lectin conjugates, *Neurosci. Lett.* **17:**1–6.

Carson, K. A., and Mesulam, M. M., 1982, Electron microscopic tracing of neuronal connections with horseradish peroxidase, in: *IBRO Handbook Series: Methods in the Neurosciences, Tracing Neural Connections with Horseradish Peroxidase* (M.-M. Mesulam, ed.), John Wiley & Sons, New York, pp. 153–185.

Chalmers, J. P., White, S. W., Gefen, L. B., and Rush, R., 1978, the role of central catecholamines in the control of blood pressure through the baroreceptor reflex and the nasopharyngeal reflex in the rabbit, in: *Hypertension and Brain Mechanisms, Progress in Brain Research,* Volume 47 (W. DeJong, A. P. Provoost, and A. P. Shapiro, eds.) Elsevier/North Holland, Amsterdam, pp. 85–94.

Chan, J., Velley, L., Milner, T. A., Morrison, S., and Pickel, V. M., 1988, Identity of vagal afferents and efferents in relation to neurons containing enkephalin-like immunoreactivity, *Soc. Neurosci. Abstr.* **14:**1317.

Courville, J., and Saint-Cyr, J. A., 1978, Modification of the horseradish peroxidase method avoiding fixation, *Brain Res.* **142:**551–558.

Cowan, W. M., and Cuenod, M. (eds.), 1975, *The Use of Axonal Transport for Studies of Neuronal Connectivity,* Elsevier, Amsterdam, New York.

Cowan, W. M., Gottlieb, D. I., Hendrickson, A. E., Price, J. L., and Woolsey, T. A., 1972, The autoradiographic demonstration of axonal connections in the central nervous system, *Brain Res.* **37:**21–51.

Cuello, A. C. (ed.), 1983, *Immunohistochemistry, IBRO Handbook Series: Methods in Neurosciences,* Volume 3, John Wiley & Sons, Chichester.

Cuello, A. C., and Kanazawa, I., 1978, The distribution of substance P immunoreactive fibers in the rat central nervous system, *J. Comp. Neurol.* **178:**129–156.

Dahlström, A., and Fuxe, K., 1964, Evidence for the existence of monoamine-containing neurons in the central nervous system, *Acta. Physiol. Scand.* **62:**1–55.

DeJong, W., 1974, Noradrenaline: Central inhibitory control of blood pressure and heart rate, *Eur. J. Pharmacol.* **29:**178–181.

DeMey, J., 1983, A critical review of light and electron microscopic immunocytochemical techniques used in neurobiology, *J. Neurosci. Methods* **7:**1–18.

DeOlmos, J., and Heimer, L., 1977, Mapping of collateral projections with the HRP-method *Neurosci. Lett.*, **6:**107–114.

Descarries, L., and Beaudet, A., 1983, Use of radioautography for investigation of transmitter-specific neurons, in: *Handbook of Chemical Neuroanatomy*, Volume 3 (A. Bjorklund and T. Hökfelt, eds.), Elsevier, Amsterdam, pp. 286–364.

Eckenstein, F., and Thoenen, H., 1982, Production of specific antisera and monoclonal antibodies to choline acetyltransferase: Characterization and use for identification of cholinergic neurons, *EMBO J.* **1:**363–368.

Elde, R., Hökfelt, T., Johansson, O., and Terenius, L., 1976, Immunohistochemical studies using antibodies to leucine-enkephalin: Initial observations of the nervous system of the rat, *Neuroscience* **1:**349–351.

Falls, W. M., 1988, Synaptic organization of primary axons in trigeminal nucleus oralis, *J. Electron Micros. Tech.* **10:**213–228.

Fertuck, H. C., and Salpeter, M. M., 1974, Sensitivity in electron microscopic autoradiography for ^{125}I, *J. Histochem. Cytochem.* **22:**80–87.

Glazer, E. J., Ramachandran, J., and Basbaum, A. I., 1984, Radioimmunocytochemistry using a tritiated goat anti-rabbit second antibody, *J. Histochem. Cytochem.* **32:**778–782.

Gonatas, N. K., Harper, C., Mizutani, T., and Gonatas, J. O., 1979, Superior sensitivity of conjugates of horseradish peroxidase with wheat germ agglutinin for studies of retrograde azonal transport, *J. Histochem. Cytochem.* **27:**728–734.

Graham, R. C., Jr., and Karnovsky, M. J., 1966, The early stages of absorption of injected horseradish peroxidase in the proximal tubules of mouse kidney: Ultrastructural cytochemistry by a new technique, *J. Histochem. Cytochem.* **14:**291–302.

Groenewegen, H. J., and Russchen, F. T., 1984, Organization of the efferent projections of the nucleus accumbens to pallidal, hypothalamic, and mesencephalic structures: A tracing and immunohistochemical study in the cat, *J. Comp. Neurol.* **223:**347–367.

Heym, C., and Lang, R., Transmitters in sympathetic postganglionic neurons, in: *Neurohistochemistry: Modern Methods and Applications*, Alan R. Liss, Inc., New York, pp. 493–525.

Higgins, G. A., Hoffman, G. E., Wray, S., and Schwaber, J. S, 1984, Distribution of neurotensin-immunoreactivity within baroreceptive portions of the nucleus of the tractus solitarius and the dorsal vagal nucleus of the rat, *J. Comp. Neurol.* **226:**155–164.

Howe, P. R. C., Costa, M., Furness, J. B., and Chalmers, J. P., 1980, Simultaneous demonstration of phenylethanolamine N-methyl-transferase immunofluorescent and catecholamine fluorescent nerve cell bodies in the rat medulla oblongata, *Neuroscience* **5:**2229–2238.

Hunt, S. P., and Mantyh, P. W., 1984, Radioimmunohistochemistry with ^3H-biotin, *Brain Res.* **291:**203–217.

Isaacson, L. G., and Tanaka, D., 1988, Cholinergic innervation of canine thalamostriatal projection neurons: an ultrastructural study combining choline acetyltransferase immunocytochemistry and WGA-HRP retrograde labeling, *J. Comp. Neurol.* **227:**529–540.

Joh, T. H., Gegham, C., and Reis, D. J., 1973, Immunochemical demonstration of increased tyrosine hydroxylase protein in sympathetic ganglia and adrenal medulla elicited by reserpine, *Proc. Natl. Acad. Sci. U.S.A.* **70:**2767–2771.

Kalia, M., and Mesulam, M.-M., 1980, Brain stem and spinal cord projections of vagal sensory and motor fibers in the cat: I. The cervical vagus and nodose ganglion, *J. Comp. Neurol.* **193:**435–466.

Karlsson, J.O., and Sjöstrand, J., 1969, The effect of colchicine on the axonal transport of protein in the optic nerve and tract of rabbit, *Brain Res.* **13:**617–619.

Katz, D. M., and Karten, H. J., 1979, The discrete anatomical localization of vagal aortic afferents within a catecholamine-containing cell group in the nucleus solitarius, *Brain Res.* **171:**187–195.

Khachaturian, H., and Watson, S. J., 1982, Some perspectives on monoamine–opioid peptide interactions in rat central nervous system, *Brain Res. Bull.* **9:**441–462.

Kim, C. C., and Strick, P. L., 1976, Critical factors involved in the demonstration of horseradish peroxidase retrograde transport, *Brain Res.* **103:**356–361.

King, J. C., Lechan, R. M., Kugel, G., and Anthony, E. L. P., 1983, Acrolein: a fixative for immunocytochemical localization of peptides in the central nervous system, *J. Histochem. Cytochem.* **31**:62–68.

Larsson, L.-I., 1981, A novel immunocytochemical model system for specificity and sensitivity screening of antisera against multiple antigens, *J. Histochem. Cytochem.* **29**:408–410.

LaVail, J. H., and LaVail, M. M., 1974, The retrograde intra-axonal transport of horseradish peroxidase in chick visual system: A light and electron microscopic study, *J. Comp. Neurol.* **157**:303–358.

Leranth, C., and Pickel, V. M., 1989, Electron microscopic pre-embedding double immuno-staining methods, in: *Neuroanatomical Tract-Tracing Methods 2: Recent Progress* (L. Heimer and L. Zaborszky, eds.), Plenum, New York, Chapter 6.

Ljungdahl, A., Hökfelt, T., and Nilsson, G., 1978, Distribution of substance P-like immuno-reactivity in the central nervous system of the rat. I. Cell bodies and nerve terminals, *Neuroscience* **3**:861–943.

Loewy, A. D., and Burton, H., 1978, Nuclei of the solitary tract: Efferent projections to the lower brainstem and spinal cord of the cat, *J. Comp. Neurol.* **181**:421–450.

MacMillan, F. M., and Cuello, A. C., 1986, Monoclonal antibodies in neurohistochemistry: The state of the art, in: *Neurohistochemistry: Modern Methods and Applications* (P. Panula, H. Paivarinta, and S. Soinila, eds.), Alan R. Liss, New York, pp. 49–74.

Maley, B., and Elde, R., 1982, Immunohistochemical localization of putative neurotransmitters within the feline nucleus tractus solitarii, *Neuroscience* **7**:2469–2490.

Masurovsky, E. R., and Bunge, R. P., 1968, Fluoroplastic coverslips for long-term nerve tissue culture, *Stain Technol.* **43**:161–165.

McLean S., Skirboll, L. R., and Pert, C. B., 1983, Opiatergic projection from the bed nucleus to the habenula: Demonstration by a novel radioimmunohistochemical method, *Brain Res.* **278**:255–257.

Mesulam, M.-M., 1976, The blue reaction product in horseradish peroxidase histochemistry: Incubation parameters and visibility, *J. Histochem. Cytochem.* **24**:1273–1280.

Mesulam, M.-M., 1978, Tetramethyl benzidine for horseradish peroxidase histochemistry: A non-carcinogenic blue reaction product with superior sensitivity for visualizing neural afferents and efferents, *J. Histochem. Cytochem.* **26**:106–117.

Mesulam, M.-M., 1982, Principles of horseradish peroxidase neurohistochemistry and their applications for tracing neuronal pathways—Axonal transport, enzyme histochemistry, and light microscopic analysis, in: *Tracing Neuronal Connections with Horseradish Peroxidase* (M. M. Mesulam, ed.), John Wiley & Sons, New York, pp. 1–152.

Mesulam, M.-M., and Mufson, E. J., 1980, The rapid anterograde transport of horseradish peroxidase, *Neuroscience.* **5**:1277–1286.

Mesulam, M.-M., and Rosen, D. L., 1979, Sensitivity in horseradish peroxidase neurohistochemistry: A comparative and quantitative analysis of nine methods, *J. Histochem. Cytochem.* **27**:763–773.

Mesulam, M.-M., Hegarty, E., Barbas, H., Carson, K. A., Gower, E. C., Knapp, A. G., Moss, M. B., and Mufson, E. J., 1980, Additional factors influencing sensitivity in the tetramethyl benzidine method for horseradish peroxidase neurohistochemistry, *J. Histochem. Cytochem.* **28**:1255–1259.

Milner, T. A., and Pickel, V. M., 1986a, Neurotensin in the rat parabrachial region: Ultrastructural localization and extrinsic sources of immunoreactivity, *J. Comp. Neurol.* **247**:326–343.

Milner, T. A., and Pickel, V. M., 1986b, Ultrastructural localization and afferent sources of substance P in the rat parabrachial region, *Neuroscience* **17**:687–707.

Milner, T. A., Joh, T. H., Miller, R. J., and Pickel, V. M., 1984, Substance P, neurotensin, enkephalin and catecholamine-synthesizing enzymes: Light microscopic localization compared with autoradiographic label in solitary efferents to the rat parabrachial region, *J. Comp. Neurol.* **226**:434–447.

Milner, T. A., Morrison, S., Abate, C., and Reis, D. J., Phenylethanolamine N-methyltransfer-ase-containing terminals synapse directly on sympathetic preganglionic neurons in the rat, *Brain Res.* **448**:205–222.

Mogensen, G. J., Jones, D. L., and Yim, C. Y., 1980, From motivation to action: Functional interface between the limbic system and the motor system, *Prog. Neurobiol.* **14:**69–97.

Molin, S. O., Nygren, H., and Dolonius, L., 1978, A new method for the study of glutaraldehyde-induced cross-linking properties in proteins with special reference to the reaction with amino groups, *J. Histochem. Cytochem.* **26:**412–414.

Nauta, W. J. H., Smith, G. P., Faull, R. L. M., and Domesick, V., 1978, Efferent connections and nigral afferents of the nucleus accumbens septi in the rat, *Neuroscience* **3:**385–401.

Norgren, R., 1978, Projections from the nucleus of the solitary tract in the rat, *Neuroscience* **3:**207–218.

Oldfield, B. J., Hou-Yu, A., and Silverman, A. J., 1983, Techniques for the simultaneous ultrastructural demonstration of anterogradely transported horseradish peroxidase and immunocytochemically identified neuropeptides, *J. Histochem. Cytochem.* **31:**1145–1150.

Palkovits, M., and Jacobowitz, D. M., 1974, Topographic atlas of catecholamine and acetylcholinesterase-containing neurons in the rat brain. I: Hindbrain (mesencephalon, rhombencephalon), *J. Comp. Neurol.* **157:**29–42.

Paxinos, G., and Watson, C., 1986, *The Rat Brain in Stereotaxic Coordinates*, Academic Press, Orlando, FL.

Pickel, V. M., 1981, Immunocytochemical methods, in: *Neuroanatomical Tract-Tracing Methods* (L. Heimer and M. J. Robards, eds.), Plenum Press, New York, pp. 483–509.

Pickel, V. M., 1985, Ultrastructure of central catecholaminergic neurons, in: *Neurohistochemistry Today* (P. Panula, H. Paivarinta, and S. Soinilal, eds.), Alan R. Liss, New York, pp. 397–423.

Pickel, V. M., and Beaudet, A., 1984, Combined use of autoradiography and immunocytochemical methods to show synaptic interactions between chemically defined neurons, in: *Immunolabelling for Electron Microscopy* (J. M. Polak and I. M. Varenell, eds.), Elsevier, Amsterdam, pp. 259–265.

Pickel, V. M., Chan, J., and Milner, T. A., 1986, Autoradiographic detection of (^{125}I)-secondary antiserum: A sensitive light and electron microscopic labeling method compatible with peroxidase immunocytochemistry for dual localization of neuronal antigens, *J. Histochem. Cytochem.* **34:**707–718.

Polak, J. M., and Van Noorden, S. (eds.), 1983, *Immunocytochemistry: Practical Applications in Pathology and Biology*, Wright, Bristol.

Priestley, J. V., Somogyi, P., and Cuello, A. C., 1981, Neurotransmitter-specific projection neurons revealed by combining peroxidase–antiperoxidase immunocytochemistry with retrograde transport of horseradish peroxidase, *Brain Res.* **220:**231–240.

Rosene, D. L., and Mesulam, M.-M., 1978, Fixation variables in horseradish peroxidase neurohistochemistry. I. The effects of fixation time and perfusion procedures upon enzyme activity, *J. Histochem. Cytochem.* **26:**28–39.

Ross, C. A., Armstrong, D. M., Ruggiero, D. A., Pickel, V. M., Joh, T. H., and Reis, D. J., 1981, Adrenaline neurons in the rostral ventrolateral medulla innervate thoracic spinal cord: A combined immunocytochemical and retrograde transport demonstration, *Neurosci. Lett.* **25:**257–262.

Ross, M. E., Reis, D. J., and Joh, T. H., 1981, Monoclonal antibodies to tyrosine hydroxylase: Production and characterization, *Brain Res.* **208:**493–498.

Rye, D. B., Saper, C. B., and Warner, B. H., 1984, Stabilization of the tetramethyl benzidine (TMB) reaction product: Application for retrograde and anterograde tracing and combination with immunohistochemistry, *J. Histochem. Cytochem.* **32:**1145–1153.

Sakumoto, T., Tohyama, M., Satoh, K., Kimoto, Y., Kinugasa, T., Tanizawa, O., Kurachi, K., and Shimuzu, N., 1978, Afferent fibre connections from lower brain stem to hypothalamus studies by the horseradish peroxidase method with special reference to noradrenaline innervation, *Exp. Brain Res.* **3:**81–94.

Sakumoto, T., Nagai, T., Kimura, H., and Maeda, T., 1980, Electron microscopic visualization of tetramethyl benzidine reaction product on horseradish peroxidase neurohistochemistry, *Cell. Mol. Biol.* **26:**211–216.

Salpeter, M. M., Bachman, L., and Salpeter, E. E., 1969, Resolution in electron microscopic autoradiography, *J. Cell Biol.* **41**:1–20.

Salpeter, M. M., Fertuck, H. C., and Salpeter, E. E., 1977, Resolution in electron microscopic autoradiography III. Iodine-125, the effect of heavy metal staining and reassessment of critical parameters, *J. Cell Biol.* **72**:161–173.

Sawchenko, P. E., and Swanson, L. W., 1981, A method for tracing biochemically defined pathways in the central nervous system using combined fluorescence retrograde transport and immunocytochemical techniques, *Brain Res.* **210**:31–51.

Sawchenko, P. E., and Swanson, L. W., 1982, The organization of noradrenergic pathways from the brainstem to the paraventricular and supraoptic nuclei in the rat, *Brain Res. Rev.* **4**:275–325.

Schachner, M., Hedley-Whyte, E. T., Hse, D. W., Schoonmaker, G., and Bignami, A., 1977, Ultrastructural localization of glial fibrillary acidic protein in mouse cerebellum by immunoperoxidase labeling, *J. Cell Biol.* **75**:67–73.

Schwab, M. E., Javoy-Agid, F., and Agid, Y., 1978, Labeled wheat germ agglutinin (WGA) as a new, highly sensitive retrograde tracer in the rat brain hippocampal system, *Brain Res.* **152**:145–150.

Sofroniew, M. V., Madler, M., Muller, O. A., and Scriba, P. C., 1978, A method for the consistent production of high quality antisera to small peptide hormones, *Fresnius Z. Anal. Chem.* **290**:163.

Steinbusch, H. W. M., Verhofstad, A. A. J., and Joosten, H. W. J., 1978, Localization of serotonin in the central nervous system by immunohistochemistry: Description of a specific and sensitive technique and some applications, *Neuroscience* **3**:811–819.

Sternberger, L. A., 1979, *Immunocytochemistry*, John Wiley & Sons, New York.

Storm-Mathisen, J., Leknes, A. K., Bare, A. T., Vaaland, J. L., Edminson, P., Huang, F.-M. S., and Ottersen, O. P., 1983, First visualization of glutamate and GABA in neurons by immunocytochemistry, *Nature* **301**:517–520.

Sturmer, C., Bielenberg, K., and Spatz, W. B., 1981, Electron microscopical identification of 3,3′,5,5′-tetramethyl benzidine reacted horseradish peroxidase after retrograde axonal transport, *Neurosci. Lett.* **23**:1–6.

Sumal, K. K., Blessing, W. W., Joh, T. H., Reis, D. J., and Pickel, V. M., 1983 Synaptic interaction of vagal afferents and catecholaminergic neurons in the rat nucleus tractus solitarius, *Brain Res.* **277**:31–40.

Uhl, G. R., Goodman, R. R., Kuhar, M. J., Childers, S. R., and Snyder, S. H., 1979a, Immunohistochemical mapping of enkephalin-containing cell bodies, fibers and nerve terminals in the brainstem of the rat, *Brain Res.* **166**:75–79.

Uhl, G. R., Goodman, R. R., and Snyder, S. H., 1979b, Neurotensin-containing cell bodies, fibers and nerve terminals in the brain stem of the rat: Immunohistochemical mapping, *Brain Res.* **167**:77–91.

Venegas, H., Hollander, H., and Distel, H., 1978. Early stages of uptake and transport of horseradish peroxidase by cortical structures and its use for the study of local neurons and their processes, *J. Comp. Neurol.* **177**:193–212.

Velley, L., Milner, T. A., Chan, J., Morrison, S., and Pickel, V. M., 1989, Synaptic interactions between neurons containing enkephalin-like immunoreactivity and vagal afferents and efferents, *J. Comp. Neurol.* (in preparation).

Zaborszky, L., and Leranth, C., 1985, Simultaneous ultrastructural demonstration of retrogradely transported horseradish peroxidase and choline acetyltransferase immunoreactivity, *Histochemistry* **82**:529–537.

6

Electron Microscopic Preembedding Double-Immunostaining Methods

CSABA LERANTH and VIRGINIA M. PICKEL

I. INTRODUCTION

During the last decade, immunocytochemistry has become one of the major tools for the light and electron microscopic identification of neurons containing classical transmitters and neuropeptides (e.g., Cuello, 1983; Polak and Van Noorden, 1983; Steinbush *et al.*, 1978). The immunocytochemical studies have provided a complete characterization of the regional distributions and ultrastructural morphology of a variety of chemically specific neurons (Elde *etal.*, 1976; Pickel, 1981). More recently, dual immunocytochemical labeling of two antigens in the same section prepared for electron microscopy has permitted the characterization of transmitters within pre- and post synaptic junctions in the central nervous system (Leranth *et al.*, 1984; van den Pol, 1985a; Milner *et al.*, 1987).

Electron-dense markers have been used in different combinations to localize two antisera in sections either before (preembedding) or after (postembedding) tissues are infiltrated with plastic for eletron miscroscopy. Many of the postembedding methods appear to be more appropriate for the local-

CSABA LERANTH • Section of Neuroanatomy and Department of Obstetrics and Gynecology, Yale University School of Medicine, New Haven, Connecticut 06510. VIRGINIA M. PICKEL • Department of Neurology and Neuroscience, Laboratory of Neurobiology, Cornell University Medical College, New York, New York 10021.

ization of antigens in peripheral tissues. For example, in certain endocrine tissues where the antigens are highly concentrated in secretory granules, colloidal gold particles of varying sizes have been used for the differential localization of antigens after plastic embedding (see references in Larsson, 1983; van den Pol, 1984). Alternatively, immunoperoxidase labeling has been used before and immunogold labeling after embedding of endocrine tissues in plastic (Slot and Gueze, 1981; Bendayan, 1982; Roth, 1982; Tapia *et al.*, 1983). The generally poor success with application of these methods for localization of antigens in the CNS may be attributable either to low quantities or diffuse distribution of neuronal antigens or to less cross reactivity or accessibility of the antigenic sites after plastic embedding (Pickel, 1981).

The most commonly used dual-labeling methods for ultrastructural studies of synaptic interactions in brain have relied on immunolabeling of Vibratome sections prior to embedding of the tissue in plastic. In the dual-labeling methods described in this chapter, at least one or both of the antigens are localized by immunoperoxidase techniques including the peroxidase–antiperoxidase (Sternberger *et al.*, 1970) and the avidin–biotin peroxidase complex (ABC) according to Hsu *et al.* (1981). The immunoperoxidase method has been successfully combined with colloidal gold (Pickel *et al.*, 1986b; Milner *et al.*, 1987), silver-intensified colloidal gold (van den Pol, 1985a), and avidinated ferritin (Leranth *et al.*, 1984). These three electron-dense markers are readily distinguished from the more diffuse black precipitate formed by the interaction of osmium tetroxide with the peroxidase reaction product. Silver intensification also renders the peroxidase product formed by diaminobenzidine (DAB) distinguishable from the unintensified DAB reaction product and thus has been employed as a fourth differential labeling method (Liposits *et al.*, 1983).

A number of other dual-labeling methods now being used extensively for light and electron microscopic localization of neuronal antigens are based on the distinction between autoradiographic silver grains and the immunoperoxidase reaction product. The autoradiographic markers include tritium-labeled primary antibodies (Cuello *et al.*, 1982; Priestley and Cuello, 1982) as well as tritiated (Glazer *et al.*, 1984) and iodinated (McLean *et al.*, 1983, 1985; Picket *et al.*, 1986a) secondary immunoglobulins (IgGs) and tritiated biotin (Hunt and Manthy, 1984). Internally labeled primary antisera have been the least widely used autoradiographic markers, largely because of the relative scarcity of radiolabeled monoclonal antisera (MacMillan and Cuello, 1986). Tritiated and iodinated IgGs are applicable to the localization of a wide variety of unlabeled primary antisera. Furthermore, the radioiodinated IgG has the added advantage of giving higher resolution for electron microscopy (Fertuck and Salpeter, 1974; Salpeter *et al.*, 1969, 1977).

In order to present a nearly complete overview of preembedding double immunostaining procedures that have been used in the central nervous system, we must mention a recently described light and electron microscopic double immunostaining method of Levey *et al.* (1986). This method employs sequential unlabeled immunoperoxidase staining using diaminobenzidine (DAB) and the very sensitive (Mesulam and Rosene, 1979; Lakos and Basbaum, 1986) benzidine dihydrochloride (BDHC) as two contrasting electron-dense immunomarkers. The procedure has been used to localize simultaneously choline acetyltransferase and either substance P or tyrosine hydroxylase in the central nervous system (Levey *et al.*, 1986; Bolam *et al.*, 1986). The advantage of this method is that it can be used for correlated light and electron microscopic experiments, since the brown diffuse DAB reaction product is easily distinguished from the blue, granular BDHC deposit at the light microscopic level. Other applications and technical aspects of this double-labeling procedure are discussed in Chapter 3 by Zaborszky and Heimer. Other double-labeling techniques are available, but they do not necessarily use two distinct markers at the ultrastructural level (e.g., Kohno *et al.*, 1988).

The protocols described in the present chapter for dual ultrastructural localization of neuronal antigens are based on the procedures currently in use in our laboratories or those that are now well established in the literature. The specific methods for tissue preparation and immunolabeling with each of the combined electron-dense markers are described.

II. TISSUE PREPARATION

Preparation of tissue for single or double immunostaining for electron microscopy reflects a compromise between the mutually exclusive requirements of good preservation of cellular membranes and deep penetration of the antisera and electron-dense markers. Anesthetics, vascular rinsing, fixation procedures, and penetration enhancement methods are especially important when conditions must be met for labeling two different antigens while allowing penetration of two electron-dense markers.

A. Anesthesia

Preservation of ultrastructural morphology and immunocytochemical labeling appear to be unaltered by the use of different types of anesthetic (e.g., ether, ketamine hydrochloride, sodium pentobarbital, chloropent). However, the depth of anesthesia is an important variable. Because of individual differences in sensitivity and rate of absorption, physiological clues such as the diameter of the pupils, rate and depth of respiration, and activity of reflexes must be evaluated in order to determine that the animal is appropriately anesthetized (Friedrich and Mugnaini, 1981). Either excessive or marginal levels of anesthesia can result in poor perfusion.

B. Vascular Rinsing

In order to remove red blood cells, which contribute to nonspecific peroxidase reactions and also may block the flow of fixative in small capillaries, the vascular system should be rinsed with saline (0.9% NaCl in water) prior to perfusion with aldehydes. However, the vascular rinsing may contribute to loss of immunocytochemically detectable antigens through either anoxic damage to the cellular membranes or diffusion of more soluble substances such as monoamines or GABA prior to cross linking by aldehyde fixative (Molin *et al.*, 1978). Three techniques have been most commonly employed to circumvent this problem.

In the first method, the saline solution is saturated with oxygen by bubbling with Carbogen (95% O_2 and 5% CO_2). The gas cylinder is connected to a cannula, which is placed in the rinsing solution for 20–30 min immediately prior to initiation of the vascular perfusion. In the second method, the animal is artificially ventilated during the vascular rinsing and the first few seconds of perfusion with the fixative solution. A simple artificial respiratory method described by Williams and Jew (1975) consists of delivery of low-pressure Carbogen through a plastic tube (8–10 mm inner diameter) that is connected to a thin (1.8–2.5 mm outer diameter), short (4–5 cm) cannula inserted in the trachea of a tracheotomized animal. Closing and opening a hole on the side of the plastic tubing simulates inspiration and respiration. A third method is to deliver rapidly (30 sec) only a small (10-cc) volume of heparin saline immediately before the fixative, which also is initially delivered at a rapid rate using a Masterflex pump. The necessity for speed in all aspects of this procedure probably accounts for the fact that it is not as widely used as the first two methods. However, if properly executed, there is potentially much less opportunity for diffusion of antigens with the rapid perfusion (Pickel *et al.*, 1986c).

C. Fixation

For many years, buffered solutions containing paraformaldehyde and high (1–2%) concentrations of glutaraldehyde have been known to provide excellent preservation of ultrastructural morphology (Graham and Karnovsky, 1966). These fixatives also harden the tissue so that sectioning with a Vibratome is greatly facilitated. Unfortunately, the higher glutaraldehyde concentrations reduce the detection of immunoreactivity for most antigens. The reduction of immunolabeling generally is attributed to loss of antigenicity or failure of the antisera to reach antigenic sites in well-fixed tissues. The localization of transmitters such as γ-aminobutyric acid (GABA) and norepinephrine (NE) is an important exception. In contrast to most antigens, which are no longer detectable with glutaraldehyde concentrations greater than 0.2%, GABA (Hudgson *et al.*, 1985) and NE (unpublished observation of C. Leranth and M. Palkovits, using the antibody of Verhofstaad *et al.*, 1983) show better immunocytochemical labeling with glutaraldehyde concentrations as high as 0.7–0.8%. Thus, for dual labeling of these transmitters with other, more glutaraldehyde-sensitive antigens such as the neurotransmitter-synthesizing enzymes, the most appropriate concentration or duration of exposure to the glutaraldehyde must be a compromise between the optimal conditions for each antigen.

Four major types of fixatives are in current use for single or dual immunocytochemical labeling for electron microscopy. The choice of fixative depends on both the antigen and the type of immunolabel, since some of the larger markers may not permeate intact membranes.

1. Paraformaldehyde–Glutaraldehyde Fixative

A solution containing 4% paraformaldehyde and 0.1–0.2% glutaraldehyde in 0.1 M phosphate buffer (pH 7.4) has been used for fixation of neural tissues for the immunocytochemical localization of a variety of single antigens (DeMey, 1983; Pickel, 1981; Pickel and Teitelman, 1983). More recently this fixative has also been used for the dual localization of some of the same antigens (van den Pol, 1985a). Specifically, the paraformaldehyde–glutaraldehyde fixative has been used for the dual labeling of TH, GAD, and neurophysin with immunoperoxidase and silver-intensified gold as contrasting electron-dense markers (van den Pol, 1985a,b; Van den Pol and Görcs, 1986; van den Pol *et al.*, 1985). The fixative also can be used for the dual localization of tyrosine hydroxylase (TH) and choline acetyltransferase (ChAT), the respective synthesizing enzymes for catecholamines and acetylcholine (Pickel *et al.*, 1988a). For these specific antisera, 200 ml of the fixative was delivered by vascular perfusion over a 10-min interval immediately following a brief 10-ml saline rinse. The brains were then removed, coronally cut in 1 to 2-mm slices, and placed in the same fixative for an additional 1 hr at room temperature or for 2–3 hr at 4°C. The most appropriate concentration of aldehydes, volume of the perfusate, and duration of post fixation should be experimentally determined for each antigen prior to dual localization.

2. Paraformaldehyde–Glutaraldehyde–Picric Acid Fixative

A fixative containing 4% paraformaldehyde, 0.08% glutaraldehyde, and 15.0% saturated picric acid in 0.1 M phosphate buffer, pH 7.3 (Somogyi and Takagi, 1982), is applicable to dual localization of a variety of antigens, particularly when immunoperoxidase and avidinated ferritin (Leranth *et al.*, 1985a–c, 1986, 1988a,b; Zaborszky *et al.* 1986; Leranth and Frotscher, 1987; MacLusky *et al.*, 1988) or silver-intensified and unintensified DAB (Görcs *et al.*, 1986; Leranth and Frotscher, 1986b) are used as electron-dense markers. The fixative (150–200 ml for a 200- to 250-g rat) is perfused through the brain tissue immediately following the saline rinse. The brains are then removed, dissected into selected areas of interest, and postfixed for 4–12 hr in an ice-cold solution containing only paraformaldehyde and picric acid in phosphate buffer.

3. Acrolein–Paraformaldehyde Fixative

Acrolein is known both for its capacity to produce excellent preservation of ultrastructure and for its extreme toxicity (King *et al.*, 1983; Pickel *et al.*, 1986b). Thus, preparation of the fixative and perfusions of the animals must be carried out in a well-ventilated hood, preferably while wearing goggles and rubber gloves. The animal also should be placed on a rack so that the perfusate can be collected for safe disposal. A rapid 10-cc vascular rinse with heparin saline followed successively by 40–70 ml of a solution containing 3.75% acrolein and 2% paraformaldehyde in 0.1 M phosphate buffer (pH 7.2) and 200 ml of 2% paraformaldehyde in the same buffer provides good ultrastructural morphology and labeling of one (Pickel, 1985; Pickel et al., 1985; 1986c) or two (Pickel *et al.*, 1986b) antigens by immunoperoxidase and immunoautoradiography methods. These volumes apply to the fixation of the brain of a rat weighing 200–250g. Immersion of 1 to 2-mm slices of the tissue in buffered 2% paraformaldehyde after completion of the perfusion also appears to improve the ultrastructural morphology without compromising immunoreactivity.

The potency of acrolein as a fixative makes it necessary to determine carefully the concentrations and volumes needed for each antiserum (King *et al.*, 1983). Excessive exposure can result in complete loss of immunocytochemical labeling. Some antigens, for example, ChAT, are difficult to localize with even minute (0.5–1%) concentrations and small (50 ml) volumes of acrolein. In the above protocol, one of the advantages of the continued perfusion with paraformaldehyde appears to be the removal of the acrolein mixture within the blood vessels and brain tissues.

4. Double Fixation at Variable pH

Use of two fixatives at different pHs (Berod *et al.*, 1981) has been shown to provide excellent ultrastructural preservation while permitting good penetration of immunoreagents in dual-labeling studies of PNMT and CRF with silver-intensified and nonintensified diaminobenzidine reactions (Liposits *et al.*, 1986a). After vascular rinsing, the brains are perfused with a solution of 4% paraformaldehyde in 2% sodium acetate buffer at pH 6.5 (adjusted with 10% acetic acid), followed by a solution of 4% paraformaldehyde in 0.1 M sodium carbonate–bicarbonate buffer at pH 10.5–10.8. The volumes used for a 200 to 300-g rat are 150 ml of each solution. The dissected brain areas can be stored for 1–2 days in the second fixative at 4°C.

5. Remarks

The type of fixative that is most appropriate for obtaining the best preservation of morphology while providing the most intense immunostaining must be experimentally tested for each antiserum prior to initiation of dual labeling.

Removal of residual fixatives in the tissue improves the detection of specific immunoreactivity while reducing nonspecific, background labeling. Rinsing the tissue through several changes of phosphate or Tris buffer over periods ranging from 24–48 hr for thick blocks (2–3mm) to 2–6 hr for thin Vibratome sections (25–40 μm) usually effectively removes the residual fixatives. The inclusion of a 30-min incubation with 1% sodium borohydride decreases the duration of the rinse procedure by reducing the dialdehydes to their corresponding alcohols (Abdel-Akher et al., 1952; Schachner et al., 1977; Pickel et al., 1986b).

To minimize possible degradation, the post fixation and washes usually are carried out at 4°C. However, more frequent changes of buffer at room temperature increase the rate at which the aldehydes diffuse from the tissue and appear not to alter the immunocytochemical labeling of most antigens. Under these conditions, the washing period often can be reduced to 1 hr or less.

For preparation of fixatives and washing solutions, both phosphate and Tris buffers appear to be compatible with electron microscopic immunocytochemistry of one or two antigens. However, since Tris contains amino groups and aldehyde fixatives are known for their capacity to cross link amines (Molin et al. 1978; Graham and Karnovsky, 1966), Tris usually is not used in the preparation of the fixatives but is considered to be more effective in removing the aldehydes in wash solutions. The buffer used for the dilution of the primary antiserum also may be of some importance. For example, dilution of the antiserum against cholecystokinin (CCK) with 0.1 M potassium (pH 7.4) rather than sodium phosphate buffer at the same molarity and pH significantly improves the detection of immunocytochemical labeling (Leranth and Frotscher, 1986a,b).

D. Penetration

To achieve substantial penetration of primary antisera or relatively large secondary markers such as ferritin or protein A or immunoglobulin (IgG) conjugates of colloidal gold, the cellular membranes must be made permeable. Detergents such as Triton X-100 or saponin or protease have been used to permeate sections, thus allowing for greater penetration of immunoreagents for light microscopy. However, even at low concentrations, these compounds have an extremely damaging effect on ultrastructural morphology. In addition, Triton X-100 interferes with avidin–biotin binding.

Two other methods for enhancing penetration of immunoreagents in tissues prepared for electron microscopy include osmotic shock and freeze–thaw treatments.

In the osmotic shock treatment, low osmotic concentrations (0.03 M) of phosphate buffer are used to prepare the fixatives (Leranth et al., 1980a,b,

1981). This initial osmotic shock damages the cytoplasmic membranes, thus allowing for better penetration of the antisera and secondary markers. A limitation of this approach is the possibility that the osmotic shock may also dislocate some of the antigens in the tissue.

Freeze–thaw treatments offer a milder but effective method for enhancing penetration. In this procedure, previously washed Vibratome sections of fixed tissues are transferred to a vial (10–12 mm diameter) containing 0.5–0.8 ml of 10% sucrose in phosphate buffer. The vial is first dipped into liquid nitrogen and then allowed to thaw to room temperature. Two or three repetitions of the freeze–thaw treatment enhance the penetration of immunoreagents but compromise the ultrastructural morphology. The sucrose is removed by three 15-min washes in phosphate buffer prior to the immunocytochemical labeling procedure.

III. DOUBLE IMMUNOSTAINING

Four major combinations of electron-dense markers have been applied for dual labeling of two antigens in single sections of nervous tissue prior to plastic embedding. Each of these is described below.

A. Immunoperoxidase–Colloidal Gold

Colloidal gold particles were used more than 15 years ago for immunocytochemical labeling of single antigens (Faulk and Taylor, 1971). However, gold particles have begun to be used only recently as second electron-dense markers with immunoperoxidase for the simultaneous detection of neural antigens (Pickel et al., 1984; van den Pol, 1984, 1985a,b; van den Pol and Görcs, 1986; van den Pol et al., 1985). These studies used either double labeling of Vibratome sections prior to plastic embedding or immunoperoxidase before and immunogold labels after the tissues were embedded and sectioned for electron microscopy. The most commonly used immunoperoxidase methods for combined studies are the peroxidase–antiperoxidase (PAP) method of Sternberger (1979) or the ABC technique of Hsu et al. (1981).

1. Preparation and Protein Adsorption of Colloidal Gold

A detailed description of the methods for production of colloidal gold particles and the procedure of adsorption of gold particles to IgG or protein A are beyond the scope of this chapter. However, a brief outline of the procedure is given to provide the basic information needed for the successful application of colloidal gold as a second electron-dense marker in dual-labeling studies.

Colloidal gold particles of larger sizes (20–40 nm) can be produced by reduction of gold chloride with sodium citrate (Ferns, 1973; Horisberger and Rosset, 1977; Horisberger, 1982), whereas medium-sized particles (10–20 nm) are formed with sodium ascorbate (Horisberger, et al., 1978; Stathis and Fabrikanos, 1958). Recently, Aleppo tannin has been shown to produce colloidal gold particles of diameters 3–17 nm depending on the amount of tannic acid present during the reduction of gold chloride. Smaller particles (5–10 nm) are the most useful for immunocytochemical labeling of Vibratome sections because of the limited penetration of the larger colloidal gold–protein complexes.

Adsorption of colloidal gold to large protein molecules such as IgG or protein A depends on the negative charge of the particles (DeMey *et al.*, 1981; Roth *et al.*, 1978). The pH, which is determined by the pI of the protein, is an important determinant in the adsorption of the gold particles. For heterologous antisera and protein A, a pH of 9.0 in a 2 mM borax buffer adjusted to proper pH by K_2CO_3 can be used. In this case the protein will adsorb to the gold particles within a few seconds after their combination. The product is fairly stable, and the adsorbed protein prevents flocculation of the gold particles following addition of salts. Since unadsorbed gold particles precipitate with addition of 10% NaCl, a simple way to determine the correct amount of protein needed to stabilize the gold particles is by addition of 100 μl of 10% NaCl to 1 ml of adsorbed gold. If any color change is seen, either more protein must be added to stabilize the gold or the particular protein may not be suitable for adsorption. In general, smaller gold particles require more protein to stabilize them than larger particles (van den Pol, 1984). An additional 10% of the protein should be added after the titration necessary to stabilize the gold has been reached (DeMey *et al.*, 1981). Centrifugation can be used for removal of the aggregates of particles and unadsorbed proteins in the solution prior to storage and use for immunocytochemistry (DeMey, 1983; Slot and Gueze, 1981). The gold solution can be stored at −20°C if glycerol is added to prevent freezing. The optimal working dilution of colloidal gold adsorbed to proteins has to be tested in each sample. Commercial gold adsorbed to proteins varies greatly in concentration, which may be deduced from spectrophotometric analysis (DeMey, 1983).

2. Silver Intensification of Immunogold

Colloidal gold adsorbed to IgG or protein A can be used for the ultrastructural detection of neuronal antigens in Vibratome sections immunolabeled prior to their being embedded in plastic for electron microscopy (Pickel *et al.*, 1986a; van den Pol, 1984). However, because of the small size of particles that effectively penetrate the tissue, the immunocytochemical labeling is difficult to detect by light microscopy and requires considerable perseverance to locate with relatively high magnification (×20–30,000) electron microscopy.

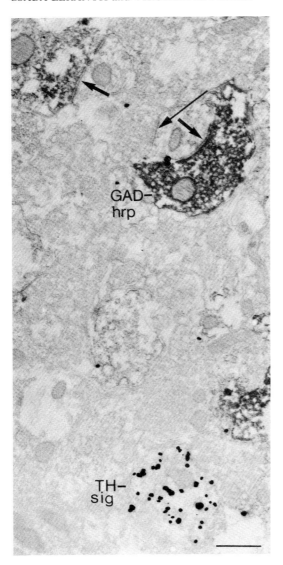

Figure 1. Electron micrograph demonstrates the result of a silver-intensified gold (SIG) and immunoperoxidase double-immunostaining experiment. In a section from the rat arcuate nucleus, a single TH-immunoreactive dendrite labeled with the SIG procedure is seen in the same thin section as two GAD-immunoreactive boutons making synaptic contact (short arrows) with unlabeled dendrites. One unlabeled dendrite is also in synaptic contact with a second unlabeled axon (long arrow). No peroxidase label is seen in the SIG-stained dendrite, and, vice versa, peroxidase-stained axons are free of silver particles. The photomicrograph is printed light to facilitate identification of HRP and silver particles. Bar scale, 0.45 μm. From van den Pol (1985b), courtesy of Dr. A. N. van den Pol and the Society for Neuroscience.

Recently a simple method of silver intensification was introduced to enhance the detection of colloidal gold particles (Fig. 1) adsorbed to IgG (van den Pol, 1985a,b) or protein A (van den Pol, 1985b). The principle of the technique is based on the well-known capacity of silver salts to intensify the staining of heavy metals in histological preparations (Brunk *et al.*, 1966; Danscher, 1981; Haug, 1967; Pearson and O'Neil, 1958; Phil, 1967; Tryer and Bell, 1974). The silver intensification of colloidal gold (SIG) enables a correlated light and electron microscopic recognition of the same immunolabeled neuronal profile. Furthermore, the silver precipitate surrounding the immunoglobulins bound to the tissue, in principle, may prevent the nonspecific attachment of antisera used to label the second antigen (van den Pol, 1985a).

The silver intensification of colloidal gold has been used for dual labeling of TH and glutamic acid decarboxylase (GAD) in unembedded Vibratome sections that were previously freeze–thawed to enhance penetration (van den Pol *et al.*, 1985). The GAD antiserum is localized selectively in axon terminals that are presynaptic to TH-labeled perikarya and dendrites in the rat substantia nigra.

As described in these studies by van den Pol (1985b), the dual-labeling protocol consists of the following incubations, which are separated by three 15-min washes in phosphate buffer:

1. A 30-min incubation at 20°C in a solution containing 0.1% lysine, 0.1% glycine, and 1% bovine serum albumin in phosphate buffer. This incubation at least partially reduces nonspecific attachments of primary and secondary antisera.

2. Incubation for 24–48 hr at 4°C in an experimentally determined optimal dilution of the first, primary antiserum (in this case rabbit antiserum to TH).

3. Incubation for 2–16 hr at 20°C in a solution of gold bound to protein A or IgG (against the species of the primary antiserum). The duration of the incubation and the dilutions should be determined experimentally to achieve maximal specific and minimal nonspecific binding.

4. Incubation in a silver solution in the dark at room temperature for periods ranging from a few minutes to several hours. The time required for optimal intensification without enhanced nonspecific staining of the tissue is determined by light microscopic examination of test sections that are removed from the silver solution and washed in citrate buffer. If the reaction is not sufficiently enhanced, the same sections can be returned to the silver solution, and the process repeated. The reaction should be stopped before the silver solution turns dark.

The silver solution is prepared in a darkened room by the sequential addition of 12.0 ml of stock solution A, 1.0 ml of solution D, 3.0 ml of solution B, and 3.0 ml of solution C in a container wrapped with aluminum foil. The stock solutions are prepared on the day they are used, using clean glass or plastic dishes and nonmetallic tools.

Solution A: 2 M citrate buffer, pH 4.0

Citric acid	25.5 g
Trisodium citrate	23.5 g
Distilled water	100 ml

Solution B

| Hydroquinone | 5.6% in distilled water |

Solution C

AgNO₃   07.5% in distilled water

Solution D

Gum acacia 1 : 2 dilution in water (A few hours are necessary to dissolve)

5. Three 15-min rinses in citrate buffer (0.15 M, pH 4.0) and a 10-min wash in phosphate buffer (0.1 M, pH 7.4)
6. Incubation for 30 min in 10–20% normal rabbit serum in phosphate buffer. This blocking step is used to reduce the possible binding of unsaturated antirabbit binding sites of the antirabbit IgG or protein A to rabbit antisera used in the second stage of labeling. This incubation is followed by three 15-min washes in phosphate buffer.
7. Incubation for 24–48 hr at 4°C in a previously determined optimal dilution of the second antiserum (i.e., GAD, raised in sheep). This is followed by three 15-min washes in phosphate buffer.
8. Incubation for 2 hr at room temperature in biotinylated rabbit anti-sheep IgG. The use of a species (e.g., swine) other than that used for production of the first primary antiserum also helps to eliminate problems of nonspecific cross reactions with immunoreagents of the first series of labeling steps. This incubation also is followed by three 15-min washes in phosphate buffer.
9. Incubation for 2 hr at 20° C in ABC complex, 1 : 250 dilution (Vector Lab, Burlingame, California).
10. Reaction for 5-10 min a solution containing:

DAB	15.0 mg
0.3% H₂O₂	165.0 μl
Phosphate buffer	25.0 ml

11. Processing for electron microscopy (see Section III.E)

B. Immunoperoxidase–Avidinated Ferritin

Ferritin-conjugated antibodies were introduced about 20 years ago (Singer and Schick, 1961) as specific electron-dense markers for immunolabeling macromolecules in complex biological structures. In the intervening years, ferritin conjungates have been used successfully to immunolabel a variety of extracellular as well as intracellular antigens (McLean and Singer, 1970; Painter *et al.*, 1973; Doerr-Schott and Garaud, 1981). These studies employed immunolabeling after embedding tissue for electron microscopy. However, this method was limited by the copious and nonspecific binding of ferritin–IgGh to most embedding media, presumably through hydrophobic interactions between the embedding polymer and the antibody (McLean and Singer, 1970).

Hydrophilic cross-linked polyampholate embedding medium has been proposed to solve the problem of nonspecific attachment to the plastic sections McLean and Singer, 1970).

A second approach is to immunolabel sections with the ferritin conjugates prior to embedding for electron microscopy. Initially, this method also had limited success. In well-fixed Vibratome sections, we observed a virtual complete lack of penetration and dissociation of ferritin molecules from IgG even after repeated freeze–thawing. In these sections, immunocytochemical labeling with peroxidase revealed that the dissociated IgG was selectively bound to antigenic sites. Use of avidinated ferritin in combination with a biotinylated second antibody resulted in less dissociation of the ferritin except after prolonged (1 year) storage of the stock solution. In this case the dissociated avidin D also was shown to be selectively localized in the tissue by labeling with biotinylated peroxidase and reaction with diaminobenzidine.

A 1 : 1 molar solution of avidin D and 7.0nm iron-core horse spleen ferritin (Vector Laboratories, Burlingame, California) specifically labels bound antisera via the bridge of the second biotinylated IgG (Leranth et al., 1984, 1985a, b,c, 1986; Zaborszky et al., 1986). After one or two freeze–thaw treatments of aldehyde-fixed Vibratome sections, the penetration of the avidinated ferritin is nearly equivalent to that of the immunoreagents for peroxidase labeling (Fig. 2). Furthermore, in studies of transmitter-related substances presumed to be in synaptic vesicles, the selective localization of ferritin over these organelles and not around mitochondria or plasma membranes as usually seen with the peroxidase reaction product indicates that the ferritin label may give a more selective subcellular localization (Fig. 3).

1. Single Immunolabeling with Avidinated Ferritin

Before dual immunolabeling is attempted, the optimal dilution of primary and secondary antisera, the fixation conditions necessary for each antiserum, and, most importantly, the quality of the avidinated ferritin must be established in single labeling studies. Vibratome sections of aldehyde-fixed tissues that have been permeabilized by freeze–thawing are processed through the incubations for single labeling with avidinated ferritin (Fig. 2). These include:

1. Incubation for 24–48 hrs at 4°C in experimentally determined optimal dilutions of primary antiserum.
2. Incubation for 8–12 hr at 4°C or for 2–4 hr at 20°C in the second biotinylated antibody (directed against the species in which the primary antiserum was raised).
3. Incubation for 8–12 hr at 4°C in avidinated ferritin.

The sections are washed through three 15-min changes of phosphate buffer between each incubation. Optimal dilutions of the biotinylated secondary IgG and the avidinated ferritin are experimentally determined and prepared in

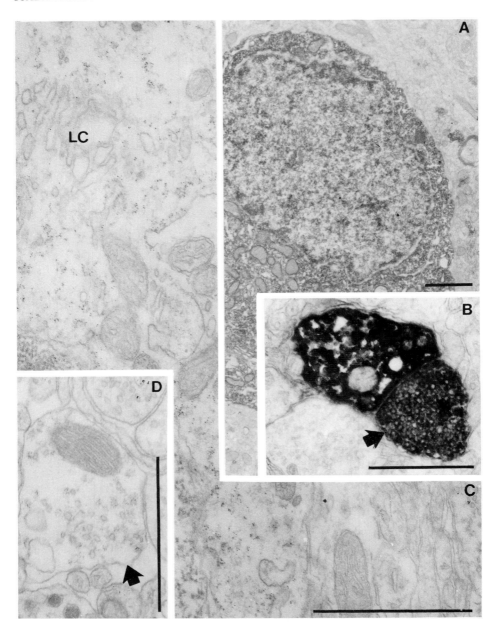

Figure 2. Electron micrographs representing immunolabeling with avidinated ferritin (panels C and D) and immunoperoxidase (panels A and B) for TH in the rat medial preoptic area demonstrate the difference between the localization of the two electron-dense immunolabels. The ferritin immunolabel is connected to ribosomes in a TH-immunoreactive cell (LC) and to synaptic vesicles in a TH-immunoreactive bouton (arrowhead on panel D), whereas the immunoperoxidase labeling for TH immunoreactivity is homogeneously distributed in the cytoplasm (panel A), dendrite, and axon terminal (arrowhead on panel B) and seems to connect to all types of neuronal membranes. Bar scales, 1 μm.

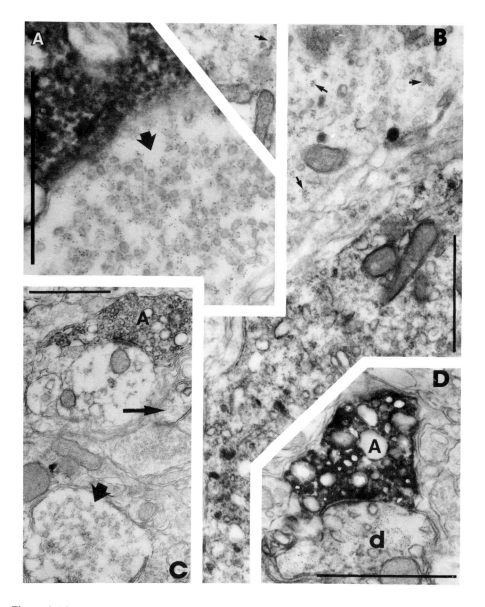

Figure 3. Electron micrographs demonstrate dual immunolabeling for TH (immunoperoxidase) and GAD (avidin–ferritin) in the arcuate nucleus (panels A, B, and C) and for choline acetyltransferase (ChAT) (immunoperoxidase) and GAD (avidin–ferritin) in the hippocampal dentate area (panel D) of a colchicine-pretreated rat. Panels A and B are taken from a material processed according the sequential double-immunostaining procedure (see Fig. 5); over the immunoperoxidase labeling occasional ferritin molecules are seen. Panels C and D represent the result of a sequential immunostaining performed according to the steps of Fig. 4; the immunoperoxidase-labeled profiles, axons (A), are free from ferritin immunolabel. Small arrows on panel B point to accumulations of ferritin immunolabel in a GAD-immunoreactive cell body. Arrowheads on panels A and C point to ferritin-immunolabeled GAD axons, and a large arrow on panel C points to a ferritin-immunolabeled GAD dendrite; d on panel D is a ferritin-labeled GAD-immunopositive dendrite postsynaptic to an immunoperoxidase-labeled ChAT-immunoreactive axon terminal (A). Bar scales, 1 μm.

phosphate buffer. When the biotinylated-IgG and the ferritin avidin D from Vector Co. (Burlingame, California) are used, the dilutions are in the range of 1 : 250 and 1 : 40–80 respectively. After completion of the final incubation, the sections are washed in phosphate buffer and processed for electron microscopy (Section III.E).

2. Double Immunostaining with Avidinated Ferritin and Immunoperoxidase

The detailed protocol for double immunolabeling with avidinated ferritin and immunoperoxidase is described. In addition, two methods are described for intensification of the ferritin molecule for easier microscopic detection.

a. Double-Immunostaining Procedure. Avidinated ferritin and immunoperoxidase can be used as two contrasting electron-dense markers with either sequential (Figs. 4 and 5) (Leranth *et al.*, 1985b, 1986; Leranth and Frotscher,

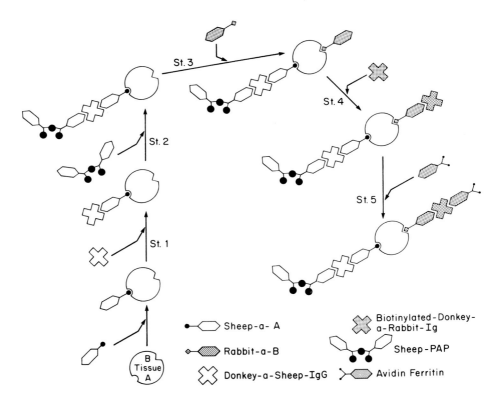

Figure 4. Schematic representation of sequential double immunostaining. The procedure using primary antibodies generated in different species and second antibodies (one of them biotinylated) generated in the same animal results in single ferritin labeling for tissue antigen B and single immunoperoxidase labeling for tissue antigen A.

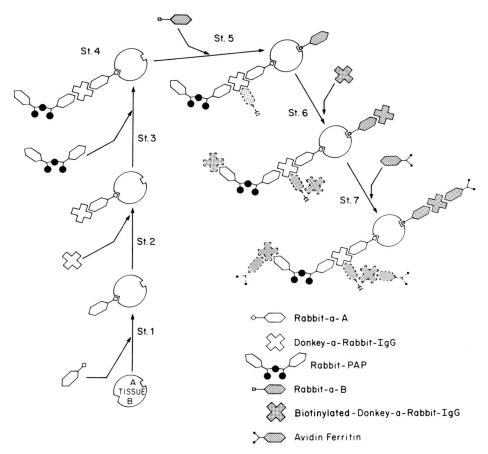

Figure 5. Schematic representation of the sequential double-immunostaining procedure using primary antibodies raised in the same species. The procedure will result in single ferritin immunolabeling for tissue antigen B and immunoperoxidase with occasional ferritin immunolabeling for tissue antigen A.

1987; Zaborszky *et al.*, 1986) or simultaneous (Figs. 6 and 7) double-staining procedures (Leranth *et al.*, 1985a).

Sequential Double Immunostaining. In the sequential method, two groups of antigenic sites are recognized by two consecutive series of incubations with the primary and secondary markers. The tissue antigen that is more likely to deteriorate during long incubations is immunolabeled in the first immunostaining procedure with peroxidase, using either PAP (Sternberger *et al.*, 1970) or ABC (Hsu *et al.*, 1981) methods. After reaction of the bound peroxidase with DAB, the Vibratome sections are rinsed (three times for 30 min) in phosphate buffer at 4°C, and then incubated with an experimentally determined optimal dilution of the second antiserum, which is immunolabeled with avidinated ferritin as described in Section III.B.1. The peroxi-

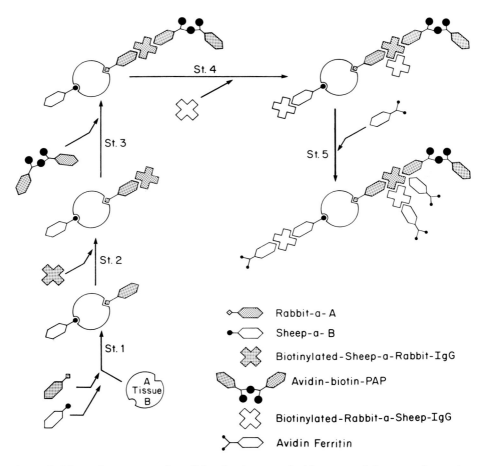

Figure 6. Schematic representation of the simultaneous dual-immunostaining procedure using primary antibodies generated in the same species. The procedure results in double immunolabeling (immunoperoxidase with occasional ferritin) for tissue antigen A and single ferritin immunolabeling for tissue antigen B.

dase product formed by reaction with DAB at least partially protects the immunoglobulins of the first labeling series from reaction with the second series (Sternberger and Joseph, 1979). Thus, the sequential labeling procedure is appropriate for double immunostaining using two primary antisera generated in the same species.

Simultaneous Double Immunostaining. The simultaneous double immunostaining procedure has the advantage of requiring less time than the sequential method. In addition, ferritin labeling of the second antigen appears to be more intense, and the ultrastructural morphology is slightly improved because of a more rapid processing of the tissue in the simultaneous labeling method. However, in this procedure there is a greater possibility of nonspe-

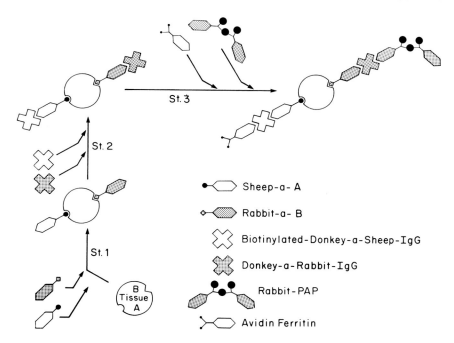

Sheep-a- A

Rabbit-a- B

Biotinylated-Donkey-a-Sheep-IgG

Donkey-a-Rabbit-IgG

Rabbit-PAP

Avidin Ferritin

Figure 7. Schematic representation of a simultaneous double-immunostaining procedure using primary antibodies raised in different species and second antibodies generated in the same species. Since the PAP method is applied to label one of the tissue antigens, the procedure will result in a single ferritin labeling for tissue antigen B and single immunoperoxidase labeling for tissue antigen A.

cific cross reactions between the different IgGs because of the lack of the protective effects of the DAB reaction product (Sternberger and Joseph, 1979). Thus, the use of antisera from separate species is essential.

For simultaneous double immunostaining, freeze–thawed Vibratome sections of aldehyde-fixed brains are processed through the following series:

1. Incubation for 24–48 hr at 4°C with two combined and optimally diluted primary antisera from separate, non-cross-reacting species. The dilution of each antiserum is half of that used for single labeling in order to compensate for the increased dilution produced by the addition of the other antiserum. For example, if the optimal dilution for single labeling is 1 : 1000, a 1 : 500 dilution is used in combination with an equal volume of the second primary antiserum.
2. Reagents for localizing the more sensitive tissue-bound primary antibody using either the PAP (Sternberger *et al.*, 1970) or the ABC (Hsu *et al.*, 1981) method.
3. Incubation for 6–8 hr at 4°C in the biotinylated secondary IgG produced against the remaining unlabeled antiserum bound to the tissue.
4. Incubation for 6–8 hr at 4°C in the avidinated ferritin.

All incubations and reactions are separated by at least three 15-min washes in phosphate buffer.

b. Remarks. Both the sequential and simultaneous double-immunostaining procedures result in single immunoperoxidase labeling of antigen A and single ferritin labeling of antigen B in sections processed under the following conditions:

1. If the antisera to A and B were raised in different species (Figs. 4 and 7).
2. If the secondary IgGs produced against the primary antisera to A and B are generated in the same third, non-cross-reacting species, e.g., donkey antisheep IgG and donkey antirabbit IgG (Fig. 7).
3. If the PAP method is used instead of the ABC method for detection of the antiserum to antigen A (Figs. 4 and 7).

Both double-staining methods will result in the detection of peroxidase reaction product and occasional ferritin molecules at the sites of antigen A and single ferritin labeling of antigen B in the following conditions:

1. If the ABC method is used rather than the PAP method for detecting one of the antigenic sites (Fig. 6).
2. If the two primary antisera to A and B were raised in the same species (Fig. 5).
3. If both the primary and secondary antisera were raised in different species (Fig. 6).

3. Intensification of Ferritin Immunolabel

For better visualization, the bound ferritin can be intensified by reaction of ultrathin plastic-embedded sections with bismuth subnitrate or by reaction of immunolabeled, unembedded Vibratome sections with a silver solution.

a. Bismuth Subnitrate Intensification of Ferritin. An ultrastructural staining method for enhancing the size and electron density of ferritin in thin sections was described by Aimsworth and Karnovsky (1972). This procedure also can be used to increase the size (approximately 1.5 to twofold) of the ferritin core of the avidinated ferritin immunolabel (Fig. 8a). The stock solution is made as follows:

1. Sodium tartrate, 400.0 mg, is dissolved in 10 ml 2 N sodium hydroxide.
2. This solution is added in drops to 200.0 mg bismuth subnitrate while being stirred with a magnetic bar. The solution begins to clear after addition of 6–8 ml and becomes completely clear after the addition of the entire 10 ml of sodium tartrate.

The solution is stable at 4°C for at least 1 month. For intensification of immunoferritin labels, aliquots of the stock solution are diluted from 1 : 20

to 1 : 50 in distilled water, filtered, and placed in small drops on dental wax. Formvar-coated single-slot grids containing the ferritin-labeled sections are floated on the drops of solution for 30–60 min at room temperature. These grids then are washed in several changes of distilled water. The bismuth subnitrate not only enhances the electron density of the bound ferritin but also increases the contrast of the cellular membranes. If even more contrast is desired, the sections can additionally be counterstained with uranyl acetate and Reynold's lead citrate standard protocols.

b. Silver Intensification of Ferritin. The silver intensification procedure, which was developed by Dr. T. Görcs (Tulane University, Louisiana), has been used in our laboratory for enhancing the detectability of avidinated ferritin only in single-labeling studies of GAD in unembedded Vibratome sections (Fig. 8b). However, the method also should be applicable to dual-labeling studies employing avidinated ferritin and immunoperoxidase. For silver intensification, Vibratome sections previously labeled with avidinated ferritin (Section II.b.1) and washed through several changes of phosphate buffer, are processed through the following steps:

1. A 20- to 30-min incubation at room temperature in solution I or solution II, which was prepared at least 4 hr prior to use.

   Solution I

Sodium ferricyanide	30.0 gr
Distilled water	93.0 ml
Glacial acetic acid	7.0 ml

   Solution II

Sodium ferricyanide	2.0 gr
Sodium ferrocyanide	1.2 g
Distilled water	93.0 ml
Glacial acetic acid	7.0 ml

2. Three 10-min rinses in 2% sodium acetate in water.
3. A 3- to 10-min reaction in a filtered solution containing:

DAB	50.0 mg
2% Na acetate in water (pH 5.5)	100.0 ml
(adjusted with acetic acid)	
30% Hydrogen peroxide	60.0 ml

4. Silver intensification as detailed in Section III.C.1.

These sections are then processed for electron microscopy (Section III.E).

C. Silver-Intensified and Unintensified Diaminobenzidine

Silver intensification by a physical developer was introduced by Gallyas (1971) and was applied to the light microscopic localization of two antigens

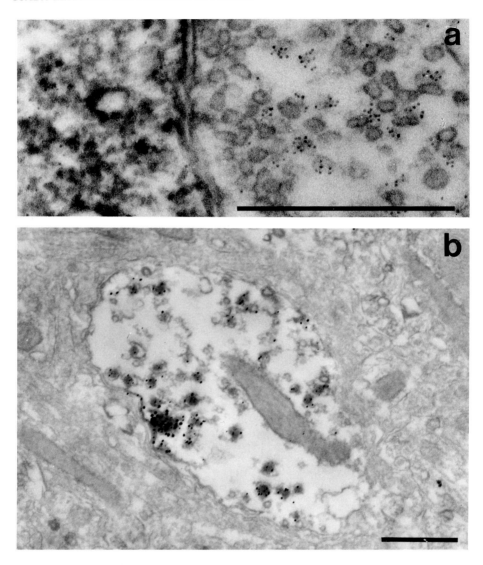

Figure 8. Electron micrographs demonstrate the result of the ferritin intensification procedures using the bismuth subnitrate (Section III.B.2a) (panel a) or silver intensification (Section III.B.2b) (panel b) techniques. The silver intensification of the ferritin immunolabel provides easy recognition of the labeling because of its size and electron opacity; however, the ultrastructure is damaged. Bar scales, 0.5 μm.

in the same section of tissue using the differential colors afforded by intensified (black) and nonintensified (brown) DAB reactions for immunoperoxidase labeling (Liposits *et al.*, 1983). The intensified DAB reactions also were detectable by electron microscopy (Liposits *et al.*, 1984) and, furthermore, were structurally distinct from the nonintensified DAB reactions as seen in dual immunoperoxidase labeling of two antigens in the same section (van den Pol and Görcs, 1985, 1986; Liposits *et al.*, 1986a,b; Görcs *et al.*, 1986; Leranth and Frotscher, 1986b). The use of the intensified and nonintensified DAB labeling of two antigens in the same section is illustrated in the light and electron micrographs of Figs. 9–11.

1. Labeling Procedures

Two variations of the immunolabeling sequence have been developed that differ primarily with regard to whether silver intensification is carried out before or after the sections are incubated with the second antiserum. These two methods are described.

a. Method I: Silver Intensification Prior to Second Antiserum. Vibratome sections from the brains of animals fixed either by perfusion with paraformaldehyde–glutaraldehyde–picric acid solution (Section I.C.2; Görcs *et al.*, 1986; Leranth and Frotscher, 1986b) or by the dual-pH fixative (Section I.C.4a, Liposits *et al.*, 1986a,b) are processed through the following series:

1. Incubation with appropriate dilution of primary antiserum for 24–48 hr at 4°C. The first antiserum is chosen based on the relative stability of the antigen to long incubations and/or the deleterious effects of silver intensification on subsequent binding of the antiserum.
2. Incubation with reagents for immunoperoxidase labeling of the first antiserum using either the PAP (Sternberger *et al.* 1970) or ABC method (Hsu *et al.*, 1981).
3. Silver intensification of the DAB reaction product (Fig. 11a) according to the protocol of Section III.C.2.
4. Incubation with the second primary antiserum.
5. Incubation with reagents for immunoperoxidase labeling of the second antiserum using either PAP (Sternberger *et al.*, 1970) or ABC methods (Hsu *et al.*, 1981).

All incubations are separated by appropriate washes as described previously. After the final DAB reaction in step 5, the sections are processed for electron microscopy (Section III.E). This technique, which is illustrated in Fig. 10, has allowed the elucidation of the catecholaminergic innervation of CRF immunoreactive neurons at both light and electron microscopic levels.

b. Method II: Silver Intensification after Incubation with Second Antiserum. This procedure is usually considered more appropriate when both antigens may be lost from the tissue during prolonged incubations or when the second antigen–antibody interactions may be altered by silver intensification. Silver intensification after incubation with the second antiserum has been used successfully for the simultaneous immunolabeling of cholecystokinin and GAD in the rat hippocampus (Leranth and Frotscher, 1986a; Fig.

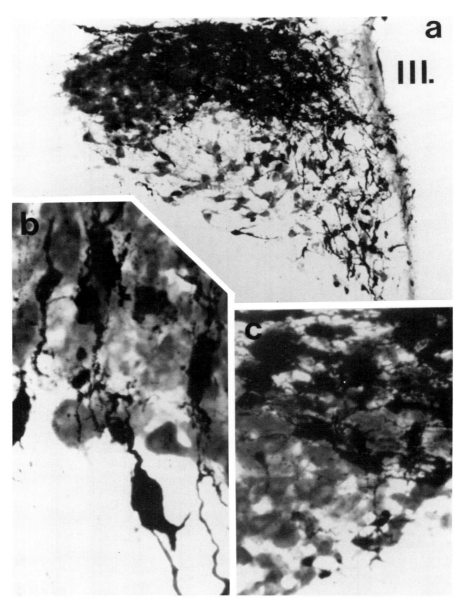

Figure 9. Low- (panel a) and high-power (panels b and c) light micrographs taken from the rat paraventricular nucleus immunostained for vasopressin and CRF using the silver-intensified DAB–unintensified DAB double-immunostaining technique. The black, silver-intensified DAB-immunolabeled CRF neurons are well contrasted from the single DAB-immunolabeled vasopressin neurons. (Courtesy of Dr. T. Görcs.) A color reproduction of this figure appears following p. 352.

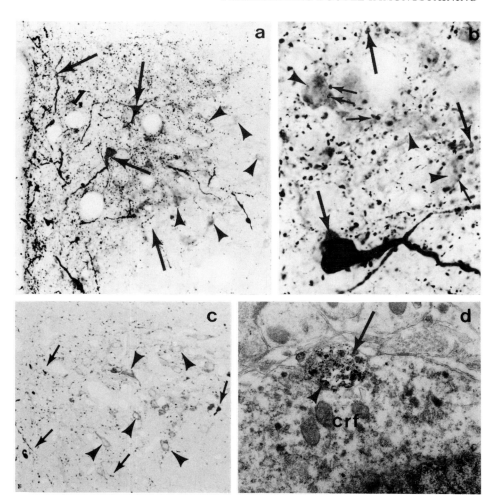

Figure 10. Light (a,b,c) and electron microscopic (d) demonstration of the immunocytochemical double-labeling technique utilizing silver-intensified gold (SIG) and nonintensified diamino-benzidine (DAB) chromogens. a and b: 40-μm Vibratome sections; c: 1-μm-thick plastic section; d: ultrathin section. On panel a, black-colored, SIG DAB-labeled TH-immunoreactive elements (arrows) are simultaneously visualized with CRF-containing structures (arrowheads) labeled with gray-colored nonintensified DAB end product in the hypothalamic paraventricular nucleus of the rat. Panel b (enlarged area of panel a) shows the distinct appearance of TH- (arrows) and CRF- (arrowheads) immunoreactive neuronal elements. Double arrows indicate sites suspected to represent interaction between the two different systems. Panel c demonstrates that the different physicochemical properties of the chromogens used for labeling of TH (arrows) and CRF (arrowheads) positive structures allow them to be distinguished even in semithin sections. On panel d a TH-immunoreactive axon (arrow) labeled by silver–gold particles is seen terminating (arrowhead) on a CRF-synthesizing neuron (crf). Note the marked difference between the electron densities of the pre- and postsynaptic labels. Asterisks indicate immunonegative structures. (Courtesy of Drs. Z. Liposits and W. K. Paull.)

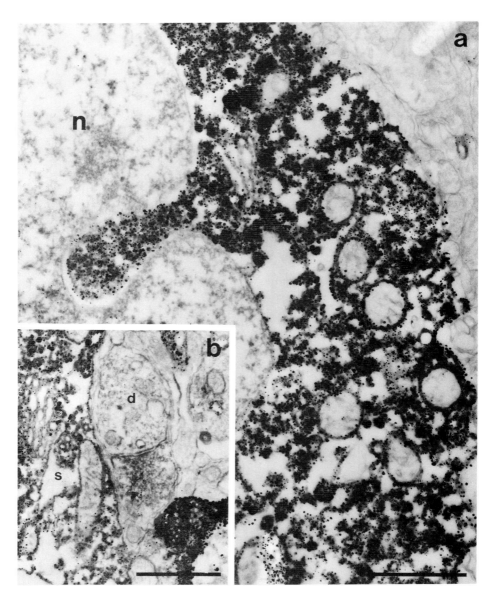

Figure 11. Electron micrographs demonstrate the result of the gold-substituted silver-intensified DAB–DAB double immunostaining for CCK and GAD in the rat hippocampal dentate hilar area. Panel a shows a detail of a neuron (immunoreactive for CCK) after the first immunostaining and the silver intensification of the DAB chromogen. Note that all of the DAB labels are covered with gold particles. Panel b was photographed after the second immunostaining for GAD using DAB. In addition to the silver–DAB labeling of CCK-immunoreactive profiles, the figure shows a single DAB-labeled GAD axon (asterisk) forming a symmetrical synaptic connection with an unlabeled dendrite (d). s, soma of a silver-intensified DAB-labeled CCK-immunoreactive neuron. Bar scales, 0.5 μm on panel a and 1 μm on panel b.

11b). In this procedure, Vibratome sections prepared as for method I are processed through the following series:

1. Incubation with the first primary antiserum.
2. Incubation with reagents for immunolabeling the first antiserum by the PAP method (Sternberger *et al.*, 1970).
3. Incubation with the second primary antiserum.
4. Incubation in biotinylated IgG directed against the second primary antiserum.
5. Silver intensification of the DAB reaction product for the first antiserum (Section III.C.2).
6. Incubation in avidin–biotin–peroxidase complex (ABC).
7. Incubation in DAB solution for visualization of the second bound peroxidase.

All incubations are separated by appropriate washes. The sections are processed for electron microscopy at the end of the last DAB reaction (Section III.E).

2. Silver Intensification and Gold Toning of DAB Product

Silver intensification and subsequent gold toning of the DAB reaction product in single or dual immunoperoxidase labeling studies consists of three consecutive procedures.

a. Preincubation. A preincubation procedure is necessary to suppress the argyrophil III reaction in sections of neural tissue (Gallyas, 1982). The Vibratome sections are washed through three 10-min changes of phosphate buffer following step 2 in method I or step 4 in method II and then transferred for 2 hr at room temperature or for 4–8 hr at 4°C into a 10.0% solution of thioglycolic acid in distilled water. The shorter (2-hr) incubation may be beneficial with regard to preservation of ultrastructural morphology (Liposits *et al.*, 1986b). The preincubation is followed by four 10-min washes in an isotonic (2%) solution of sodium acetate made in distilled water with pH adjusted to 8.7.

b. Silver Intensification. Following the preincubation and washes, the sections are transferred on the ends of clean glass rods to a physical developer prepared from solutions A–C.

Solution A

Sodium carbonate, anhydrous 5%, freshly prepared in distilled water

Solution B

Ammonium nitrate	2.0 gr
Silver nitrate	2.0 gr

| Tungstosilicic acid (Merck) | 10.0 gr |
| Distilled water | 100.0 ml |

The first three compounds should be dissolved in the order given. The tungstosilicic acid should be of high quality and stored with silica gel under vacuum to prevent absorption of water by the amorphous powder.

Solution C

| Paraformaldehyde | 35.0% in distilled water |

In preparation of the developer, 40 μl of solution C is added to 10.0 ml of solution B while stirring vigorously. This mixture is added by drops to 10.0 ml of solution A with continued stirring. If the developer becomes cloudy or forms a white precipitate during this procedure, a new solution should be prepared. The bottom of the Petri dish also should be checked with the light microscope to insure the absence of a silver precipitate before the sections are added to the solution. The precipitates generally can be eliminated by using well-cleaned glass or plastic utensils. After addition of solution C, the developer is stable for only about 30 min. Thus, solution C should be added immediately before use; if prolonged incubations are required, the sections should be transferred to freshly prepared solutions at intervals of less than 30 min. Decanting the developer into new plastic dishes immediately after preparation also seems to extend the usable period (Liposits *et al.*, 1986b; Görcs *et al.*, 1986).

The extent of the silver intensification can be determined by examining the sections with a dissecting or light microscope to verify when the brown DAB reaction product has been changed to a black precipitate. Uncontrolled variables in the reaction make it necessary to examine each Vibratome section separately. The usual time for development is 8–15 min. However, if the preincubation with thioglycolic acid is shortened or prolonged, the silver intensification period is either abbreviated or extended appropriately. Excessively long incubations in the developer result in nonspecific silver deposits throughout the tissue.

The silver intensification reaction is terminated by transferring the sections for 5 min into a solution containing 1.0% acetic acid in distilled water, followed by a 10-min rinse in 2% sodium acetate in distilled water.

c. Gold Toning. The silver precipitate embedded in the DAB polymer is replaced by gold chloride in order to obtain better-quality ultrathin sections and also to protect the diamond knife used for collecting the sections for electron microscopy. Following the above rinse in sodium acetate, the sections are incubated in 0.05% gold chloride ($HAuCl \cdot 4H_2O$) in distilled water for 10 min at 4°C. The low temperature is important for controlling the speed of the reaction.

After the gold-toning procedure, the Vibratome sections are transferred sequentially for 10 min each into a 2% sodium acetate solution, a freshly prepared 3% sodium thiosulfate solution to remove the unbound silver, a 2% sodium acetate solution, and phosphate buffer. The sections are then prepared for electron microscopy (Section III.E).

d. Remarks. The procedure is highly reproducible if the following precautions are taken:

1. The components of the stock solution should be added in the described order.
2. Tungstosilicic acid should be of high quality and stored in an amorphous state.
3. Mechanical damage to Vibratome sections, which may cause nonspecific deposits of silver, should be controlled as much as possible. Specifically, the chatter marks produced by the Vibratome can be minimized by adjustments of speed, frequency of vibration, and angle of the knife. If necessary, the quality of the Vibratome sections can be microscopically established by examining a few test sections after exposure to osmium tetroxide (Liposits *et al.*, 1986b).
4. Solutions, with the exception of thioglycolic acid, which is preferably kept in a glass container, are prepared and used in clean, disposable plastic containers while the utmost care is taken in cleanliness during their preparation. Contact of sections or solutions with metal results in nonspecific silver deposits.

The silver intensification procedure can also be used for intensification of retro- or anterogradely transported HRP (visualized by the DAB reaction) (Fig. 12a) or even for intensification of endogenous peroxidase granules (Fig. 12b).

D. Immunoperoxidase and Immunoautoradiography

The autoradiographic localization of iodinated secondary immunoglobulins provides a marker that is readily distinguishable from the reaction product of peroxidase immunocytochemistry (Picket *et al.*, 1986a). The method is applicable to dual localization of two antisera from the same or separate species. The underlying principle for the differential labeling of two antisera from the same species (e.g., rabbit) is based on the greater sensitivity of the autoradiographic labeling for ^{125}I, which allows the detection of the first antiserum at dilutions that are poorly recognized by the PAP or conjugated peroxidase methods (Pickel *et al.*, 1986a). The effective working dilutions depend on the titer of the first primary and secondary antisera. Therefore, the optimal dilutions for differential localizations must be experimentally determined. With a rabbit antiserum to TH produced and characterized by Dr. Tong Joh, Cornell University Medical College (Joh *et al.*, 1973), a dilution of 1 : 30,000 was recognized by immunoautoradiographic but not by immunoperoxidase methods (Pickel *et al.*, 1986a). One disadvantage of using

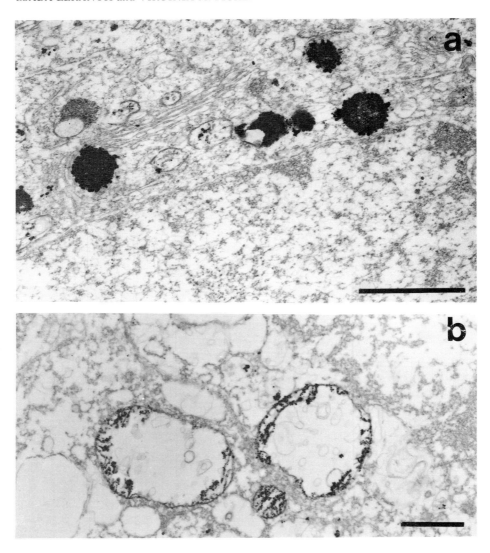

Figure 12. Electron micrographs demonstrate retrogradely transported (panel a, taken from the rat hippocampus after a contralateral HRP injection) and endogenous (panel b, taken from embryonic tissue) peroxidase granules. In both cases the HRP was visualized by the glucose oxidase reaction, and the final DAB chromogen was silver intensified. (Panel b courtesy of Dr. E. Pinter.) Bar scales, 1 μm.

the high dilution of antiserum is that the autoradiographic exposures are much longer than with more optimal (e.g., 1 : 2000) dilutions. In contrast to the 4 to 6-month exposure needed for electron microscopic autoradiographs at 1 : 30,000 dilution of TH antiserum, only 2–3 months are needed at 1 : 2000. The lower dilutions are applicable to dual-labeling studies of two antisera from different species. Using the rabbit TH antiserum and a mouse monoclonal antiserum to ChAT from Boehringer-Mannheim (Eckenstein and Theonen, 1982), we have differentially labeled cholinergic and catecholaminergic terminals in the striatum of the adult rat using the same dilutions as those of single-labeling methods with no apparent cross reactions among the various antisera (Pickel *et al.*, 1988a; Fig. 13). Similar methods also were used for dual localization of a rabbit antiserum against the epinephrine-synthesizing enzyme phenylethanolamine N-methyl transferase (PNMT) and a rat polyclonal antibody against GABA (Pickel *et al.*, 1988b). The GABAergic terminals formed symmetrical synapses with PNMT-containing perikarya in the medial nuclei of the solitary tracts (NTS) (Fig. 14).

1. Labeling Method

Vibratome sections of aldehyde-fixed brains are processed through the following steps:

1. A 24-hr incubation in an empirically derived dilution of the first antiserum (e.g., rabbit TH).
2. A 2-hr incubation in a 1 : 100 dilution of ^{125}I-labeled donkey anti-species-1 immunoglobulin (IgG) (Amersham, Arlington Heights, Illinois) with a radioactive concentration of 100 μCi/ml. The incubations are carried out at room temperature with continuous agitation. The solutions and washes (three times for 15 min between step 1 and 2 and at least three for 30 min after step 2) are in 0.1 M Tris-saline at pH 7.6. The wash after step 2 should be continued until negligible radioactivity is detected in the wash solutions.
3. A 24-hr incubation with a previously determined optimal dilution of the second antiserum (e.g., mouse monoclonal ChAT).
4. Incubation with anti-species-2 IgG, PAP, and DAB reaction for the standard PAP labeling procedure.
5. A 10-min reaction with 1% glutaraldehyde in phosphate buffer.

The incubations in steps 3–5 are separated by washes in Tris-saline followed by phosphate buffer. Reversal of the labeling procedure such that the immunoperoxidase precedes the radioactive labeling results in silver grains superimposed nonspecifically on the DAB reaction product. After step 5, the sections are washed through three 10-min rinses in phosphate buffer and then processed for light or electron microscopic autoradiography.

2. Processing for Light and Electron Microscopic Autoradiography

For light microscopy, the labeled sections are mounted on slides previously cleaned with acid and coated with 0.25% gelatin. The sections dried on the slides are then defatted by processing through two 15-min changes

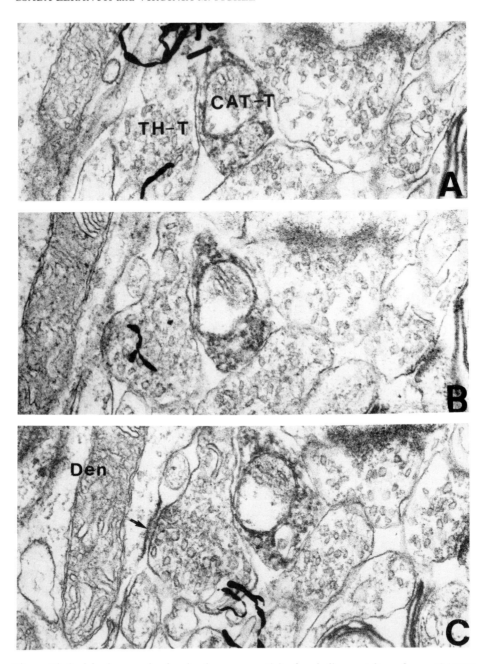

Figure 13. Serial micrographs showing immunoreactivity for choline acetyltransferase (CAT-T) in an axon terminal immediately apposed to a second terminal containing immunoautoradiographic labeling for tyrosine hydroxylase (TH-T) in the rat caudate nucleus. The TH-labeled terminal forms a symmetrical synapse (arrow) with unlabeled dendrite (Den) in C. Autoradiographic exposure was 3 months. Bar scale, 0.5μm.

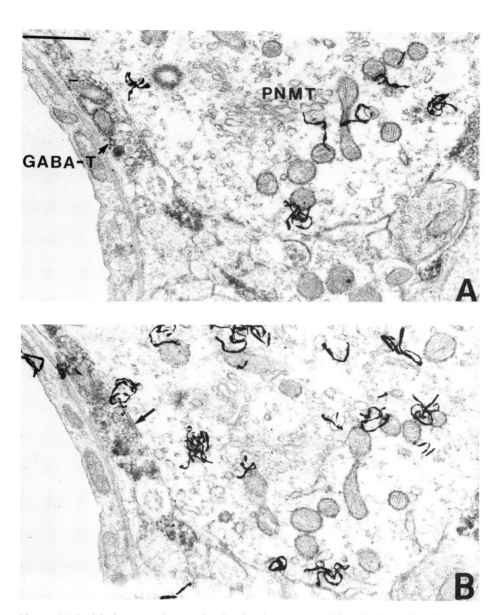

Figure 14. Serial electron micrographs showing immunoperoxidase labeling of GABA in an axon terminal (GABA-T) that forms a symmetrical junction (arrow) with a perikaryon containing autoradiographic labeling for PNMT. The perikaryon is located in the caudal and medial nuclei of the solitary tracts of a rat. Autoradiographic exposure was 2.5 months. Bar scale, 0.5 μm.

of chloroform–100% ethanol (1 : 1) followed by a graded ethanol series to deionized water. The slides then are dipped in a 1 : 1 dilution of Ilford L4 emulsion (at 50°C). These slides are dried and exposed in light-proof boxes with desiccant at 4°C for periods of 4–30 days. At the end of the exposure periods, they are developed for 2 min at 17°C using Kodak D-19 developer, rinsed in water, and then placed in Kodak Ektaflo fixer for 8 min, washed in running water for 1 hr, dehydrated, and examined with a light microscope.

For electron microscopy, the dually labeled sections are processed as described in Section III.E. The autoradiographic procedure is the same as that described in detail by Beaudet (1982), Descaries and Beaudet (1983), and Pickel and Beaudet (1984). In brief, ultrathin sections are collected from the outer surface of the flat-embedded Vibratome sections and deposited with a loop on slides coated with 2% parlodion in amyl acetate. These slides are counterstained with uranyl acetate and lead citrate, coated with a silver-gray layer of carbon (Varian Vacuum Evaporator), and dipped in a 1 : 4 dilution of Ilford L4 emulsion at 50°C. They are then air dried and stored with a desiccant in light-proof boxes for 1–4 months. The autoradiographs are developed 1–2 min at 17°C with Kodak Microdol X developer, rinsed in water, fixed in 30% sodium thiosulfate, and washed in deionized water. The parlodion coating with autoradiographic thin sections is then collected on grids, and the film is removed by amyl acetate. The localization of reduced silver grains to specific neuronal profiles in electron microscopic autoradiographs is confirmed by the detection of labeling over the same neuronal profile in consecutive or semiconsecutive serial sections. The need for serial sections for confirmation that selected profiles are labeled by immunoautoradiography is considerably greater when the labeling is over small structures such as axon terminals (e.g., Fig. 13) than when over large perikarya (e.g., Fig. 14). Sometimes only one silver grain is detected in single sections of small axons or terminals. These can be easily mistaken for background labeling without serial sections.

E. Processing for Electron Microscopy

Following the final incubations for dual labeling, the sections are postfixed for 1–2 hr in 2% OsO_4 and then washed in phosphate buffer, dehydrated and embedded in plastic. Because of excellent stability and tolerance for humid conditions, we suggest the use of Epon 812 or Durcupan (Fluka). Flat embedding the Vibratome section between sheets of plastic or aluminum foil and a glass coverslip (Leranth and Fehér, 1983) with a small lead weight on top of the plastic sheets or the coverslip provides extremely flat sections, which can be examined and photographed by light microscopy. Following light microscopic analysis, the areas of interest in the flat-embedded sections are cut with scissors, and the small pieces then embedded in Beam capsules for ultrathin sectioning (Pickel, 1981).

F. Controls

Some of the controls needed in double immunostaining are the same as for single labeling (Larsson, 1981; DeMey, 1983; Petrusz, 1983) whereas others, particularly those involving nonspecific cross reactions between immunoreagents, are unique to dual labeling.

1. Specificity of Antiserum

One of the primary concerns for both single- and double-labeling immunocytochemistry is the specificity of the antiserum. If an antiserum is specific for a given antigen or a conjugate of a smaller molecule that has been rendered antigenic by binding to a larger protein such as serum albumin, adsorption of the diluted antiserum with the antigen or conjugate should remove the observed immunocytochemical reaction. For example, addition of 0.5 μg of substance P to 0.1 ml of 1 : 1000 diluted rabbit antiserum against the peptide, centrifugation, and substitution of the supernatant in the immunocytochemical labeling procedure effectively removes all detectable immunoreactivity. Such blocking experiments are not always possible when the antigen is difficult to purify or present in small amounts. In these cases the adsorption controls may be used only in the original publication describing the purification and specificity of the antisera. In other routine studies using the same antiserum, the specificity of the labeling method can be tested by replacing the specific antiserum with either normal or preimmune serum from the same species or by using infinitely high dilutions of the specific antiserum.

In the first use of antisera, particularly those against the neuropeptides, their cross reactivities within larger peptide families also should be established by the immunoblot method (Larsson, 1981). Many of the available antisera to the peptides cross react to limited degrees with a variety of related peptide fragments other than the ones used to produce the original antiserum. We have shown, for example, that the rabbit polyclonal antiserum against NT obtained from Immunotech, Inc. principally recognizes NT, NT_{8-13}, and $[Gln^4]$-NT but also cross reacts with angiotensin I (ANG-I) (Milner and Pickel, 1986). For immunoblots, the peptides or other antigenic substances are dissolved in water to yield a concentration of 1 mg/ml and then spotted on Whatman No. 1 filter paper held by a filtration manifold (Schleicher and Schuell, Inc.). Each well in the filtration unit contains 10 μl of the peptides at concentrations ranging from 1 to 1000 ng/10μl. These are air dried on the paper and exposed to paraformaldehyde vapors at 80°C for 1 hr. The papers are then stained immunocytochemically with a 1 : 1000 dilution of the anitserum being tested (Larsson, 1981).

Neither adsorption nor immunoblotting excludes the possibility that the antisera to the peptides may cross react with longer-chain precursors or smaller fragments. Thus, the term "-like immunoreactivity" should be used or implied in all descriptions of localization.

2. Nonspecific Interactions of Immunoreagents in Dual Labeling

Immunostaining for two antigens on single sections is fraught with possibilities for nonspecific interactions between the immunoreagents used in each labeling series. In particular, primary or secondary antisera or the second series may cross react with those of the first. One simple and direct approach is to process alternate sections for dual labeling with omission of the second primary antiserum. For example, in sections radiolabeled for rabbit TH antiserum and peroxidase labeled for mouse antiserum to ChAT, there should be no detectable peroxidase immunoreactivity when ChAT antiserum is omitted and the sections are processed by the PAP method. Detection of immunoperoxidase labeling in this case would indicate that a secondary IgG or PAP of the second series recognized a primary or secondary antiserum from the first series. When two antisera from the same species are used, such cross reactions are difficult to avoid and thus must be dealt with in an effective manner. At least three approaches have been used.

The sections may be processed first with immunoperoxidase, since the DAB reaction product reportedly blocks interactions with antisera of the second series (Sternberger and Joseph, 1979). This method has been unsuccessful in the described autoradiographic method largely because of nonspecific attachments to the DAB product.

One of the antisera can be localized by a method such as autoradiography, where the signal can be amplified by longer exposures to detect dilutions of the antiserum that are not seen by immunoperoxidase methods (Pickel *et al.,* 1986a).

From the sequence of incubations, the differential identity of the two antigens can be inferred from observation of both labels for the first and single labeling for the second antiserum. Caution is necessary for the successful application of either of these methods. Possible pitfalls include changes in optimal dilution of the antiserum as a result of changes in the temperature, method of agitation, or titer of primary or secondary antisera (applicable to method 2) and differential penetration of different antisera or reagents, which may result in failure of the DAB reaction product to cover all of the cross-reacting antigenic sites (applicable to method 1) or erroneous interpretations with regard to whether some single labeled profiles actually contain antigen 2 versus 1 (applicable to method 3). The alternative, of course, is always to use primary antisera from two separate, non-cross-reacting species and anti-IgG for a common third species (Figs. 4, 5, and 7).

3. Controls in Autoradiography

A possible source of artifact that is specific to autoradiographic dual immunolabeling with peroxidase as the second marker is the possible exposure to the overlying emulsion by the dense DAB reaction. Autoradiographic processing of tissues labeled only for immunoperoxidase can be used to de-

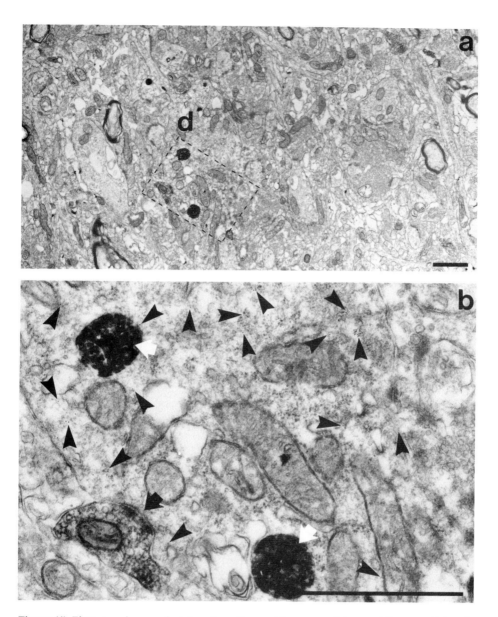

Figure 15. Electron micrographs taken from the rap hippocampal dentate hilar area 48 hr after a contralateral HRP injection demonstrate the result of a triple-labeling study consisting of a double immunostaining (using avidin–ferritin and immunoperoxidase) and retrograde HRP tracer technique. Dendrite (d) of a commissural ferritin-labeled (arrowheads) neuron immunoreactive for GAD establishes a symmetrical synaptic connection (arrow) with an immunoperoxidase labeled ChAT-immunoreactive axon terminal. Note the retrogradely transported HRP granules (white arrows) in the commissural GAD-immunoreactive neuron. The visualization of the traced HRP has been performed by a glucose oxidase reaction prior to the double immunostaining. The relative low intensity of ferritin immunolabeling in the commissural GAD-immunoreactive neuron results from the lack of a colchicine pretreatment. Panel b is a high-power magnification of the indicated area on panel a. Bar scales, 1 μm.

termine whether this type of kymography is occurring. This problem has been encountered most frequently near the surface of the tissue, where the DAB reaction is most intense.

The differentiation of specific labeling from scattered silver grains also is unique to the autoradiographic dual-labeling methods. The profile expected to be the source of the radiation must be identified by the presence of silver grains in at least two and frequently three or more adjacent thin sections.

IV. CONCLUDING REMARKS

Four major protocols have been given for the immunocytochemical labeling of two antigens in the same section prepared for electron microscopy. Satisfactory dual immunolabeling can be obtained with any of the described methods when adequate precautions are taken. The choice often depends on the specific antigen being investigated and the requirement for immediate results. The duration of autoradiographic exposure (2–3 months) frequently is considered excessive compared to the few days required for dual labeling with most other methods. However, the cellular organelles within the autoradiographically labeled profiles usually are distinguished readily, and the silver grains bear absolutely no resemblance to any of the other reaction products. Thus, the autoradiographic marker is an ideal third marker for use with any of the other electron-dense products described in this chapter.

All of the double-immunolabeling procedures, in principle, can be combined with the tract-tracing techniques described in other chapters of this volume. Specifically, they are most applicable for combination with acute axonal degeneration and anterograde and retrograde tracing using autoradiographic or peroxidase markers (Leranth and Frotscher, 1987; Fig. 15).

ACKNOWLEDGMENTS. The authors gratefully acknowledge the support provided by grants from NIH (HL18974), NIMH (MH00078 and MH40342), NS (BNS 8320120), NIH (NS 22807), NIH (NS 26068), and the Andrew Mellon Foundation as well as the excellent technical support from Marya Shanabrough, June Chan, and Melinda Carson.

REFERENCES

Abdel-Akher, M., Hamilton, J. K., Montgomery, R., and Smith, F., 1952, A new procedure for the demonstration of the fine structure of polysacharide, *J. Am. Chem. Soc.* **74**:4970–4971.

Aimsworth, S. K., and Karnovsky, M. J., 1972, An ultrastructural staining method for enhancing the size and electron opacity of ferritin in the sections, *J. Histochem. Cytochem.* **20**:225–229.

Beaudet, A., 1982, High resolution radioautography of central 5-hydroxytryptamine (5-HT) neurons, *J. Histochem Cytochem.* **9**:765–768.

Bendayan, M., 1982, Double immunocytochemical labeling applying to protein A-gold technique, *J. Histochem. Cytochem.* **30**:81–85.

Berod, A., Hartman, B. K., and Pujol, J. F., 1981, Importance of fixation in immunohistochemistry: use of formaldehyde solutions at variable pH for the localization of thyrosine hydroxylase, *J. Histochem. Cytochem.* **29**:844–850.

Bolam, J. P., Ingham, C. A., Izzo, P. N., Levey, A. I., Rye, D. B., Smith, A. D., and Wainer, B. H., 1986, Substance P-containing terminals in synaptic contact with cholinergic neurons in the neostriatum and basal forebrain: A double immunocytochemical study in the rat, *Brain Res.* **397**:279–289.

Brunk, U., Brun, A., and Skold, G., 1966, Histochemical demonstration of heavy metals with the sulphide-silver method. Methodological study, *Acta Histochem.* **31**:345–357.

Cuello, A. C. (ed.), 1983, *IBRO Handbook Series: Methods in Neurosciences*, Volume 3, *Immunohistochemistry*, John Wiley & Sons, Chichester.

Cuello, A. C., Priestley, J. V., and Milstein, C., 1982, Immunocytochemistry with internally labeled monoclonal antibodies, *Proc. Natl. Acad. Sci. U.S.A.* **79**:665–669.

Danscher, G., 1981, Histochemical demonstration of heavy metals. A revised version of the sulphid silver method suitable for both light and electron microscopy, *Histochemistry* **71**:1–16.

DeMey, J., 1983, A critical review of light and electron microscopic immunocytochemical techniques used in neurobiology, *J. Neurosci. Methods* **7**:1–18.

DeMey, J., Moermans, M., Guens, G. Nuydens, R., and DeBrabender, M., 1981, High-resolution light and electron microscopic localization of tubulin with the IGS (immuno gold staining) method, *Biol. Int. Rep.* **5**:889–899.

Descaries, L., and Beaudet, A., 1983, Use of radioautography for investigation of transmitter-specific neurons, in: *Handbook of Chemical Neuroanatomy*, Volume 3 (A. Bjorklund and T. Hokfelt, eds.), Elsevier, Amsterdam, pp. 286–364.

Doerr-Schott, J., and Garaud, J. C., 1981, Ultrastructural identification of gastrin-like immunoreactive nerve fibers in the brain of *Xenopus laevis* by means of colloidal gold or ferritin immunocytochemical methods, *Cell Tissue Res.* **216**:581–589.

Eckenstein, F., and Theonen, H., 1982, Production of specific antisera and monoclonal antibodies to choline acetyltransferase: Characterization and use for identification of cholinergic neurons, *EMBO J.* **1**:363–368.

Elde, R., Hokfelt, T., Johansson, O., and Terenius, L., 1976, Immunohistochemical studies using antibodies to leucine-enkephalin: Initial observations of the nervous system of the rat, *Neuroscience* **1**:349–351.

Faulk, V. P., and Taylor, G. P., 1971, An immunocolloid method for electron microscope, *Immunochemistry* **8**:1081–1083.

Ferns, G., 1973, Controlled nucleation for the regulation of the particle size in nondisperse gold solutions, *Nature* **241**:20–22.

Fertuck, H. C., and Salpeter, M. M., 1974, Sensitivity in electron microscopic autoradiography for ^{125}I, *J. Histochem. Cytochem.* **22**:80–87.

Friedrich, V. L., and Mugnaini, E., 1981, Electron microscopy: Preparation of neural tissues for electron microscopy, in: *Neuroanatomical Tract-Tracing Methods* (L. Heimer and M. J. Robards, eds.), Plenum Press, New York, pp. 345–377.

Gallyas, F., 1971, A principle for silver staining of tissue elements by physical development, *Acta Morphol. Acad. Sci. Hung.* **19**:57–71.

Gallyas, F., 1982, Suppression of argyrophil III reaction by mercaptocompounds. Prerequisite for intensification of histochemical reactions by physical developers, *Acta Histochem.* **70**:99–105.

Glazer, E. J., Ramachandran, J., and Basbaum, A. I., 1984, Radioimmunocytochemistry using a tritiated goat anti-rabbit second antibody, *J. Histochem. Cytochem.* **32**:778–782.

Görcs, T., Leranth, C., and MacLusky, N. J., 1986, The use of gold substituted silver-intensified diaminobensidine (DAB) and non-intensified DAB for simultaneous electron microscopic labeling of tyrosine hydroxylase and glutamic acid decarboxylase immunoreactivity in the rat medial preoptic area, *J. Histochem. Cytochem.* **34**:1439–1447.

Graham, R. C., Jr., and Karnovsky, M. J., 1966, The early stages of a absorption of injected horseradish peroxidase in the proximal tubules of mouse kidney: Ultrastructural cytochemistry by a new technique, *J. Histochem. Cytochem.* **14**:291–302.

Haug, F. M., 1967, Electron microscopic localization of the zinc in hippocampal mossy fibre synapses by a modified sulfide procedure, *Histochemie* **8:**355–368.

Horisberger, M., 1982, Evaluation of colloidal gold as a cytochemical marker for transmission and scanning electron microscopy, *Biol. Cell.* **36:**253–258.

Horisberger, M., and Rosset, J., 1977, Colloidal gold, a useful marker for transmission and scanning electron microscopy, *J. Histochem. Cytochem.* **25:**295–305.

Horisberger, M., Farr, D. R., and Vonlanthen, M., 1978, Ultrastructural localization of D-galactan in the nuclei of the myxomycete *(Physarum polycephalum)*, *Biochim. Biophys. Acta* **542:**308–314.

Hsu, S. M., Raine, L., and Fayer, H., 1981, The use of avidin–biotin–peroxidase complex (ABC) in immunoperoxidase technique: A comparison between ABC and unlabeled antibody (peroxidase) procedures, *J. Histochem. Cytochem.* **29:**577–590.

Hudgson, A. J., Penke, B., Erdei, A., Chubb, I. W., and Somogyi, P., 1985, Antisera to gamma amino butyric acid. I. Production and characterization using a new model system, *J. Histochem. Cytochem.* **33:**229–239.

Hunt, S. P., and Mantyh, P. W., 1984, Radioimmunohistochemistry with ³H-biotin, *Brain Res.,* 291:203–217.

Joh, T. H., Gegham, C., an Reis, D. J., 1973, Immunochemical demonstration of increased tyrosine hydroxylase protein in sympathetic ganglia and adrenal medulla elicited by reserpine, *Proc. Natl. Acad. Sci. U.S.A.* **70:**2767–2771.

King, J. C., Lechan, R. M., Kugel, G., and Anthony, E. L. P., 1983, Acrolein: A fixative for immunocytochemical localization of peptides in the central nervous system, *J. Histochem. Cytochem.* **31:**62–68.

Kohno, J., Shinoda, K., Kawai, Y., Ohuchi, T., Ono, K., and Shiotani, Y., 1988, Interaction between adrenergic fibers and intermediate cholinergic neurons in the rat spinal cord: A new double-immunostaining method for correlated light and electron microscopic observations, *Neuroscience* **25:**113–121.

Lakos, S., and Basbaum, A. I., 1986, Benzidine dihydrochloride as a chromogen for single- and double-label light and electron microscopic immunocytochemical studies, *J. Histochem. Cytochem.* **34:**1047–1056.

Larsson, L.-I., 1981, A novel immunocytochemical model system for specificity and sensitivity screening of anitsera against multiple antigens, *J. Histochem. Cytochem.* **29:**408–410.

Larsson, L.-I., 1983, Methods for immunocytochemistry of neurohormonal peptides, in: *Handbook of Chemical Neuroanatomy*, Volume 1, *Methods in Chemical Neuroanatomy* (A. Bjorklund and T. Hokfelt, eds.), Elsevier, Amsterdam, pp. 147–209.

Leranth, C., and Fehlér, E., 1983, Synaptology and sources of vasoactive intestinal polypeptide (VIP) and substance P (SP) containing axons of the cat celiac ganglion. (An experimental electron microscopic immunohistochemical study), *Neuroscience* **10:**947–958.

Leranth, C., and Frotscher, M., 1986a, Synaptic connections of cholecystokinin-immunoreactive neurons and terminals in the rat fascia dentata: A combined light and electron microscopic study, *J. Comp. Neurol.* **254:**51–64.

Leranth, C., and Frotscher, M., 1986b, GABAergic input of cholecystokinin-immunoreactive neurons in the hilar region of the rat hippocampus: An electron microscopic double immunostaining study, *Histochemistry* **86:**287–290.

Leranth, C, and Frotscher, M., 1987, Cholinergic innervation of hippocampal GAD- and somatostatin-immunoreactive commissural neurons: Electron microscopic double immunostaining combined with retrograde tracer technique, *J. Comp. Neurol.* **261:**33–47.

Leranth, C., Williams, T. H., Chretien, M., and Palkovits, M., 1980a, Ultrastructural investigation of ACTH immunoreactivity in arcuate and supraoptic nuclei of the rat, *Cell. Tissue Res.* **210:**11–19.

Leranth, C., Williams, T. H., Jew, J. Y., and Arimura, A., 1980b, Immuno-electron microscopic identification of somatostatin cells and axons of guinea pig sympathetic ganglia, *Cell. Tissue Res.* **212:**83–89.

Leranth, C., Jew, J. Y., Williams, T. H., and Palkovits, M., 1981, Stria terminalis axons ending on substance P and neurotensin-containing cells of rat central amygdaloid nucleus: An electron microscopic immunocytochemical study, *Neuropeptides* **1:**261–272.

Leranth, C., Sakamoto, H., MacLusky, N. J., Shanabrough, M., and Naftolin, F., 1985a, Application of avidin–ferritin and peroxidase as contrasting electron-dense markers for simultaneous electron microscopic immunocytochemical labelling of glutamic acid decarboxylase and tyrosine hydroxylase in the rat arcuate nucleus, *J. Histochem.* **82:**165–168.

Leranth, C., MacLusky, N. J., Sakamoto, H., Shanabrough, M., and Naftolin, F., 1985b, Glutamic acid decarboxylase-containing axons synapse on LHRH neurons in the rat medial preoptic area, *Neuroendocrinology* **40:**536–539.

Leranth, C., MacLusky, N., and Naftolin, F., 1985c, Synaptic inter-connections between LHRH, GAD, TH and ACTH hypothalamic neurons involved in the control of gonadotrophin release in the rat, *Neurosci. Lett. Suppl.* **22:**598.

Leranth, C., MacLusky, N. J., and Naftolin, F., 1986, Inter-connections between neurotransmitter and neuropeptide containing neurons involved in gonadotrophin release in rat, in: *Neural and Endocrine Peptides and Receptors* (T. W. Moody, ed.), Plenum Press, New York, pp: 177–193.

Leranth, C., MacLusky, N. J., Shanabrough, M., and Naftolin, F., 1988a, Immunohistochemical evidence for synaptic connections between proopiomelanicortin immunoreactive axons and LHRH neurons in the preoptic area of the rat, *Brain Res.* **449:**167–176.

Leranth, C., MacLusky, N. J., Sharabrough, M., and Naftolin, F., 1988b, Catecholaminergic innervation of LHRH and GAD immunoreactive neurons in the rat medial preoptic area: an electron microscopic double immunostaining and degeneration study, *Neuroendocrinology* **48:**591–602.

Levey, A. I., Bolam, J. P., Rye, D. B., Hallanger, A. E., Demuth, R. M., Mesulam, M. M., and Wainer, B. H., 1986, A light and electron microscopic procedure for sequential double antigen localization using diaminobenzidine and benzidine dihydrochloride, *J. Histochem. Cytochem.* **34:**1449–1457.

Liposits, Z., Görcs, T., Török, A., Dómány, S., and Sétáló, G., 1983, Simultaneous localization of two different tissue antigens based on the silver intensified PAP–DAB and the traditional PAP–DAB methods, *Acta Morphol. Acad. Sci. Hung.* **31:**356–369.

Liposits, Z., Sétáló, G., and Flerkó, B., 1984, Application of the silver–gold intensified 3,3'-diaminobenzidine chromogen to the light and electron microscopic detection of the LH-RH system of the rat brain, *Neuroscience* **13:**513–525.

Liposits, Z., Phelix, C., and Paull, W. K., 1986a, Adrenergic innervation of corticotropin releasing factor (CRF)-synthesizing neurons in the hypothalamic paraventricular nucleus of the rat. A combined light and electron microscopic immunocytochemical study, *Histochemistry* **84:**201–205.

Liposits, Z., Sherman, D., Phelix, C., and Paull, W. K., 1986b, A combined light and electron microscopic immunocytochemical method for the simultaneous localization of multiple tissue antigens: TH immunoreactive innervation of CRF synthesizing neurons in the paraventricular nucleus of the rat, *Histochemistry* **85:**95–106.

MacMillan, F. M., and Cuello, A. C., 1986, Monoclonal antibodies in neurohistochemistry: The state of the art, in: *Neurohistochemistry: Modern Methods and Applications* (P. Panula, H. Paivarinta, and S. Soinila, eds.), Alan R. Liss, New York, pp. 49–74.

McLean, D. C., and Singer, S. J., 1970, A general method for the specific staining of intracellular antigens with ferritin–antibody conjugates, *Proc. Natl. Acad. Sci. U.S.A.* **65:**122–128.

McLean S., Skirboll, L. R., and Pert, C. B., 1983, Opiatergic projection from the bed nucleus to the habenula: Demonstration by a novel radioimmunohistochemical method, *Brain Res.* **278:**255–257.

McLean, S., Skirboll, L. R., and Pert, C. B., 1985, Comparison of substance P and enkephalin distribution in rat brain: An overview using radioimmunocytochemistry, *Neuroscience* **14:**837–852.

Mesulam, M.-M., and Rosene, D. L., 1979, Sensitivity in horseradish peroxidase neurohistochemistry: A comparative and quantitative analysis of nine methods, *J. Histochem. Cytochem.* **27:**763–773.

Milner, T. A., and Pickel, V. M., 1986, Neurotensin in the rat parabrachial region: Ultrastructural localization and extrinsic sources of immunoreactivity, *J. Comp. Neurol.* **247:**326–343.

Milner, T. A., Pickel, V. M., Chan, J., Massari, V. J., Oertel, W. H., Park, D. H., Joh, T. H., and Reis, D. J., 1987, Adrenaline neurons in the rostral ventrolateral medulla: II. Synaptic relationships with GABAergic terminals, *Brain Res.* **411**:46–57.

Molin, S.-O., Nygren, H., and Dolonius, L., 1978, A new method for the study of glutaraldehyde-induced cross-linking properties in proteins with special reference to the reaction with amino groups, *J. Histochem. Cytochem.* **26**:412–414.

Painter, R. G., Tokuyasu, K. T., and Singer, S. J., 1973, Immunoferritin localization of intracellular antigens: The use of ultracryotomy to obtain ultrathin sections suitable for direct immunoferritin staining, *Proc. Natl. Acad. Sci. U.S.A.* **70**:1649–1653.

Pearson, A. A., and O'Neil, S. L., 1958, A silver gelatine method for staining nerve fibers, *Anat. Rec.* **95**:297–301.

Petrusz, P., 1983, Essential requirements for the validity of immunocytochemical staining procedures, *J. Histochem. Cytochem.* **34**:177–179.

Phil, E., 1967, Ultrastructural localization of heavy metals by a modified sulfide silver method, *Histochemie* **10**:126–139.

Pickel, V. M., 1981, Immunocytochemical methods, in: *Neuroanatomical Tract-Tracing Methods* (L. Heimer and M. J. RoBards, eds.), Plenum Press, New York, pp. 483–509.

Pickel, V. M., 1985, Ultrastructure of central catecholaminergic neurons, in: *Neurohistochemistry Today* (P. Peuula, H. Paivarimpa, and S. Soiuila, eds.), Alan R. Liss, New York, pp. 379–424.

Pickel, V. M., and Beaudet, A., 1984, Combined use of autoradiography and immunocytochemical methods to show synaptic interactions between chemically defined neurons, in: *Immunolabeling for Electron Microscopy* (J. M. Polak and J. M. Varnell, eds.), Elsevier, Amsterdam, pp. 259–265.

Pickel, V. M., and Teitelman, G., 1983, Light and electron microscopic localization of single and multiple antigens, in: *Histochemical and Ultrastructural Identification of Monoamine Neurons* (J. Furness and M. Costa, eds.), John Wiley & Sons, New York, pp. 79–109.

Pickel, V., Chan, J., Joh, T., and Massari, V., 1984, Catecholaminergic neurons in the medial nuclei of the solitary tracts receive direct synapses from GABA-gabaergic terminals: Combined colloidal gold and peroxidase labeling of synthesizing enzymes, *Soc. Neurosci. Abstr.* **1**:537.

Pickel, V. M., Chan, J., and Milner, T. A., 1986a, Autoradiographic detection of (^{125}-I)-secondary antiserum: A sensitive light and electron microscopic labeling method compatible with peroxidase immunocytochemistry for dual localization of neuronal antigens, *J. Histochem. Cytochem.* **34**:707–718.

Pickel, V. M., Chan, J., and Ganten, D., 1986b, Dual peroxidase and colloidal gold-labeling study of angiotensin converting enzyme and angiotensin-like immunoreactivity in the rat subfornical organ, *J. Neurosci.* **6**:2457–2469.

Pickel, V. M., Chan, J., Park, D. H., Joh, T. H., and Milner, T. A., 1986c, Ultrastructural localization of phenylethanolamine N-methyltransferase in sensory and motor nuclei of the vagus nerve, *J. Neurosci. Res.* **15**:439–455.

Pickel, V. M., Joh, T. H., and Chan, J., 1988a, Dual ultrastructural localization of choline acetyltransferase and tyrosine hydroxylase in the rat caudate nucleus, *Brain Res.* (in preparation).

Pickel, V. M., Chan, J., and Milner, T. A., 1988b, Cellular substrates for interactions between neurons containing PNMT and GABA in the nuclei of solitary tracts, *J. Comp. Neurol.* (in press).

Polak, J. M., and Van Noorden, S. (eds.), 1983, *Immunocytochemistry: Practical Applications in Pathology and Biology*, Wright, Bristol.

Priestley, C. V., and Cuello, A. C., 1982, Co-existence of neuroactive substances as revealed by immunohistochemistry with monoclonal antibodies, in: *Cotransmission* (A. C. Cuello, ed.), Macmillan, London, pp. 117–128.

Roth, J., 1982, The preparation of protein A-gold complexes with 3 nm and 15 nm gold particles and their use in labeling multiple antigens on ultrathin sections, *Histochem J.* **14**:791–801.

Roth, J., Bendayan, M., and Orci, L., 1978, Ultrastructural localization of intracellular antigens by the use of protein A–gold complex, *J. Histochem. Cytochem.* **26**:1074–1081.

Salpeter, M. M., Bachman, L., and Salpeter, E. E., 1969, Resolution in electron microscopic autoradiography, *J. Cell Biol.* **41**:1–20.

Salpeter, M. M., Fertuck, H. C., and Salpeter, E. E., 1977, Resolution in electron microscopic autoradiography III. Iodine-125, the effect of heavy metal staining and reassessment of critical parameters, *J. Cell. Biol.* **72**:161–173.

Schachner, M., Hedley-Whyte, E. T., Hse, D. W., Schoonmaker, G., and Bignami, A., 1977, Ultrastructural localization of glial fibrillary acidic protein in mouse cerebellum by immunoperoxidase labeling, *J. Cell Biol.* **75**:67–73.

Singer, R. S., and Schick, A. I., 1961, The properties of specific stains for electron microscopy prepared by conjugation of antibody with ferritin, *J. Biophys. Biochem. Cytol.* **9**:519–537.

Slot, J., and Gueze, H., 1981, Sizing of protein A-colloidal gold probes for immuno-electron microscopy, *J. Cell. Biol.* **90**:533–536.

Somogyi, P., and Takagi, H., 1982, A note on the use of picric acid paraformaldehyde–glutaraldehyde fixative for correlated light and electron microscopic immunocytochemistry, *Neuroscience* **7**:1779–1784.

Stathis, E. C., and Fabrikanos, A., 1958, Preparation of colloidal gold, *Chem. Ind.* **27**:860–861.

Steinbusch, H. W. M., Verhofstaad, A. A. J., and Joosten, H. W. J., 1978, Localization of serotonin in the central nervous system by immunohistochemistry: Description of a specific and sensitive technique and some applications. *Neuroscience* **3**:811–819.

Sternberger, L. A., 1979, *Immunocytochemistry*, John Wiley & Sons, New York, Chicago, Brisbane, Toronto.

Sternberger, L. A., and Joseph, S. H., 1979, The unlabeled antibody method. Contrasting color staining of paired pituitary hormones without antibody removal, *J. Histochem. Cytochem.* **27**:1424–1429.

Sternberger, L. A., Hardy, P. H., Cuculis, J. J., and Meyers, H. G., 1970, The unlabeled antibody enzyme method of immunohistochemistry preparation and properties of soluble antigen–antibody complex (Horseradish peroxidase–antiperoxidase) and its use in identification of spirochetes. *J. Histochem. Cytochem.* **18**:315–333.

Tapia, F., Varndell, I., Robert, M., DeMey, J., and Polak, J., 1983, Double immunogold staining method for simultaneous ultrastructural localization of regulatory peptides, *J. Histochem. Cytochem.* **31**:977–981.

Tryer, N. M., and Bell, E. M., 1974, The intensification of cobalt-filled neuron profiles using a modification of Timm's sulphide silver method, *Brain Res.* **73**:151–155.

van den Pol, A. N., 1984, Colloidal gold and biotin–avidin conjugates as ultrastructural markers for neural antigens, *Q. J. Exp. Physiol.* **69**:1–33.

van den Pol, A. N., 1985a, Silver-intensified gold and peroxidase as dual ultrastructural immunolabels for pre- and postsynaptic neurotransmitters, *Science* **228**:332–335.

van den Pol, A. N., 1985b, Dual ultrastructural localization of two neurotransmitter-related antigens: Colloidal gold-label neurophysin-immunoreactive supraoptic neurons receive peroxidase-labeled glutamate decarboxylase- or gold-labeled GABA-immunoreactive synapses, *J. Neurosci.* **11**:2940–2954.

van den Pol, A. N., and Görcs, T., 1985, Suprachiasmatic nucleus, synaptic relationships: a dual ultrastructural immunocytochemistry study with peroxidase and gold substituted silver peroxidase, *Soc. Neurosci. Abstr.* **11**:34.

van den Pol, A. N., and Görcs, T., 1986, Synaptic relationships between neurons containing vasopressin, gastrin releasing hormone, VIP, and GAD immunoreactivity in the rat suprachiasmatic nucleus: Dual ultrastructural immunocytochemistry with gold substituted silver peroxidase, *J. Comp. Neurol.* **252**:507–521.

van den Pol, A. N., Smith, A. D., and Powell, J. F., 1985, GABA axons in synaptic contact with dopamine neurons in the substantia nigra: Double immunocytochemistry with biotin–peroxidase and protein A–colloidal gold, *Brain Res.* **348**:146–154.

Verhofstaad, A. A. J., Steinbusch, H. W. M., Joosten, H. W. J., Penke, B., Varga, J., and Goldstein, M., 1983, Immunocytochemical localization of noradrenaline, adrenaline and serotonin, in: *Immunocytochemistry. Practical Applications in Pathology and Biology* J. M. Polak and S. Van Noorden, eds.), Wrigle, Bristol, pp. 143–167.

Williams, T. H., and Jew, J. Y., 1975, An improved method for perfusion fixation of neural tissues for electron microscopy, *Tissue Cell* **7:**407–418.

Zaborszky, L., Heimer, L., Eckenstein, F., and Leranth, C., 1986, GABAergic input to cholinergic forebrain neurons: An ultrastructural study using retrograde tracing of HRP and double immunolabeling, *J. Comp. Neurol.* **250:**282–295.

7

Intracellular Labeling and Immunocytochemistry

STEPHEN T. KITAI, G. RICHARD PENNY, and HOWARD T. CHANG

I. INTRODUCTION

Since its introduction in 1976 (Cullheim and Kellerth, 1976; Jankowska *et al.*, 1976; Kitai *et al.*, 1976; Light and Durkovic, 1976; Snow *et al.*, 1976), the method of intracellular injection of horseradish peroxidase (HRP) has established itself as an enormously productive tool for neurobiology (Kitai and Bishop, 1981; Kitai and Wilson, 1982). The fundamental advantage of the technique is that it allows direct correspondence between cellular physiology and morphology to be established. First, as a physiological tool, the HRP-filled microelectrode is suitable for the analysis of any neurophysiological property of a neuron that can be assayed by intracellular recording. Second, as a morphological tool, intracellular iontophoresis of HRP fills and labels the entire extent of a neuron, including soma, dendrites, dendritic specializations such as spines, and as much of the axon, axonal collaterals, and terminals as survival time permits. The morphological rendition of the HRP-filled neuron revealed by enzyme histochemistry is equal to or better than the results of the very best Golgi stains.

STEPHEN T. KITAI, G. RICHARD PENNY, and HOWARD T. CHANG • Department of Anatomy and Neurobiology, College of Medicine, University of Tennessee, Memphis, Tennessee 38163.

The many advantages offered by intracellular labeling are now exploited by many laboratories around the world, using a variety of preparations including both *in vivo* animals and the *in vitro* brain slice. Since the HRP reaction product is permanent, sections processed for HRP-labeled neurons can be stored archivally. Another major advantage is that the material containing neurons intracellularly filled by HRP is subsequently compatible with processing for immunocytochemistry. The combination of intracellular HRP labeling with immunocytochemistry offers the possibility of determining the neurotransmitter of an identified neuron (Chang *et al.*, 1986; see also Section V) or of identifying the neurotransmitter contained within terminals contacting an identified neuron (Penny *et al.*, 1986). We have also used this combination for visualizing the neuronal processes arising from single identified neurons and for defining their relationship to tissue boundaries revealed by immunocytochemical techniques. Some examples from our study of the striatum are presented following a description of the methodologies. The two techniques, intracellular labeling and immunocytochemistry, can also be applied in conjunction with ultrastructural analysis; techniques for preparation and electron microscopic examination of tissue are described in the next two chapters of this volume.

II. METHODOLOGY

A. Intracellular Labeling with Horseradish Peroxidase

1. The Recording Apparatus

The apparatus for intracellular recording and HRP injection includes (1) a biological bridge amplifier with the capability for capacitance compensation, transient suppression, and intracellular current injection, (2) oscilloscopes, (3) an audio amplifier, (4) an EKG amplifier, (5) a stimulator consisting of a timing device and two or more stimulus isolation units, each with a capability of constant-current and constant-voltage stimulation, (6) a micromanipulator (e.g., Narishige Canberra type), and (7) a mechanism for storing the electrophysiological traces. For this latter function, we use a Nicolet digital oscilloscope to digitize the traces. These are subsequently fed to a PDP 11-23 computer for storage and later analysis (Park, 1985). Publication-quality reproductions of the traces can be obtained using an *X–Y* plotter such as the HP7470A. A digital voltmeter with a range of ±0–200 mV is also useful for monitoring resting potentials. A typical apparatus is shown in Fig. 1. The electronic components of the apparatus are usually mounted for convenience in standard 19-inch electronics racks (e.g., Amco Engineering); signal paths can be interconnected on the front panel by standard BNC cables or can be carried to the back for a cleaner look. Advice for arranging the grounds and shields is provided in Brown *et al.* (1973) and Morrison (1986).

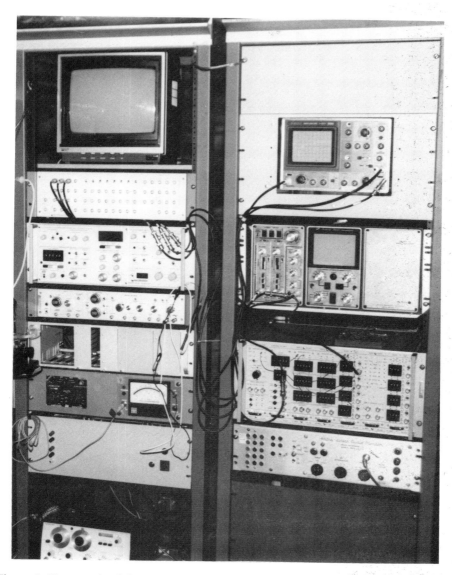

Figure 1. Photograph of the electronic components of typical electrophysiological apparatus. Left rack from top to bottom: video monitor (NEC), digital interface (Axon Instrument), voltage/current-clamp electrometer (amplifier and current injector)(Axon Instrument), intracellular electrometer (amplifier and current injector)(NeuroData), empty panel, calibrator (Stoelting)(left side), telemetric thermometer (YSI)(right side), DC power supply, waveform generator (Wave Tek). Right rack from top to bottom: monitor analogue oscilloscope (Hitachi), digital oscilloscope (Nicolet), electrical pulse generator (stimulator)(Hi-med), audio monitor amplifier (Grass Instrument).

2. The Preparation

a. *In Vivo* Preparation. Adult male hooded rats are anesthetized with intraperitoneal injection of urethane (1 g/kg) supplemented with intramuscular injection of ketamine (70 mg/kg) as needed. Strict precautions must be taken with the use of urethane, as it is a suspected carcinogen. Administration of dexamethasone at least 1 hr prior to the experiment may serve to reduce edema. The animal is placed in a stereotaxic frame (Kopf) and suspended with clamps at C2 and the tail root from a spinal stand (Fig. 2) placed on a gymbal–piston vibration-resistant table (e.g., Technical Manufacturing Corp.). Suspension of the animal avoids transfer of vascular and respiratory pulsation to the cranium. It is often necessary to readjust the suspension if pulsation becomes a problem. The spinal stand is useful both for suspending the animal and for arranging ancillary devices such as the amplifier head stage, a small box for connecting stimulator leads, and a light

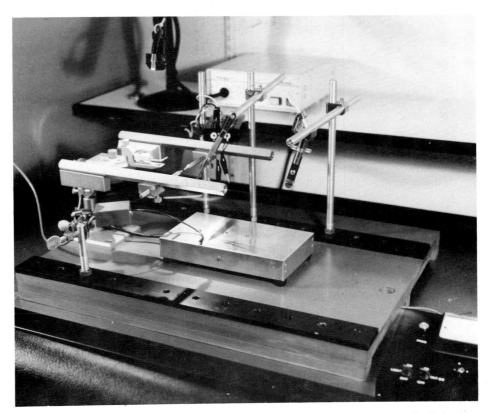

Figure 2. Photograph of a spinal stand with attached stereotaxic instrument, C2 and tail clamps, amplifier head stage, stimulator lead box, and animal thermoregulator. A fiberoptic light source provides illumination.

source. The stereotaxic frame and the micromanipulator should be attached firmly to the spinal stand. Spinal stands are available commercially from Narishige or can be manufactured from a 1-inch-thick sheet of PVC plastic (18 × 24 inches) with steel bar stocks attached at the edges and with rows of 1/2-inch–12 holes drilled and tapped at 2-inch intervals in the bar stocks. A boom-arm dissection microscope with a × 0.5 auxiliary lens to increase working distance is adequate for viewing the preparation.

The bone and dura overlying the stimulation and recording sites are removed, and bipolar stimulating electrodes (epoxylite-insulated steel insect pins bared 0.2 to 0.5 mm at the tips) are stereotaxically positioned in afferent areas (e.g., in the case of neostriatum, the cortex, substantia nigra, and thalamus) and affixed in place with skull screws and dental cement (e.g., Durelon carboxylate cement). A recording well is constructed of dental cement around the exposed recording site, and this recording well is sealed with melted paraffin (prepared by mixing paraffin wax with paraffin oil to yield a melting point slightly above 40°C) after each insertion of a microelectrode in order to reduce cerebral pulsations. Prior to recording, the cisterna magna is pierced to relieve CSF pressure; this procedure also helps to reduce cerebral pulsations. The temperature of the animal is maintained between 37 and 38°C by a feedback control device. Monitoring the EKG helps to assay the depth of anesthesia.

b. *In Vitro* Slice Preparation. For the experiments combining intracellular recording and labeling, slices are prepared from ether-anesthetized animals perfused through the heart with a small volume (20 to 50 ml) of cold (5 to 10°C) oxygenated Krebs–Ringer's solution. The perfusion is helpful in reducing staining of erythrocytes in blood vessels, which often obscure the HRP-labeled neurons. Perfusion prior to decapitation does not seem to alter electrophysiological activities of the slice. Immediately after perfusion, the rat is decapitated, and the brain gently removed from the skull. Slices are prepared using a tissue chopper, Vibratome, or Vibroslicer. With the tissue chopper method, the structure to be sectioned is initially supported by a small piece of filter paper. The tissue is sectioned with the tissue chopper in parasagittal planes of a thickness of about 350 μm. It is important to use a clean and sharp razor blade on the tissue chopper to ensure better survival of the slice. With the Vibratome sectioning method, the brain is placed immediately in a small Petri dish containing cold (~5°C) oxygenated Krebs–Ringer. The brain is cut by hand into an appropriately oriented block (i.e., frontal, sagittal, etc.) with a razor blade. The tissue block is then glued to the cutting stage of a Vibratome using a cyanoacrylic cement. The Vibratome bath is filled with cold Krebs–Ringer's solution, and the block is sectioned to approximately 350-μm thickness. Four to six slices are stored in a beaker containing continuously oxygenated Krebs–Ringer at room temperature until each slice is ready to be used for recording. We have usually found it best to store the tissue in this manner at least 1–2 hr prior to recording. For both tissue chopper and Vibratome sectioning methods, the

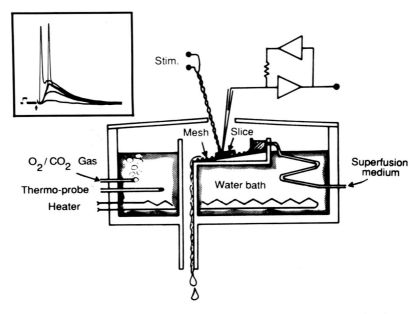

Figure 3. A schematic diagram of a slice chamber and intracellular records showing an anti-dromic action potential and monosynaptic EPSPs with an action potential evoked by stimulation locally applied to the slice preparation. Five traces with different stimulus intensities are super-imposed. Calibration pulse: 5 mV in amplitude and 2 msec in duration. An arrow indicates stimulation onset. Stimulation duration is 0.2 msec.

entire operation from decapitation to placement of the slices in oxygenated Krebs–Ringer should be carried out within 15 to 20 min.

In vitro recording (Fig. 3) requires a chamber in which the slice is maintained. Most of the slice chambers are constructed of acrylic plastic (Plexiglas). The chamber consists of a recording well and a water bath. A suitable bath can readily be custom constructed or is available commercially from Stoelting. The temperature of the water bath is kept constant at 37°C with a thermostatic heater. The O_2/CO_2 gas is pumped continuously through the waterbath to create a warm, moist environment over the recording chamber. The superfusing Krebs–Ringer passes by gravity feed to the recording well via a heat exchanger in the water bath. One end of the recording chamber is raised so that the Krebs–Ringer can run past at a rate of 1.0 ml/min. The slice surface is free of Krebs–Ringer and is directly exposed to the warm and moist O_2/CO_2 gas mixture. A boom-arm dissection microscope is placed over the slice chamber for visualization of stimulation and recording electrode placements. Further details on the slice preparation and chamber can be found in Dingledine (1984).

The Krebs–Ringer's solution is composed as follows: NaCl 124.0 mM, KCl 5.1mM, $MgSO_4$ 1.3 mM, $CaCl_2$ 2.5 mM, KH_2PO_4 1.25 mM, $NaHCO_3$ 26.0 mM, and D-glucose 10.0 mM. The pH of the Krebs–Ringer is maintained at

7.3 to 7.4 by bubbling a gas mixture of 95% O_2/5% CO_2 through the perfusate. The osmolarity of the Krebs–Ringer is checked prior to the experiment with an osmometer and adjusted to 305 ± 5 mOsm. It is noteworthy to mention that the Ca^{2+} concentration of the Krebs–Ringer is a factor in determining patterns of synaptic response in neostriatal slice preparations; using a Krebs–Ringer of a similar composition to that above except with only 1.2 mM $CaCl_2$ (Misgeld and Bak, 1979) prevents the recording of inhibitory responses. On the other hand, inhibition was observed when the concentration of $CaCl_2$ was raised to 2.3 to 2.5 mM (Lighthall *et al.*, 1981).

3. The Microelectrode and Marker

Microelectrode fabrication for both the *in vivo* and *in vitro* preparation is the same. The characteristics of the microelectrode are determined by the need for acceptable intracellular recordings rather than by any special requirements for injection of HRP. Glass microelectrodes with tip diameter less than 1 μm (probably in the range between 0.5 and 0.1 μm) are necessary to penetrate CNS neurons successfully; these microelectrodes are pulled immediately before use from 10cm blanks of 2- or 3-mm Pyrex glass using a Narishige vertical puller. The microelectrodes are then bumped under microscopic observation and epiillumination by using the microscope stage to manipulate the electrode tip into contact with a roughened glass surface. Bands of interference colors produced near the electrode tip can be used to provide an indication of resultant tip size. A scanning electron micrograph of an electrode tip is shown in Fig. 4.

The electrodes are filled with 4% HRP in 0.5 M potassium methylsulfate or 0.5 M KCL and 0.05 M Tris buffer, pH 7.6, yielding electrodes with resistances in the range between 50 and 100 MΩ. The electrodes are filled by placing several μl of solution in the barrel of the microelectrode with a Hamilton syringe and then using a fine glass filament to work the solution into and bubbles out of the shaft and tip of the electrode. Further descriptions of microelectrodes and their uses can be found in Purves (1981) and in Brown and Flaming (1986).

4. Recording and Injection Procedures

a. *In Vivo* Procedure. Care must be taken as the electrode is inserted through the relatively tough surface of the brain to not break or clog the tip. It may be necessary to carry out a suction ablation of overlying tissues to avoid this problem. As the electrode is advanced by the micromanipulator through the tissue, an 0.5-nA, 10-msec hyperpolarizing square-wave pulse is passed across the electrode once each sweep and used initially to balance the amplifier bridge and subsequently to monitor electrode impedance. An increase in electrode impedance (signaled by an increase in the voltage drop across the

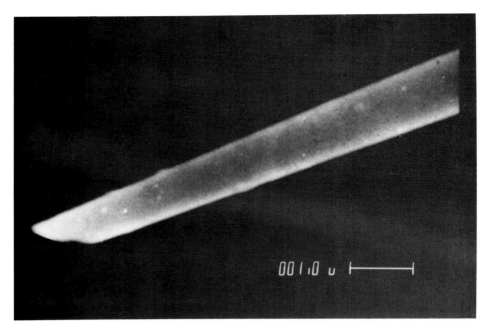

Figure 4. A scanning electron micrograph of an electrode tip after bumping to suitable size.

electrode during this constant-current pulse) is often an indication that the electrode tip is in contact with somatic membrane of a neuron. The "cell penetrator" is used to establish brief potentials across the electrode tip (10–50 V, 2–50 msec), facilitating the penetration of neurons. It is equally effective to use constant-current pulses or oscillations because of excess capacitance compensation ("ringing the electrode") to achieve penetration. Successful penetrations are signaled by a potential drop to a stable resting potential, the presence of postsynaptic potentials in response to stimulation, and action potentials of at least 45 mV. Recordings that fail to meet these standards are discarded, and the penetration is continued. After completion of a protocol of neurophysiological analysis, the neuron receives an injection of HRP via iontophoresis. We use an injection current of 2 to 5 nA square-wave depolarizing pulses, 100–150 msec in length, delivered 5/sec. A hyperpolarizing current of up to 1.0 nA may be maintained during the off period of the cycle. Typically 5–10 min of injection is sufficient to recover a well-filled neuron; 30 min facilitates the tracings of axons over longer distances, and injection times as short as 3 min allow lightly stained neurons to be recovered. Such lightly stained neurons are valuble for electron microscopic studies, as the cellular organelles are less likely to be obscured by a dense accumulation of osmiophilic HRP reaction product.

   For reliable recovery of an intracellularly labeled neuron, it is crucial that the penetration remain secure and stable and that the injection current be terminated on deterioration of the cell. It is much easier to recover a well-stained profile from a healthy neuron than from one that displayed little resting potential or that lost its spikes or passive membrane potentials. The diffusion of HRP through the dendrites and proximal axonal arborization occurs swiftly, and only a few minutes of survival is sufficient to recover a neuron excellently filled to this extent. However, to trace axons for more than a few millimeters, longer survival times of 12 to 24 hr may be necessary. When neurons have been recovered after such survival times, it has sometimes been possible to trace axons for long distances. Unfortunately, it is difficult to recover neurons after long survival; in most cells that are recovered after survival times of this duration, the cell body and dendrites have undergone a considerable degree of degeneration. Degeneration of the axon appears to proceed more slowly, and it is often possible to gather useful information about the axonal arborization of a neuron whose soma and dendrites are severely degenerated.

b. *In Vitro* Slice Procedure. The following procedures are used for intracellular labeling of neurons with HRP (Kitai and Kita, 1984). When a neuron is penetrated and has a stable resting potential of -40 mV or lower, HRP is iontophoretically injected using 1- to 3-mA rectangular depolarizing pulses of 150-msec duration at 3.3 Hz for 3 to 5 min. After the injection is completed, the slice containing the labeled neuron is carefully placed on a small piece of lens paper saturated with the Krebs–Ringer's solution. The paper with the slice is gently floated onto fixative solution containing 0.5 to 4.0% formaldehyde and 1.0 to 2.0% glutaraldehyde in standard isotonic buffer for 30 sec to 1 min. The lens paper is then upturned, and the slice immersed in the fixative. This procedure of transporting the slice on the lens paper prevents it from curling during fixation. Slices with injected neurons are allowed to remain 3 to 12 hr in the fixative. Following fixation, each slice is sectioned at 50 μm using either a sliding freezing microtome or a Vibratome. For Vibratome sectioning, the slice is embedded in warm agar (2%), and the agar is cut into a block prior to sectioning. The sections are processed according to the standard HRP procedures.

B. Histology and Immunocytochemistry

1. Fixation and Sectioning

The histochemical localization of intracellularly injected HRP is surprisingly resilient with regard to changes in fixation protocols; most commonly used formaldehyde–glutaraldehyde fixations are adequate. On the other hand, high-quality immunocytochemical labeling is extremely dependent on the conditions of fixation, and the fixation of choice varies for different antisera, species, and brain structures. Moreover, the choice of fixative can be used to enhance the labeling of particular features of interest; for example, the preservation provided by one fixative may be particularly good for revealing immunoreactive cell bodies with a given antiserum, and another fixative better for revealing immunoreactive terminals with that same antiserum. It is important to assess a variety of fixatives in order to choose one that yields the optimum immunocytochemical labeling, and it is likely that whatever fixative is chosen will also serve well for the localization of intracellularly injected HRP.

Several good perfusion fixations for immunocytochemistry that are compatible with HRP histochemistry include (1) the periodate, lysine, and paraformaldehyde fixation of McLean and Nakane (1974) (0.01 M sodium periodate, 0.075 M lysine, 2% paraformaldehyde in 0.037 M phosphate buffer, pH 7.4), (2) the same solution as in (1) but with the addition of 0.02 to 0.2% glutaraldehyde, (3) the variable-pH fixation of Berod *et al.* (1981) (4% paraformaldehyde in 0.15 M acetate buffer, pH 6.5, for 5 min, followed by 4% paraformaldehyde in 0.15 M borate buffer, pH 11, for 15 min), (4) the same fixation as in (3) but with the addition of 0.05 to 0.2% glutaraldehyde to both solutions, (5) 4% paraformaldehyde in 0.15 M phosphate buffer, pH 7.4, followed by a rinse with 10% sucrose in phosphate buffer. Brief saline rinses can be used prior to any of these fixations. Use of a fixative containing at least 0.05 to 0.2% glutaraldehyde is usually necessary for adequate ultrastructural preservation for electron microscopy, but excess glutaraldehyde is to be avoided because it suppresses the immunoreactivity of many substances.

After removal, the brain may be either postfixed overnight or stored in phosphate buffer until sectioned. Sections through the block of tissue containing the HRP-filled neuron should be cut using a Vibratome or Vibroslicer; frozen sections result in loss of morphological detail in the immunocytochemical labeling. Sections of about 50-μm thickness are optimum for drawing and reconstructing intracellularly labeled neurons, and we often use sections of this thickness for combined intracellular labeling and immunocytochemistry as well. However, penetration of immunoreagents is limited in sections of this thickness (without Triton X-100 detergent treatment, terminal labeling in Vibratome sections is confined to the outer 3 μm of tissue). If increased penetration is needed, thinner sections can be cut and methods to enhance penetration applied, such as alcohol treatment, detergent treatment, or freeze–thawing. The Vibratome can reliably cut sections 20 μm in thickness, and from small blocks of very well fixed material, 10-μm sections can be achieved. Alternatively, the tissue can be embedded in polyethylene glycol prior to sectioning and histochemical processing (Scholer and Armstrong, 1982). This approach allows sections as thin as 2μm to be prepared. Thinner sections increase the amount of effort required to draw and reconstruct the sections containing intracellularly labeled neuronal processes.

2. Histochemistry for Intracellular HRP

Because of its noncrystalline reaction product, diaminobenzidine (DAB) is the best chromogen for use where preservation of morphological detail is desired, and because of its osmiophilic nature, it is the reaction substrate of choice for electron microscopic applications. Strict precautions must be taken with its use, however, as it is thought to be a carcinogen. We use the sensitive glucose-oxidase-coupled reaction of Itoh *et al.* (1979) after optional pretreatment with 0.5% cobalt chloride in Tris-buffered saline (Adams, 1977) in order to obtain a blue-black reaction product. After the reaction, the sections are washed with buffer and then examined wet under the microscope to locate labeled cells and their processes. Note that if sections reacted by the cobalt-chloride–DAB method are subsequently stained with osmium and embedded in plastic, the black reaction product becomes brown and indiscriminable in appearance from that obtained from DAB alone.

3. Blocking Steps and Treatment with the Primary Antibody

Sections to be processed for immunocytochemistry may be incubated under agitation for 2 to 12 hr in 2–10% normal serum (from the same species as that in which the secondary or linking antiserum was raised) dissolved in phosphate-buffered saline in order to reduce nonspecific or background staining; this step may be deleted if nonspecific staining is not a problem. The phosphate-buffered saline consists of 0.01 M sodium (PBS) or potassium (KPBS) phosphate buffer in 0.9% sodium chloride. Triton X-100 may be included to enhance subsequent immunoreagent penetration. Sodium azide (0.02 M) may also be included in diluted solutions of normal sera to act as a preservative, allowing them to be made up ahead of time, but should never be present in avidin–biotinylated horseradish peroxidase (ABC) or peroxidase–antiperoxidase (PAP) reagents. Disposable plastic culture tubes (10 × 75 mm) provide a convenient vessel for incubating sectins, and 500 to 1000 μl is a sufficient volume of reagent.

The sections are then incubated under agitation in diluted primary antibody or antiserum in 2% normal serum in PBS or KPBS (e.g., rabbit anti-[leu]-enkephalin serum, 1 : 3000, in KPBS containing 2% normal goat serum). The choice of PBS or KPBS may affect the quality of staining by the primary antiserum; both should be tried in initial trials. Various incubation times should be tried in the range between 2 and 72 hr; as a general rule, short incubations are better for immunolabeling of cell bodies, and long incubations are better for terminals. Incubations of 8 hr or longer are best carried out at 4°C.

4. Controls

It is necessary in every immunocytochemical experiment to include a set of control sections processed in such a way as to help confirm the validity of the results; immunocytochemical staining should be absent in such sections. Normal (or preimmune) serum control reagents, used for polyclonal antisera, are prepared identically to the primary antiserum reagent with the exception that normal serum from the same species as the one in which the primary antiserum was raised is substituted at the same dilution for the primary antiserum. Sections that serve as normal serum controls are incubated in this reagent rather than in the primary antiserum but are otherwise treated identically to standard sections. For monoclonal antibodies, which contain no serum, deletion of the primary antibody is appropriate. Control sections incubated in primary antibody or serum that has been preadsorbed with the antigenic substance are useful if that substance is readily available. Achieving blank preadsorbed controls is not altogether easy and often in fact requires a great deal of effort.

It is a good idea to determine the antibody titer prior to preadsorption; this procedure is easily carried out with a minimum in equipment by the ELISPOT assay (Czerkensky *et al.*, 1983) using a simple apparatus available from Bio-Rad Laboratories. It can be a mistake to skip this step and to attempt instead the preadsorption using an excess of antigen. In the presence of an excess of antigen, unstable triplet complexes can form, consisting of two antigen molecules and one antibody. Dissociation of one of the bonds can allow the antibody to bind the tissue. An antigen–antibody ratio of 1 : 1 favors the formation of more stable cyclic complexes consisting of two antibody molecules and two antigens; this complex remains solubilized and is removed by washes (Sternberger, 1986). Prevention of oxidation of the antigenic compound (as readily occurs for [Met]-enkephalin) and of proteolysis of the antigenic compound (prevented by bacitracin treatment) are both necessary. If the antiserum was raised against a hapten (e.g., most amino acid transmitters) linked to a carrier molecule such as bovine serum albumin (BSA), it is usually necessary to preadsorb using the hapten–carrier molecular complex. This can often be created by incubating the hapten with BSA in the prescence of glutaraldehyde (to form a hapten–BSA complex) and then dialyzing the reaction mixture to remove unbound hapten and glutaraldehyde. As an aside, antisera raised against glutaraldehyde- linked hapten–carrier complexes often provide better immunocytochemical results if used on tissue fixed with at least some glutaraldehyde. A primary antiserum dilution series also serves as a useful control. If staining results from binding of the primary antiserum rather than some other cause, intensity of staining should increase in proportion to antiserum concentration. Use of more than one antibody for a given antigen is also useful—the results should match. It should be pointed out that the controls by no means prove the specificity of the results; they are merely helpful in that regard. Hence, conservative terminology, such as "enkephalin immunoreactivity," is retained as opposed to "enkephalin localization" to emphasize the logical difference between the true distribution of the neruoactive substance and the experimental result.

It is equally important to interpret the quality and believability of the staining pattern on less formal, more intuitive grounds. This is done by ensuring that the staining includes structures described by previous workers in parts of the brain other than the particular region of interest, by ensuring that the staining pattern is crisp and well localized to appropriate biological structures, and that indiscriminate, improbable staining is absent.

The chances of achieving blank controls and high-quality immunocyto-chemical labeling are maximized by (1) using the highest dilutions of primary and secondary antisera possible, (2) using fixation protocols best for a particular antiserum and region of the brain, and (3) avoiding where possible the use of colchicine treatment because of its tendency to increase background labeling, penetrate unevenly, and cause abnormal cellular morphology.

5. Localization of the Primary Antibody by the ABC Method

After the incubation in primary antiserum, the sections should be washed well in PBS. We use six rinses of 2 min each. Porcelain Gooch crucibles, 30-ml size, provide a good vehicle for transferring the sections through the buffer washes, which can be contained in ice cube trays or in plastic egg cartons (available from purveyors of camping supplies). The ABC method (Hsu *et al.*, 1981) is used to localize the primary antiserum; this procedure is easier and generally more reliable than the PAP method. The reagents are obtained from Vector Laboratories in the form of an ABC kit, and the procedure is carried out according to their instructions. Briefly, the sections are incubated under agitation for 0.5 to 1 hr in biotinylated linking antiserum (raised against IgG molecules of the species from which the primary antiserum was obtained) diluted 1 : 100 in 2% normal serum in PBS, rinsed as above in PBS, and then incubated under agitation for 1 hr in the ABC reagent, also in PBS. After a final rinse series, the sections are ready for reaction to reveal the HRP tag in the ABC complex.

6. Histochemistry for the Horseradish Peroxidase Immunolabel

Conveniently for this technique, the HRP molecules of the first series (i.e., the intracellularly injected or transported HRP) are blocked by their accumulation of DAB and will not accumulate further reaction product. This allows the experimenter the option of choosing a second chromogen to attach to the immunolabel that can easily be distinguished in the light microscope from the brown (DAB) or black (cobalt chloride–DAB) reaction. We typically use the black cobalt-enhanced DAB reaction (Adams, 1977) for the intracellularly labeled cells and find that a brown DAB reaction (Itoh *et al.*, 1979) provides sufficient color contrast. The progress of the reaction should be monitored in the wet sections using a microscope; typically 15 to 40 min is sufficient to yield good labeling. After the reaction, sections to be processed for light microscopy are mounted from PBS onto gelatin-coated slides, optionally counterstained with cresyl violet, dehydrated in an ascending alcohol series, cleared, and coverslipped.

For purposes of double labeling to show, for example, both transported HRP and immunoreactivity in the same cell (Afsharpour *et al.*, 1985), greater color contrast is needed. The present modification of the green *o*-dianisidine reaction described earlier by Colman *et al.* (1976) is a good choice for this purpose. Prepare the reaction medium by dissolving 20 mg of *o*-dianisidine (Sigma) in 120 ml of water containing 250 μl of 1.0 M citrate buffer, pH 4.5, 20 μl of 3% hydrogen peroxide, and 2.5 ml of 5% sodium nitroferricyanide. The use of citrate buffer prevents formation of large crystals, yielding a homogeneous reaction product reminiscent of that obtained with DAB. This solution and the reaction vessel should be chilled in a freezer to about 0°C, and the reaction carried out in an ice bath. The progress of the reaction should be monitored by examining wet sections under the microscope, and usually 5 to 15 min is sufficient. After the reaction, the sections should be stabilized in a medium containing 120 ml water, 3.6 g sodium nitroferricyanide, and 250 μl of 1.0 M citrate buffer, pH 4.5. The green reaction product will withstand cresyl violet counterstaining and alcohol dehydration.

7. Alternative Methods for the Localization of the Primary Antibody: The Immunogold Method and the ABC–Alkaline Phosphatase Method

There are several alternatives to using peroxidase as the immunocytochemical marker, and these may offer advantages in certain experiments. For example, to discriminate at the electron microscopic level between structures labeled by intracellular injection of HRP and structures labeled by the antiserum, the immunogold method (van den Pol, 1984) may be useful. The immunogold method attaches to the primary antibody a secondary antibody that has been linked to a gold colloid particle of a specific size (Janssen Pharmaceutica, distributed in the United States by Ted Pella, Inc.). The 5-nm gold particle size is preferable because it penetrates the tissue readily. The gold particles are easily identified under the electron microscope or can be enhanced with silver (Holgate *et al.*, 1983) using the Janssen Silver Enhancement Kit in order to be visualized at the light microscopic level. Sections to be labeled by the immunogold method should be first treated with the primary antiserum as described above, washed in PBS, and then incubated overnight under agitation in the immunogold reagent diluted (1 : 20, 1 : 40, 1 : 80, or 1 : 160). The sections are then washed three times in PBS and then postfixed in 2% glutaraldehyde in PBS (prepared fresh). The sections can then be osmicated and embedded in plastic for electron microscopy (according to the procedure described below) or may be silver enhanced (according to the protocol distributed by Janssen) for light microscopy (Penny *et al.*, 1986).

Another useful alternative to the ABC method is the ABC–alkaline phosphatase method (ABC–AP), available in kit form from Vector Laboratories. This procedure uses alkaline phosphatase as the enzyme marker, thereby avoiding the use of two peroxidase tags when doing combined intracellular labeling and immunocytochemistry. Three chromagens are available from Vector that yield black, blue, and red reaction products. The black and red reaction products can be dehydrated with alcohols and xylene for light microscopy, but none of the three is osmiophilic, and none will withstand plastic embedment.

III. APPLICATION

The method of combining intracellular labeling and immuncytochemistry is illustrated with a few examples from our work in the striatum, where we have used the immunocytochemical method as an aid to reveal otherwise hidden tissue boundaries. The value of this application arises from the recent discovery of the heterogeneous organization of the neostriatum (Olson *et al.*, 1972a,b; Tennyson *et al.*, 1972; Nobin and Bjorklund, 1973; Graybiel and Ragsdale, 1978a,b; Kalil, 1978; Graybiel *et al.*, 1979, 1981; Herkenham and Pert, 1981; Goldman-Rakic, 1982; Graybiel, 1983; Gerfen, 1984; Herkenham *et al.*, 1984). A great deal of credit for this discovery goes to Graybiel and her collaborators, who have demonstrated by histochemical methods that the neostriatum can be divided by hidden tissue boundaries into two principal parts, striosome and matrix compartments. The striosomes are discrete islands that are relatively low in acetylcholinesterase (AChE), and the matrix in contrast is relatively rich in AChE. The histochemical distinction between striosome and matrix extends to other markers; the striosomes are relatively rich in [Leu]-enkephalin, [Met]-enkephalin, and substance P immunostaining and are embedded in a matrix that is relatively low in these substances but high in somatostatin. The histochemically defined compartments are in turn related to connections; striosome and matrix neostriatum differ in their afferents from thalamus and neocortex and their efferent connections with the substantia nigra (Goldman and Nauta, 1977; Kalil, 1978; Graybiel *et al.*, 1979; Donoghue and Herkenham, 1983; Gerfen, 1984, 1985; Ragsdale and Graybiel, 1984).

We have combined the technique of intracellular HRP labeling with immunocytochemistry for [Leu]-enkephalin in order to answer an important group of questions concerning the relationship between the cellular level of neostriatal organization and the striosome and matrix compartment system (Penny *et al.*, 1984, 1988). In particular, we wanted to know whether the spiny projection neuron (the most common neostriatal neuron) is found in both compartments, whether its dendritic field is organized in such a way as to maintain the input segregation between the two compartments, and whether its local axonal collaterals, by respecting striosome—matrix boundaries, also maintain that segregation.

Figure 5A shows the appearance of the material processed for [Leu]-enkephalin immunoreactivity. The globus pallidus (GP) appears especially densely stained because it receives a heavy enkephalinergic projection from the striatum. The distribution of [Leu]-enkephalin within the striatum (St) is heterogeneous; the arrow indicates a zone of dense [Leu]-enkephalin immunoreactivety, i.e., a striosome. The arrow in Fig. 5B indicates a neostriatal spiny projection neuron that was labeled by intracellular application of HRP. After

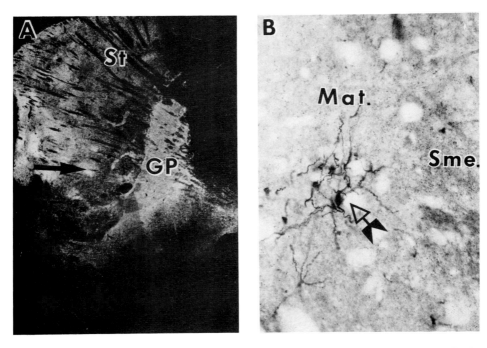

Figure 5. A: Darkfield photomicrograph of a parasagittal section through the rat forebrain stained by the immunoperoxidase method for [Leu]-enkephalin immunoreactivity. The abbreviation "St" indicates the striatum, and "GP" the globus pallidus. The arrow indicates a striosome. B: A lightfield photomicrograph of a spiny projection neuron filled by an intracellular application of HRP (arrow) on a section also processed for [Leu]-enkephalin terminal staining. The zone of dense terminals is a striosome (Sme.); the neuron falls within the less heavily stained matrix zone (Mat.).

being processed for HRP enzyme histochemistry, the sections containing the labeled neuron were processed by immunoperoxidase methods to reveal the distribution of [Leu]-enkephalin-rich striosomes and [Leu]-enkephalin-poor matrix zones. The boundary between striosome and matrix in the vicinity of the labeled neuron is apparent; clearly the neuron is found within the matrix compartment.

Figures 6 and 7 show a serial reconstruction obtained from another example of a spiny projection neuron filled by intracellular application of HRP. The reconstructed somatodendritic morphology in Fig. 6 shows that the dendrites of the neuron are confined by the striosome–matrix boundary. At places where the boundary extends close to the cell, the dendrites appear shortened and often show recurved endings as they approach the boundary (large arrow); where the boundary is farther from the cell, the dendrites have a greater extent. There is very little tendency for the dendrites to cross the border. The same is true for the local axonal collaterals, shown in Fig. 7, which also are confined by the boundary. The principal axonal branch,

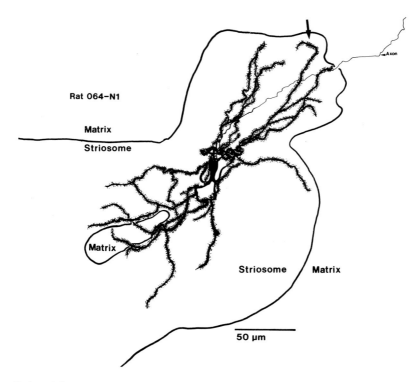

Figure 6. A serial reconstruction of the somatodendritic morphology of a spiny projection neuron filled by intracellular application of HRP. This neuron falls within the striosome compartment. A recurved dendrite is indicated by a large arrow. The main axonal branch, which is on its way out of the striatum, is indicated by a small arrow.

indicated by a small arrow in Fig. 6, leaves the striatum without further arborization. Figure 8 shows the result of filling a different class of neuron, a large aspiny type 1 cell, with HRP and simultaneously staining for [Leu]-enkephalin immunoreactivity. In contrast to the spiny projection neurons, this cell is not confined by the striosome–matrix boundaries. The cell body falls at the border, and dendrites extend from there into the matrix or into the striosome and in places (arrows) cross from striosome to matrix.

IV. SUMMARY OF ADVANTAGES AND LIMITATIONS

A. Advantages

1. The fundamental advantage of the method of intracellular injection of HRP is that it allows direct correlation between cellular physiology and morphology.

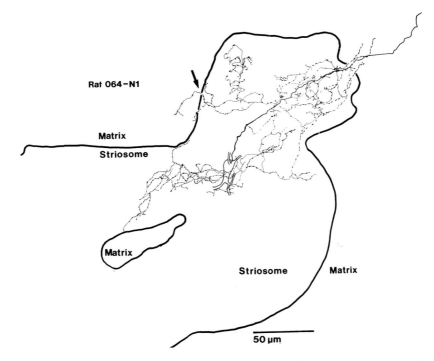

Rat 064-N1

Matrix
Striosome

Matrix

Striosome   Matrix

50 μm

Figure 7. A serial reconstruction of the local axonal collaterals of the same spiny projection neuron whose somatodendritic morphology was shown in Fig. 6. An arrow indicates a small segment of axon that leaves the striatum.

2. The intracellularly stained neuron is the only stained element in the tissue and can be easily reconstructed over many sections, as task that is often difficult or impossible in Golgi-impregnated material.
3. The method of intracellular labeling can be applied to a variety of preparations, including the *in vivo* animal, the *in vitro* brain slice (Kitai and Kita, 1984), the intact organ preparation, and tissue culture.
4. The HRP reaction product is robust and permanent, and sections processed for HRP-labeled neurons can subsequently be exposed to a variety of rigorous treatments or be stored archivally.
5. With a few minor modifications, the intracellularly labeled neuron can be prepared for electron microscopy for further analysis (see the next two chapters).

B. Limitations

1. The ease of obtaining high-quality intracellular recordings varies from experiment to experiment. Conditions within the laboratory may play a causal role in this variation; high humidity seems to interfere with the

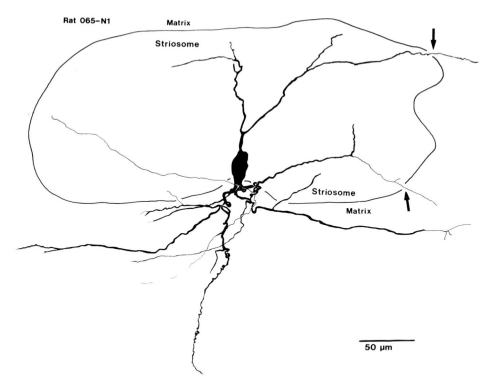

Figure 8. A serial reconstruction of the somatodendritic morphology of a large aspiny neuron filled by intracellular application of HRP. The soma of this neuron falls on the striosome–matrix boundary. Arrows indicate spots where the dendrites cross boundaries.

successful manufacture of glass microelectrodes filled with HRP solution. Vascular and respiratory pulsation are often problems in the *in vivo* preparation. Careful adjustment of the animal's suspension and maintenance of deep surgical anesthesia usually help to avoid these difficulties.

2. Recovery of neurons that have undergone intracellular injection of HRP is not automatic; chance of successful recovery varies with the overall health of the neuron during and after the injection and with the elapsed time between injection and sacrifice.

3. A third limitation, related to the second, is that neurons intracellularly labeled by HRP do not keep well in animals allowed to survive post-surgery, and this unfortunate circumstance decidedly interferes with the tracing of axons for long distances from the soma. In instances where cells do survive, the soma and dendrites are often partially degenerated.

4. The penetration of immunoreagents into thick Vibratome sections, without special treatment, is limited to about the outer 3 μm of the

section, and this penetration may be even less when immunogold reagents are used. Mechanisms to increase penetration are harsh on the tissue and may degrade ultrastructural preservation. Therefore, for combined intracellular HRP and immunocytochemical experiments that require electron microscopic analysis, penetration can be a particular problem, interfering with the immunoreagents' ability to reach particular intracellularly labeled elements of interest. Postembedding immunocytochemical methods may bypass this problem.

V. APPENDIX: IDENTIFICATION OF THE RECORDED NEURON AND ITS NEUROTRANSMITTER: INTRACELLULAR LABELING WITH BIOCYTIN COMBINED WITH IMMUNOCYTOCHEMISTRY

This section describes double-labeling procedures in which the intracellular labeling technique is combined with immunocytochemical techniques in order to identify the neurotransmitter content or other antigens of interest within the intracellularly recorded neurons.

A. Conditions Required for Double Labeling to Demonstrate the Coexistence of Intracellularly Injected Tracer and Endogenous Antigen of Interest

The intracellularly injected tracer must be easily distinguished from the labels (chromagens or fluorophores) used in the immunocytochemical reaction, and both types of labels must be clearly visible within the same section. (Because the reaction products from intracellularly injected HRP are indistinguishable from the HRP used in immunocytochemistry, the dual-labeling protocol employing different colored HRP–DAB reaction protocols cannot be used.) The most suitable combination of labels to be used for light microscopic examination includes the various fluorescent dyes. On the other hand, at the electron microscopic level a combination of different-sized colloidal gold labels and/or HRP reaction products should be used (e.g., Somogyi and Soltesz, 1986).

Endogenous intracellular content of the antigen of interest must be sufficient to be visualized by immunocytochemistry. For instance, because most striatal neurons normally do not display sufficient immunoreactivity to be visualized in single-labeling studies, it is unlikely that similar immunoreactions would be very fruitful in double-labeling studies. Although some striatal neurons do display strong immunoreactivity (e.g., cholinergic, somatostatinergic, and a minority of GABAergic neurons), they are very few and are dispersed far from each other so that there is little chance of encountering these neurons during normal *in vivo* recording experiments. These factors have remained as the major roadblocks in the general application of the combined technique (see below) in the striatum. On the other hand, other parts of the CNS have neurons containing high concentrations of endogenous antigens. For example, dopaminergic neurons of the substantia nigra are highly immunoreactive for tyrosine hydroxylase (TH), the synthetic enzyme for dopamine. Consequently, it is possible to demonstrate TH immunoreactivity within intracellularly labeled dopaminergic neurons (e.g., Fig. 9).

B. Biocytin as an Intracellular Marker

Biocytin (mol. wt. 372.48), a compound of biotin and lysine, was first used as an intracellular tracer by Horikawa and Armstrong (1988). The several advantages of biocytin used as an intracellular tracer include the following:

1. Because its biotin moiety can bind to avidin, biocytin can combine with any probes that are conjugated to avidin. The visualization of biocytin therefore depends on the types of labels conjugated to the avidin probes. Consequently, with biocytin as an intracellular tracer, the flexibility of combining intracellular labeling with other anatomic techniques increases dramatically. For example, if the avidin were linked to a fluorescent label (e.g., FITC, rhodamine, or Texas Red™), the intracellularly injected neuron would be revealed by that particular fluorescence. The same tissue sections can then be processed for immunofluorescence with a different fluorescent label to demonstrate either the spatial relationships between immunolabeled elements and intracellularly labeled neurons or the coexistence of desired antigens and intracellularly injected tracer (biocytin) within the same neurons (Fig. 9).
2. Since Fluoro-gold™ can be used effectively as a retrograde tracer, it is possible to combine Fluoro-gold™ retrograde tracing with intracellular labeling with biocytin in order to demonstrate whether the intracellularly labeled neuron is a projection neuron.
3. Intracellularly injected biocytin can be transformed into a label suitable for both light and electron microscopic analysis by reacting with avidin conjugated to various tags suitable for light and/or electron microscopic analysis. For example, HRP conjugated to avidin can be used to bind biocytin and then reacted with DAB to form conventional HRP-labeled appearance.

The only disadvantage of biocytin as an intracellular tracer is that a detergent (e.g., Triton-X) is required to enhance the penetration of probes conjugated to avidin into the tissue sections to bind to the biocytin. This is because labels conjugated to avidin (mol. wt. 66,000) have relatively large physical diameters and thus do not penetrate tissue sections very well. Consequently, the morphological preservation at the electron microscopic level will not be as good as in tissues not treated with detergent. Nevertheless, biocytin as an intracellular tracer can be used to obtain a better visualization of the macroscopic relationship between intracellularly labeled neurons and the sur-

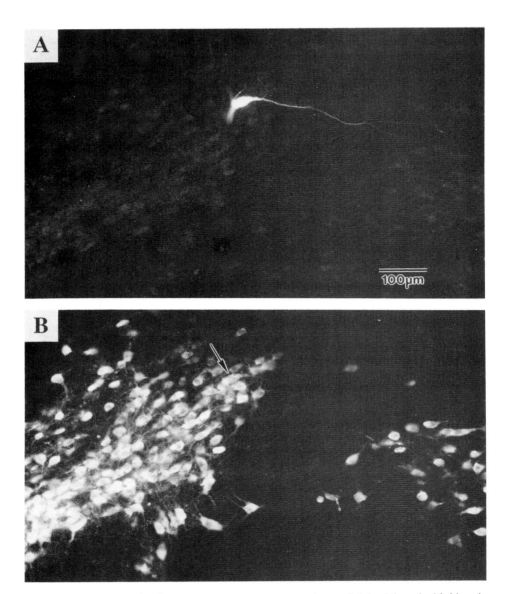

Figure 9. A: A substantia nigra pars compacta neuron was intracellulalry injected with biocytin and was labeled with avidin–Texas Red™. B: The same section was reacted to demonstrate tyrosine hydroxylase immunoreactivity. Dopaminergic neurons were revealed with FITC-labeled secondary antibodies. Arrow points to the same neuron shown in A. Calibration in A also applies to B.

rounding tissue compartment using a double-fluorescence labeling approach rather than the double HRP–DAB reactions described by Penny *et al.* (1988). In some cases, means of increasing the concentration of antigens may have to be employed to raise the concentration of endogenous antigens to immunodetectable levels (e.g., pretreating subjects with colchicine), but the impact of such treatments on the intracellularly recorded response properties of the neurons remains unclear.

C. Procedures

1. Electrolyte solution within the recording electrode consists of 1% to 4% biocytin (Sigma) dissolved in virtually any of the commonly used intracellular recording electrolyte solutions (e.g., KCl, K-acetate or K-methylsulfate). After the physiological properties of desired neurons are recorded intracellularly, biocytin is injected into the recorded neurons by passing square-wave current pulses (-1 to -5 nA, 100–300 msec duration, 50% duty cycle, 3 to 10 min) through the recording electrode. The animals are perfused with a fixative compatible with the specific antigen of interest.

2. The brains are cut on a Vibratome^{TM} into 50-μm-thick sections and then reacted to reveal the morphology of processes containing intracellularly injected biocytin using Texas Red^{TM} conjugated to avidin. Sections are rinsed with phosphate-buffered saline (PBS) and then incubated in a PBS solution containing avidin–Texas Red^{TM} (1 : 100) and 0.2% Triton X-100 for at least 2 hr at room temperature.

3. The intracellularly labeled neurons and processes can be photographed at several magnifications using a microscope equipped with fluorescence micrography attachments in order to document their appearance prior to any subsequent reactions. This step may be performed in sections wetted with buffered saline or in a solution containing 50% glycerol, which partially clears the tissue and provides better resolution of the labeled processes.

4. Serial alternate sections are washed in phosphate-buffered saline (PBS, pH 7.4) five times (total time 1 hr) and then incubated in a PBS solution containing diluted primary antibodies for 24–36 hr at 4°C with continuous gentle agitation.

5. Sections are washed five times in PBS and incubated in PBS containing fluorescein isothiocyanate (FITC)-labeled secondary antibodies (1 : 100) at room temperature for at least 2 hr.

6. Following rinses in PBS, the reacted sections are mounted in 50% glycerol in PBS on glass slides for examination on a fluorescence microscope with appropriate filter sets. Intracellularly injected processes are labeled by the red fluorescence of Texas Red^{TM}, which is different from the yellow-green FITC fluorescence produced by the immunoreactive elements.

Useful hints and comments:

1. The sections can be simultaneously incubated in a solution containing both avidin–Texas Red™ and the primary antisera in order to save time. However, because few clues are available for determining which sections would contain intracellularly labeled processes, many sections would have to be reacted for immunocytochemistry, requiring a larger expense of primary antisera.

2. For better resolution of morphological details of intracellularly labeled processes, sections containing avidin–Texas Red™-labeled processes can be incubated with a solution containing diluted HRP conjugated to biotin and subsequently reacted for visualization of HRP using DAB as the chromagen.

3. For better resolution of morphological details of immunoreactive elements, FITC-labeled immunoreactive elements can be transformed into light-stable DAB reaction products either by photocatalysis (Sandell and Masland, 1988) or by incubating with an appropriate species-specific peroxidase–antiperoxidase complex and then reacted in DAB to visualize the immunoreactive elements (Chang, 1988).

4. This method is applicable for *in vitro* brain slice preparations. For example, biocytin has been used successfully with tyrosine hydroxylase immunocytochemistry to demonstrate the dopaminergic nature of the recorded substantia nigral neurons (Bargas *et al.*, 1988).

ACKNOWLEDGMENTS. The preparation of this manuscript was supported by NIH Grant NS-20702 to S. T. Kitai and by NIH Grant NS-24897 to G. R. Penny.

REFERENCES

Adams, J. C. 1977, Technical considerations on the use of horseradish peroxidase as a neuronal marker, *Neuroscience* **2**:141–145.

Afsharpour, S., Kita, H., Penny, G. R., and Kitai, S. T., 1985, Glutamate acid decarboxylase, substance P and Leu-enkephalin-immunoreactive neurons in the neostriatum that project to the globus pallidus and substantia nigra, *Soc. Neurosci. Abstr.* **11**:362.

Bargas, J., Galarraga, E., Chang, H. T., and Kitai, S. T., 1988, Electrophysiological and double-labeling immunohistochemical analyses of neurons in the substantia nigra zona compacta of the rat, *Soc. Neurosci. Abstr.* **14**:1025.

Berod, A., Hartman, B. K., and Pujol, J. F., 1981, Importance of fixaton in immunocytochemistry: Use of formaldehyde solutions at variable pH for the localization of tyosine hydroxylase, *J. Histochem. Cytochem.* **29**:844–850.

Brown, K. T., and Flaming, D. G., 1986, *Advanced Micropipette Techniques for Cell Physiology,* John Wiley & Sons, New York.

Brown, P. G., Maxfield, B. W., and Moraff, H., 1973, *Electronics for Neurobiologists,* MIT Press, Cambridge, MA.

Chang, H. T., 1988, Dopamine–acetylcholine interaction in the striatum: A dual-labeling immunocytochemical study of tyrosine hydroxylase and choline acetyltransferase positive elements in the rat, *Brain Res. Bull.* **21**:295–304.

Chang, H. T., Waters, R. S., and Kitai, S. T., 1986, Intracellular labeling combined with immunocytochemistry in the rat substantia nigra, *Soc. Neurosci. Abstr.* **12:**654.

Colman, D. R., Scalia, F., and Cabrales, E., 1976, Light and electron microscopic observations on the anterograde transport of horseradish peroxidase in the optic pathway in the mouse and rat, *Brain Res.* **102:**156–163.

Culheim, S., and Kellerth, J. O., 1976, Combined light and electron microscopic tracing of neurons including axons and synaptic terminals after the intracellular injection of horseradish peroxidase, *Neurosci. Lett.* **2:**307–313.

Czerkensky, C. C., Nilsson, L. A., Nygran, H., Ouchterlony, O., and Tarkowski, A., 1983, A solid-phase enzyme-linked immunospot (ELISPOT) assay for enumeration of specific antibody-secretion cells, *J. Immunol. Methods* **65:**109–121.

Dingledine, R. (ed.), 1984, *Brain Slices,* Plenum Press, New York.

Donoghue, J. P., and Herkenham, M., 1983, Multiple patterns of corticostriatal projections and their relationship to opiate receptor patches in rats, *Soc. Neurosci. Abstr.* **9:**15.

Gerfen, C. R., 1984, The neostriatal mosaic: Compartmentalization of corticostriatal input and striatonigral output systems, *Nature* **314:**461–464.

Gerfen, C. R., 1985, The neostriatal mosaic: I. Compartmental organization of projections from the striatum to the substantia nigra in the rat, *J. Comp. Neurol.* **236:**454–476.

Goldman, P. S., and Nauta, W. J. H., 1977, An intracately patterned prefronto-caudate projection in the rhesus monkey, *J. Comp. Neurol.* **171:**369–386.

Goldman-Rakic, P. S., 1982, Cytoarchitechtectonic heterogenity of the primate neostriatum: Subdivisions into *island* and *matrix* cellular compartments, *J. Comp. Neurol.* **205:**398–413.

Graybiel, A. M., 1983, Compartmental organization of the mammalian striatum, in: *Progress in Brain Research,* Volume 58: *Molecular and Cellular Interactions Underlying Higher Brain Functions* (J. P. Changeux, J. Glowinski, M. Imbert, and F. E. Bloom, eds.), Elsevier, New York, pp. 247–256.

Graybiel, A. M., and Ragsdale, C. W., 1978a, Histochemically distinct compartments in the striatum of human, monkey, and cat demonstrated by acetylthiocholinesterase staining, *Proc. Natl. Acad. Sci. U.S.A.* **75:**5723–5726.

Graybiel, A. M., and Ragsdale, C. W., 1978b, Striosomal organization of the caudate nucleus. I. Acetylcholinesterase histochemistry of the striatum in the cat, rhesus monkey, and human being, *Soc. Neurosci. Abstr.* **4:**44.

Graybiel, A. M., Ragsdale, C. W., and Edley, S. M., 1979, Compartments in the striatum of the cat observed by retrograde cell labeling, *Exp. Brain Res.* **34:**189–195.

Graybiel, A. M., Ragsdale, C. W., Yoneka, E. S., and Elde, R. P., 1981, An immunohistochemical study of enkephalins and other neuropeptides in the striatum of the cat with evidence that the opiate peptides are arranged to form mosaic patterns to register with the striosomal compartments visible by acetylcholinesterase staining, *Neuroscience* **6:**377–382.

Herkenham, M., and Pert, C. B., 1981, Mosaic distribution of opiate receptors, parafascicular projections, and acetylcholinesterase in rat striatum, *Nature* **291:**415–418.

Herkenham, M., Edley, S. M., and Stuart, J., 1984, Cell clusters in the nucleus accumbens of the rat and the mosaic relationship of the opiate receptors, acetylcholinesterase and subcortical afferent termination, *Neuroscience* **11:**561–591.

Holgate, C. S., Jackson, P., Cowen, P. N., and Bird, C. C., 1983, Immunogold-silver staining: New method of immunostaining with enhanced sensitivity, *J. Histochem. Cytochem.* **31:**938–944.

Horikawa, K., and Armstrong, W. E., 1988, A versatile means of intracellular labeling: Injection of biocytin and its detection with avidin conjugates, *J. Neurosci. Methods* **25:**1–11.

Hsu, S. M., Raine, L., and Ganger, H., 1981, The use of avidin–biotin–peroxidase complex (ABC) in immunoperoxidase techniques: A comparison between ABC and unlabeled antibody (PAP) procedures, *J. Histochem. Cytochem.* **29:**577–580.

Itoh, K., Konishi, A. Nomura, S., Mizuno, N., Nakamura, Y., and Sugimoto, I., 1979, Application of coupled oxidation reaction to electron microscope demonstration of horseradish peroxidase: Cobalt–glucose oxidase method, *Brain Res.* **175:**341–346.

Jankowska, E., Rastad, R., and Westman, J., 1976, Intracellular application of horseradish peroxidase and its light and electron microscopical appearance in spino-cervical tract cells, *Brain Res.* **105**:555–562.

Kalil, K., 1978, Patch-like termination of thalamic fibers in the putamen of the rhesus monkey: An autoradiographic study, *Brain Res.* **140**:333–339.

Kitai, S. T., and Bishop, G. A., 1981, Intracellular staining of neurons, in *Neuroanatomical Tract-Tracing Methods* (L. Heimer and M. J. RoBards, eds.), Plenum Press, New York, pp. 263–277.

Kitai, S. T., and Kita, H., 1984, Electrophysiological study of the neostriatum in brain slice preparation, in: *Brain Slices* (R. Dingledine, ed.), Plenum Press, New York, pp. 285–296.

Kitai, S. T., and Wilson, C. J., 1982, Intracellular labeling of neurons in mammalian brains, in: *Cytochemical Methods in Neuroanatomy* (V. Chan-Palay and S. Palay, eds.), Alan R. Liss, New York, pp. 533–549.

Kitai, S. T., Kosis, J. D., Preston, R. J., and Sugimori, M., 1976, Monosynaptic inputs to caudate neurons identified by intracellular injection of horseradish peroxidase, *Brain Res.* **109**:601–606.

Light, A. R., and Durkovic, R. G., 1976, Horseradish peroxidase: An improvement in intracellular straining of single electrophysiologically characterized neurons, *Exp. Neurol.* **53**:847–853.

Lighthall, J. W., Park, M. R., and Kitai, S. T., 1981, Inhibition in slices of rat neostriatum, *Brain Res.* **212**:182–187.

McLean, I. W., and Nakane, P. K., 1974, Periodate–lysine–paraformaldehyde fixative: A new fixative for immunoelectron microscopy, *J. Histochem. Cytochem.* **22**:1077–1083.

Misgeld, U., and Bak, I. J., 1979, Intrinsic excitation in the rat neostriatum mediated by acetyl-choline, *Neurosci. Lett.* **12**:277–282.

Morrison, R., 1986, *Grounding and Shielding Techniques in Instrumentation*, John Wiley & Sons, New York.

Nobin, A., and Bjorklund, A., 1973, Topography of the monoamine neuron system in the human brain as revealed in fetuses, *Acta Physiol. Scand.* **88**:1–40.

Olson, L., Boreus, L., and Seiger, A., 1972a, Histochemical demonstration and mapping of 5-hydroxytryptamine and catecholamine-containing neuron systems in the human fetal brain, *Z. Anat. Entwickl. Gesch.* **139**:259–282.

Olson, L., Seiger, A., and Fuxe, K., 1972b, Heterogenity of striatal and limbic dopamine inner-vation: Highly fluorescent islands in developing and adult rats, *Brain Res.* **44**:283–288.

Park, M. R., 1985, A complete digitally neurophysiological recording laboratory, in: *The Micro-computer in Cell and Neurobiology Research* (R. R. Mize, ed.), Elsevier, New York, pp. 411–434.

Penny, G. R., Wilson, C. J., and Kitai, S. T., 1984, The influence of neostriatal patch and matrix compartments on the dendritic geometry of spiny projection neurons in the rat as revealed by intracellular labeling with HRP combined with immunocytochemistry, *Soc. Neurosci. Abstr.* **10**:514.

Penny, G. R., Chang, H. T., and Kitai, S. T., 1986, Dual localization of [Leu]enkephalin and choline acetyltransferase in the rat basal ganglia, *Soc. Neurosci. Abstr.* **12**:1328.

Penny, G. R., Wilson, C. J., and Kitai, S. T., 1988, Relationship of the axonal and dendritic geometry of spiny projection neurons to the compartmental organization of the neostria-tum, *J. Comp. Neurol.* **269**:275–289.

Purves, R. D., 1981, *Microelectrode Methods for Intracellular Recording and Ionophoresis*, Academic Press, London.

Ragsdale, C. W., and Graybiel, A. M., 1984, Further observations on the striosomal organization of frontostriatal projections in cats and monkeys, *Soc. Neurosci. Abstr.* **10**:514.

Sandell, J. H., and Masland, R. H., 1988, Photoconversion of some fluorescent markers to a diaminobenzidine product, *J. Histochem. Cytochem.* **36**:555–559.

Scholer, J., and Armstrong, W. K., 1982, Aqueous aldehyde (FAGLU) histofluorescence for catecholamines in 2 μm sections using polyethylene glycol embedding, *Brain Res. Bull.* **9**:27–31.

Snow, P. J., Rose, P. K., and Brown, A. G., 1976, Tracing axons and axon collaterals of spinal neurons using intracellular injections of horseradish peroxidase, *Science* **191**:312–313.

Somogyi, P., and Soltesz, I., 1986, Immunogold demonstration of GABA in synaptic terminals of intracellularly recorded, horseradish peroxidase-filled basket cells and clutch cells in the cat's visual cortex, *Neuroscience* **19**:1051–1065.

Sternberger, C. A., 1986, *Immunocytochemistry,* 3rd ed., John Wiley & Sons, New York.

Tennyson, V. M., Barrett, R. E., Cohen, G., Cote, L., Heikkila, R., and Mytineou, C., 1972, The developing neostriatum of the rabbit: Correlation of fluoresence histochemistry electron microscopy, endogenous dopamine levels, and [^{3}H]dopamine uptake, *Brain Res.* **46**:2541–285.

van den Pol, A. N., 1984, Colloidal gold and biotin–avidin conjugates as ultrastructural markers for neural antigens, *Q. J. Exp. Physiol.* **69**:1–33.

8

Synaptic Relationships of Golgi-Impregnated Neurons as Identified by Electrophysiological or Immunocytochemical Techniques

TAMÁS F. FREUND and P. SOMOGYI

I. INTRODUCTION

Much of our present knowledge about the cellular organization of the different brain areas derives from Golgi studies, dating back to the end of the last century when Golgi (1883), Ramon y Cajal (1891, 1911), and many others introduced the modern era of neuroanatomy. The Golgi method allows the visualization of a small proportion of the neurons present in a brain area, together with most of their dendritic and axonal processes. As a result the impregnated cells can be traced and reconstructed in great detail. To gain an overall view of the different cell types and the distribution of neuronal processes in a brain area, even today Golgi impregnation is often the method of choice. It can provide much valuable information regarding local

TAMÁS F. FREUND and PETER SOMOGYI • MRC Anatomical Neuropharmacology Unit, University Department of Pharmacology, Oxford OX1 3QT, United Kingdom. *Present address for T.F.F.:* First Department of Anatomy, Semmelweis University Medical School, H-1450 Budapest, Hungary.

circuit patterns provided the material is critically analyzed (Szentágothai, 1975; Szentágothai and Arbib, 1974; for review see Millhouse, 1981). One limitation of the Golgi technique is that generally synaptic interactions can only be predicted by indirect correlation of separately impregnated dendritic and axonal patterns. In some cases, e.g., in the cerebellum, this enabled the classical histologists to assemble correctly the wiring of the entire neuronal system, whereas in other cases the correspondence between separately impregnated pre- and postsynaptic processes is not so obvious as to predict the organization of neuronal circuits.

A new chapter in the application of the Golgi method was introduced with the electron microscopic analysis of the impregnated neurons (Blackstad, 1965, 1969; Stell, 1965, 1967). Although technically difficult, Blackstad's and Stell's pioneering work paved the way to a direct analysis of synaptic connections. Another important technical breakthrough was achieved by Peters and his colleagues (Fairen *et al.*, 1977) with the development of gold toning of Golgi-impregnated neurons. With this conversion of the original Golgi precipitate into a stable insoluble metallic deposit, the power of visualizing cells by the Golgi method could routinely be combined with electron microscopic identification of their synaptic connections.

The gold toning technique also provided an opportunity to circumvent another limitation of the Golgi method—its lack of histochemical specificity. Following gold toning, the processes of cells remain traceable, but with removal of most of the Golgi precipitate from the impregnated cells, they can be characterized by the aid of techniques such as autoradiography (Somogyi *et al.*, 1981b), immunocytochemistry (Somogyi *et al.*, 1983), and enzyme histochemistry (Bolam *et al.*, 1984a; Somogyi *et al.*, 1979; Somogyi and Smith, 1979). Through various combinations, both the impregnated cells and their synaptic input can be analyzed with histochemical methods (Freund *et al.*, 1984). With the heavy Golgi precipitate removed from the cytoplasm, it is also possible to identify the projection area of the neuron by the detection of retrogradely transported markers, e.g., HRP, in the cell body.

A further dimension was opened up in the analysis of identified circuits with the application of Golgi impregnation to brain tissue that also contained electrophysiologically characterized and intracellularly horseradish peroxidase (HRP)-injected neurons (Freund and Somogyi, 1983; Freund *et al.*, 1985b). The combined physiological, anatomic, and histochemical analysis of the same synaptic circuits became possible.

The discoveries and technical advances reviewed above provided much of the impetus for the latest revolution in the study of interneuronal connections, which is characterized by the tracing of successive links in neuronal chains with emphasis on both neuronal morphology and synaptic relations and histochemical identification of the neuronal components involved. However, before the advantages of the Golgi method could be utilized in a more systematic fashion in combination with methods that are based on histochemical markers, one additional development was needed. Most histochemical techniques require the penetration of reagents (e.g., antibodies, substrates for enzymes) into the tissue, but these usually penetrate only into thin tissue sections. The Golgi technique, on the other hand, relies on the impregnation of relatively thick slices of tissue. The seemingly incompatible requirements were resolved with the introduction of the section–Golgi impregnation procedure (Freund and Somogyi, 1983) and with the application of postembedding immunostaining of Golgi–impregnated cells (Somogyi and Hodgson, 1985).

Although there are many ways to combine neuroanatomical techniques, this chapter demonstrates how the Golgi method can be combined with tracer methods and immunohistochemical techniques in the same experiment at both the light and the electron microscopic level. This approach has greatly improved our ability to correlate directly morphology, connectivity, and histochemistry for the purpose of identifying neuronal circuits.

Figure 1 illustrates some of the questions that can be answered with this approach. For instance, by combining Golgi impregnation with histochemical and immunohistochemical techniques, it may be possible to characterize the Golgi-impregnated neuron or its synaptic input in histochemical terms (Fig. 1A,B), and the use of axonal tracers, e.g., HRP, can answer specific questions related to the projection of the Golgi-impregnated neuron or the sources of its afferent input (Fig. 1C). The combination of Golgi impregnation with intracellular recording and HRP filling allows the identification of the postsynaptic targets of electrophysiologically characterized neurons (Fig. 1D). The possibilities offered by this approach of combining various techniques are almost unlimited, as they appear dependent to a large extent on the scientist's own imagination and technical skills.

In an effort to encourage the use of this highly profitable approach, the next section features a discussion of several specific examples in which the Golgi method has been combined with other methods in the analysis of complex neuronal circuits. The subsequent Appendix (Section IV) contains detailed descriptions of the procedures involved.

II. APPLICATIONS OF THE COMBINED TECHNIQUES

A. Neurochemical Characterization of Nerve Cells Identified by Golgi Impregnation

With immunocytochemistry alone, only cell bodies, proximal dendrites, and isolated axon terminals can be revealed, and it is usually not possible to classify the neuron in morphological terms, i.e., on the basis of the appearance of the dendritic tree and axonal arborizations. However, by combining immunocytochemistry and Golgi impregnation of the same neurons, it is possible to provide a neurochemical characterization of identified cell types.

The neurochemical identification can be achieved either through preembedding or postembedding immunocytochemistry. As the name indicates, preembedding immunocytochemistry means that the immunostaining

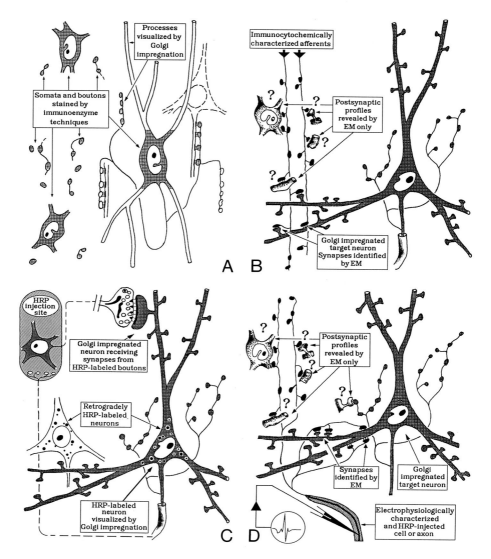

Figure 1. Schematic diagram summarizing the possible applications of combined techniques involving Golgi impregnation. (A) The combination of pre- or postembedding immunocytochemistry (or enzyme histochemistry) and Golgi impregnation of the same neurons allows the neurochemical characterization of identified cell types. The visualization of dendritic and axonal arborizations of neurons, as shown here by Golgi impregnation, is essential in many brain areas to define a particular type of neuron. Synaptic connections of the impregnated cells can be established by electron microscopy, and their immunoreactivity can be demonstrated by either light (in somata) or electron microscopy (in terminals and/or somata). (B) Postsynaptic target neurons of immunocytochemically characterized cells or pathways, visualized by Golgi impregnation. Question marks indicate that electron microscopic analysis alone reveals only minor portions of the postsynaptic neurons, which generally do not allow unequivocal identification of the cell type. (C) Axonal and dendritic processes of retrogradely HRP-labeled neurons or postsynaptic target cells of anterogradely HRP-labeled axon terminals can be revealed by Golgi impregnation. In this way it is possible to study the synaptic relationships of identified neurons with distant brain areas. (D) Postsynaptic target cells of electrophysiologically characterized and HRP-filled neurons, visualized by Golgi impregnation. Question marks as in B.

is performed on the Vibratome sections before embedding for electron microscopy, whereas in the postembedding procedure the immunostaining is done on semithin or ultrathin sections cut from the resin-embedded material. In general, postembedding staining offers some obvious advantages. For instance, there is no barrier for the penetration of antibodies. This, in turn, eliminates the need for freeze–thawing or detergent treatments, which generally decrease the quality of Golgi impregnation and tissue preservation. Furthermore, controls can be performed on the same cell bodies in adjacent plastic sections. However, a major drawback of postembedding staining is that it can only be used for localizing those antigens that survive osmium treatment and embedding. To date, we have succeeded in localizing only GABA and glutamate by the postembedding technique. For further advantages and limitations in the use of pre- and postembedding immunostaining in combination with the Golgi method, see Section III.

Figures 2–6 feature examples in which the Golgi method has been combined with an immunocytochemical or a histochemical technique. Except for the example illustrated in Fig. 4, in which the postembedding technique was used, all the other figures feature neurons identified by the aid of the preembedding immunostaining.

Figures 2, 3, and 4 demonstrate GABAergic interneurons in the cerebral cortex of the rat or cat. The axonal and dendritic patterns are revealed in great detail and on a scale far superior to any other currently used immunocytochemical technique. Although interneurons with smooth dendrites had long been suspected of being GABAergic (Ribak, 1978) and inhibitory, the combination of GAD immunocytochemistry and Golgi impregnation in the same material (Somogyi et al., 1983) provided direct evidence that most, if not all, neurons containing GAD-like immunoreactivity in the cortex belong to the class of interneurons with smooth dendrites (Fig. 2). This broad class of neurons consists of several distinct cell types. One of the most characteristic types, discovered by Szentágothai (1978; Szentágothai and Arbib, 1974), shown in Figs. 3 and 4, has a "chandelierlike" axon arborization and is also unique in the sense that it terminates exclusively on the axon initial segments of pyramidal neurons (Fig. 3C; DeFelipe et al., 1985; Fairen and Valverde, 1980; Peters et al., 1982; Somogyi, 1977; Somogyi et al., 1982; for review see Peters, 1984).

Direct evidence for the presence of GAD in the synaptic terminals of an axoaxonic cell was first obtained by the combination technique illustrated in Fig. 3 (Freund et al., 1983). The perikaryon of the neuron shown in Fig. 3A was situated deep in the 80-μm-thick section, but the preembedding immunostaining was confined to the superficial 5–10 μm as a result of the limited penetration of antibodies. Therefore, immunoreactivity could not be demonstrated in the cell body in the same way as shown in Fig. 2. However, it was possible to reveal GAD immunoreactivity at the electron microscopic level in those terminals of the neuron that could be followed to the surface of the section (Fig. 3C–E). Further evidence for the GABAergic nature of the axoaxonic cells was provided by demonstrating GABA immunoreactivity in cell bodies of Golgi-impregnated axoaxonic cells using the postembedding

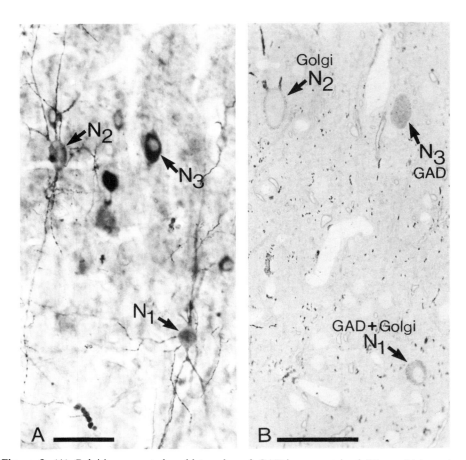

Figure 2. (A) Golgi-impregnated, gold-toned, and GAD-immunostained 80-μm-thick section from the visual cortex of the cat. A GAD-immunoreactive soma (N_3) and two Golgi-impregnated smooth dendritic neurons (N_1 and N_2) are marked. (B) Semithin section faintly stained with toluidine blue, showing that N_1 and N_3 are immunoreactive for GAD, as demonstrated by the immunoperoxidase end product (brown in the section) in their cytoplasm. Only a thin rim of Golgi/gold precipitate surrounds the immunonegative cell N_2, and the same precipitate is evident around N_1. Scales: A and B, 50 μm.

immunohistochemical procedure (Fig. 4; Somogyi *et al.,* 1985).

Clutch cells in the visual cortex of the monkey (Kisvárday *et al.,* 1986) and neurogliform and bitufted cells in the visual cortex of cat (Somogyi, 1986) have also been shown to contain immunoreactive GABA by the postembedding staining of Golgi-impregnated cells.

In another application—using a combination of preembedding immunostaining and the "single-section Golgi" method—Izzo and colleagues (1987) have shown that most neurons containing [Met]-enkephalin (Fig. 5) or sub-

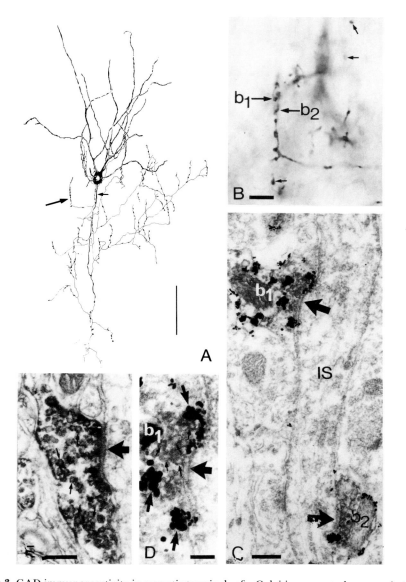

Figure 3. GAD immunoreactivity in synaptic terminals of a Golgi-impregnated axoaxonic (chandelier) cell in the cat visual cortex. (A) Drawing of the cell; the origin of the axon (small arrow) and one of its terminal segments (large arrow) are indicated. (B) Light micrograph of the same terminal segment in the GAD-immunostained and Golgi-impregnated 80-μm-thick section. Two of its boutons (b_1 and b_2) and GAD-immunoreactive varicosities (small arrows) are labeled. (C,D) Electron micrographs of the two Golgi-impregnated and GAD-immunoreactive boutons (b_1 and b_2) in synaptic contact (arrows) with an axon initial segment (IS). The homogeneous electron-dense immunoperoxidase end product (small arrows in D) surrounding synaptic vesicles can be distinguished from the more electron-dense particulate Golgi/gold precipitate (long arrows in D). (E) GAD-immunoreactive bouton in synaptic contact with an axon initial segment. The immunoperoxidase end product surrounding synaptic vesicles (small arrows) resembles that seen in the Golgi-impregnated and immunoreactive terminals (b_1 and b_2 in C and D). Thick arrows mark synaptic contacts. Scales: A, 50 μm; B, 5 μm; C,E, 0.25 μm; D, 0.1 μm.

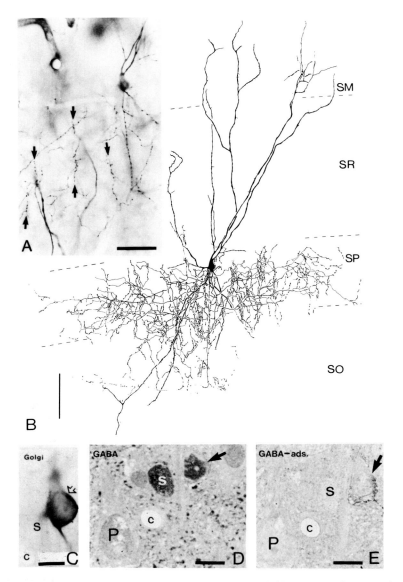

Figure 4. Demonstration of GABA immunoreactivity in a Golgi-impregnated axoaxonic (chandelier) cell of the cat hippocampus. (A,B) Light micrograph (A) and drawing of the gold-toned axoaxonic cell in an 80-μm-thick osmium-treated section. Some of its radially running rows of boutons are labelled by arrows. The dendritic tree spans all layers (SO, stratum oriens; SP, str. pyramidale; SR, str. radiatum; SM, str. moleculare). (C–E) Light micrographs of the perikaryon (open arrow) in the Golgi section (C) and in semithin (0.5-μm) sections (D,E). A capillary (c) and a nonpyramidal cell soma (s) help correlation. The section in D was immunoreacted for GABA. The dark immunoperoxidase end product is present in the soma of the axoaxonic cell (arrow) and in the nonpyramidal cell (s), whereas a pyramidal soma (P) is immunonegative. (E) A consecutive section reacted with the anti-GABA serum adsorbed to GABA. No immunostaining is present in this section; only the Golgi gold precipitate is visible in the axoaxonic cell (arrow). Data from Somogyi *et al.* (1985). Scales: A, 50 μm; B, 100 μm; C–E, 10 μm.

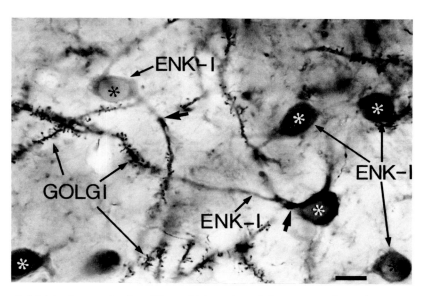

Figure 5. Light micrograph of an 80-μm-thick section of the cat neostriatum immunoreacted for [Met]-enkephalin (ENK-1) and then Golgi-impregnated by a "single section–Golgi" procedure. The immunostaining reveals only cell bodies (asterisks) with the most proximal processes. The Golgi precipitate reveals the spiny dendrites as well. The short arrows mark points where immunostained dendrites or somata become Golgi-impregnated. (Micrograph kindly provided by J. P. Bolam, P. N. Izzo, and A. M. Graybiel.) Scale: 10 μm.

stance-P-like immunoreactivities in the cat neostriatum belong to the class of medium-sized spiny neurons that are known to project to the substantia nigra or to the globus pallidus.

Distal dendrites of choline acetyltransferase-immunoreactive neurons were visualized by section–Golgi impregnation in the rat neostriatum (Bolam *et al.*, 1984b). Direct evidence was provided that the giant smooth-dendritic neurons were immunoreactive for this cholinergic marker enzyme. Examination of synaptic inputs to distal dendrites of cholinergic neurons thus became possible.

Three types of neuron in the rat neostriatum were found to contain acetylcholinesterase activity (Bolam *et al.*, 1984a) following Golgi impregnation of the AChE-positive neurons (Fig. 6). These include the giant cells, which can be recognized without Golgi impregnation on the basis of their unique soma size. However, the other two types, having medium-sized cell bodies, could not have been identified on the basis of their staining for the enzyme alone, as it reveals only the soma and most proximal dendrites (Fig. 6C). Interestingly, these latter two types are not immunoreactive for choline acetyltransferase and therefore are unlikely to be cholinergic (Bolam *et al.*, 1984a,b).

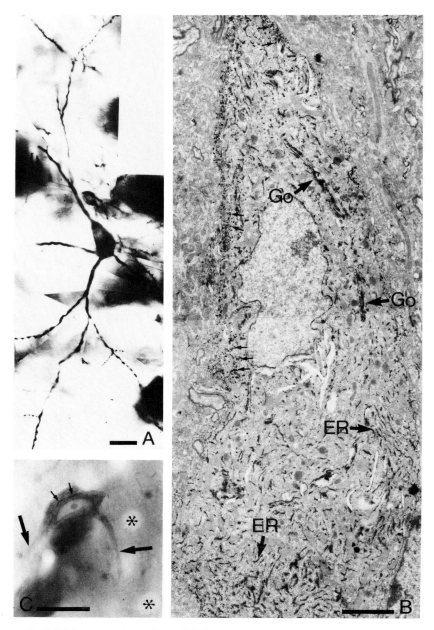

Figure 6. Golgi impregnation of acetylcholinesterase (AChE)-containing neurons in the rat neostriatum. (A) Photomontage of a Golgi-impregnated and gold-toned giant cell in an 80-μm-thick section processed to reveal AChE activity. (B) Electron micrograph of the same cell showing the electron-dense AChE end product in cisternae of the Golgi apparatus (Go) and the endoplasmic reticulum (ER). Particles of the Golgi gold precipitate are best seen in the upper left part of the cytoplasm (small arrows). (C) Light micrograph of another AChE-positive cell in the rat neostriatum as seen without Golgi impregnation. Only the most proximal parts of the dendrites are revealed. Asterisks label AChE-negative medium-sized cell bodies. (Micrographs kindly provided by J. P. Bolam, C. A. Ingham, and A. D. Smith.) Scales: A,C, 20 μm; B, 2 μm.

B. Golgi Impregnation of Neurons Postsynaptic to Immunocytochemically Identified Afferent Axons

The morphological identification of the postsynaptic cell types of immunocytochemically characterized neurons or pathways is often of crucial importance. However, the minor details of the postsynaptic elements seen during electron microscopic examination of the immunostained axons rarely allow the unequivocal identification of the target cell type. It is now possible to visualize the postsynaptic neurons by Golgi impregnation using the combination outlined in Fig. 1B.

In one of the applications of this technique, medium-sized spiny neurons projecting to the substantia nigra were identified as the major postsynaptic targets of the nigrostriatal dopaminergic projection (Freund *et al.*, 1984). These cells were retrogradely labeled with HRP from the substantia nigra and visualized in detail by Golgi impregnation using the section–Golgi procedure (Figs. 7A and 8C). The dopaminergic fibers were identified by preembedding immunocytochemistry for tyrosine hydroxylase (TH) prior to Golgi impregnation of the same material. The distribution of immunoreactive synapses on different parts of the Golgi-impregnated target neurons proved to be uneven. Nearly 60% established symmetrical synaptic contacts on the necks of dendritic spines, and the head of the same spines invariably received an asymmetric synapse from unstained boutons containing round vesicles (Fig. 9). Dendritic shafts of the same neurons were contacted by 35% (Fig. 8A,B) and cell bodies by 6% (Fig. 7) of the immunoreactive fibers.

Evidence was provided in this experiment that the nigrostriatal dopaminergic pathway can monosynaptically influence the "motor" output of the neostriatum. The results suggested that synapses on the cell body and proximal dendritic shafts might mediate a relatively nonselective inhibition, whereas the major dopaminergic input that occurs on the necks of dendritic spines is likely to be highly selective, interacting with the excitatory input to the same spines. One of the main functions of dopamine released from nigrostriatal fibers might thus be to alter the pattern of firing of striatal output neurons by regulating their input.

The same combination of techniques was applied by Bolam and colleagues to study the postsynaptic targets of glutamate decarboxylase (GAD), substance P, and choline acetyltransferase (ChAT) immunoreactive axon terminals. In contrast to the dopaminergic input, somata and proximal dendritic shafts of Golgi-impregnated medium-sized spiny neurons were the major postsynaptic sites of GAD- and substance-P-immunoreactive terminals (Bolam *et al.*, 1985; Izzo and Bolam, 1986). This suggests that GABAergic inhibitory input and substance-P-containing input to the same neurons operate in a less selective manner. The distribution of ChAT-immunoreactive synaptic terminals on striatonigral medium-sized spiny neurons—Golgi-impregnated and retrogradely labeled with HRP from the substantia nigra—was found to be similar to that of the dopaminergic input, as the distal dendrites and spines were more frequent targets than the somatic region (Bolam and Izzo, 1986).

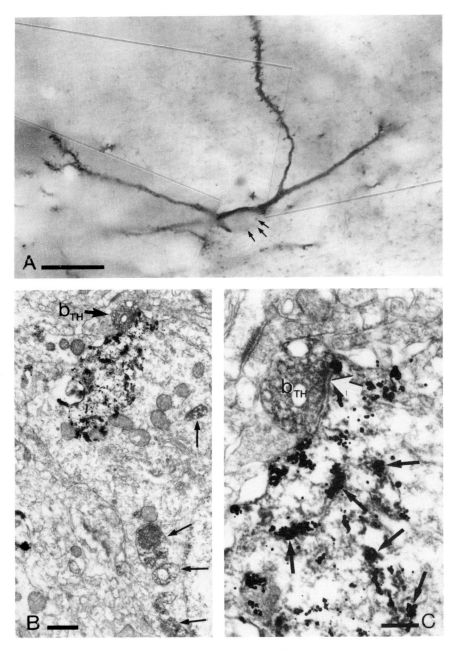

Figure 7. Postsynaptic targets of tyrosine hydroxylase (TH)-immunoreactive terminals identified by a combination of Golgi impregnation and retrograde HRP transport in the neostriatum of rat. (A) Photomontage of a Golgi-impregnated medium-sized spiny neuron retrogradely labeled with HRP from the substantia nigra (dense granules in the cytoplasm, arrows). The neuropil is densely covered by punctate TH-immunoreactive fibers and terminals (B) Electron micrograph of the neuron seen in A, containing lysosomes and multivesicular bodies (arrows) loaded with the reaction end product of retrogradely transported HRP. The highly electron-dense Golgi gold precipitate (also thin arrows in C) fills only the upper left corner of the cell body, where a TH-immunoreactive terminal (b$_{TH}$) is in symmetrical synaptic contact (thick arrow in C) with the soma. Also shown in C at higher magnification. Scales: A, 20 μm; B, 0.5 μm; C, 0.2 μm.

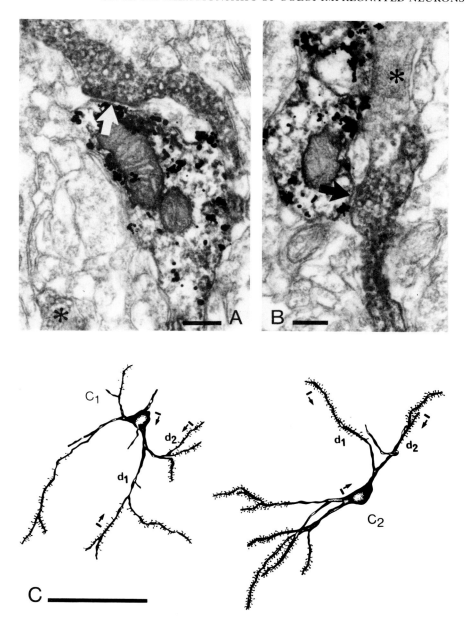

Figure 8. Further examples from the experiment illustrated in Fig. 7. (A,B) Symmetrical synaptic contacts (arrows) between TH-immunoreactive fibers and dendritic shafts of Golgi-impregnated medium-sized spiny neurons shown in C. Another immunoreactive fiber (asterisk in A) is also visible. The dendritic shaft in B is contacted by an additional immunonegative synaptic bouton (asterisk). (C) Drawings of two Golgi-impregnated and retrogradely HRP-labeled striatonigral neurons, which were shown to receive synaptic contacts from TH-immunoreactive terminals in this figure (A,B) and also in Fig. 7 and 9. Arrows label those parts of the dendritic trees ($d_{1,2}$) that have been examined in the electron microscope. Scales: A,B, 0.2 μm; C, 50 μm.

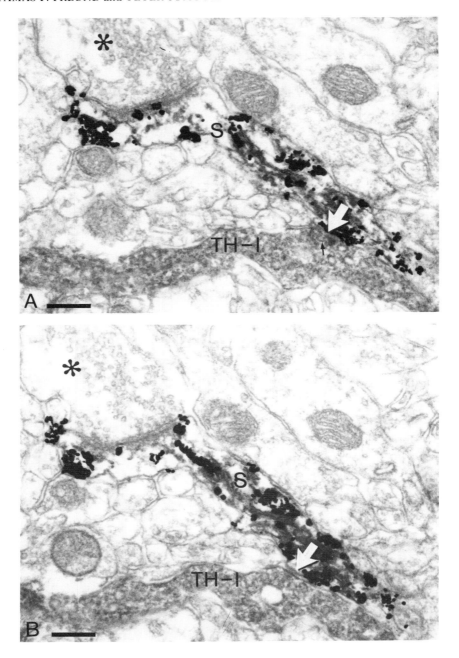

Figure 9. (A,B) Electron micrographs of serial sections cut from a spine (S) of a Golgi-impregnated striatonigral neuron. The neck of the spine is in symmetrical synaptic contact (arrow) with a TH-immunoreactive fiber (TH-I), while the head is receiving an asymmetric synapse from an unstained bouton (asterisk). In the TH-immunoreactive terminal a synaptic vesicle (small arrow in A) is fused with the presynaptic membrane. Scales: A,B, 0.2 μm.

The same approach has been applied by Frotscher and Leranth (1986) to study the distribution of cholinergic (ChAT-immunoreactive) synaptic input to granule cells of the dentate gyrus. They describe symmetrical immuno-reactive synapses on the somata and dendritic shafts of Golgi-impregnated granule cells and both symmetrical and asymmetric cholinergic synapses on the necks and heads of their dendritic spines.

C. Postsynaptic Targets of Electrophysiologically Characterized and HRP-Filled Neurons Visualized by Golgi Impregnation

The identification of cell types innervated by electrophysiologically char-acterized and HRP-filled neurons by electron microscopy alone is in most cases impossible. The difficulties are the same as described in the previous section for immunocytochemically characterized synapses; the minor pro-portion of the target neuron seen in a single ultrathin section or recon-structed from hundreds of them rarely allows the identification of the cell type. Golgi impregnation of the postsynaptic neurons, as schematically illus-trated in Fig. 1D, is a possible approach to this problem. In our hands it began to provide information not obtainable in any other way, as described in the examples below.

Physiologically characterized X- and Y-type thalamocortical axons were in-jected with HRP and shown to arborize mainly in layer IV of visual areas 17 and 18, with only a small projection to layer VI. The synaptic connections established by these afferent axons were studied by electron microscopy of the HRP-filled terminals (Freund *et al.*, 1985a). The major targets of both types of afferents were dendritic spines (80%), but more rarely cell bodies and dendritic shafts were also contacted. However, the origin of the postsyn-aptic dendritic spines and spiny dendrites was not known, since almost all types of spiny neurons in the cortex such as pyramidal cells of layers III, IV, V, and VI and spiny stellate cells have dendritic branches in layer IV. Similarly, the number of synapses between a single afferent axon and one of its target cells could not be established by electron microscopy alone.

We used Golgi impregnation to reveal neurons together with their pro-cesses that were postsynaptic to the HRP-injected thalamic afferents (Freund *et al.*, 1985b). Alternate Vibratome sections containing the filled axons were Golgi impregnated by the section–Golgi procedure, and in this way each single collateral of the axon could be followed from a section not processed for Golgi impregnation to an impregnated one, avoiding the loss of any of the branches in densely Golgi-impregnated areas. Multiple synaptic contacts from Y-type axons were identified on the basal dendrites of Golgi-impreg-nated layer III pyramidal cells in areas 17 (Fig. 10) and 18. One X axon contacted the apical dendrite of the layer V pyramidal cell, a Y axon con-tacted proximal and distal dendrites of two spiny stellate cells, and another Y axon the dendrite of a layer IV smooth-dendritic neuron, which in addi-tion was shown to be immunoreactive for GABA (Freund *et al.*, 1985b). This

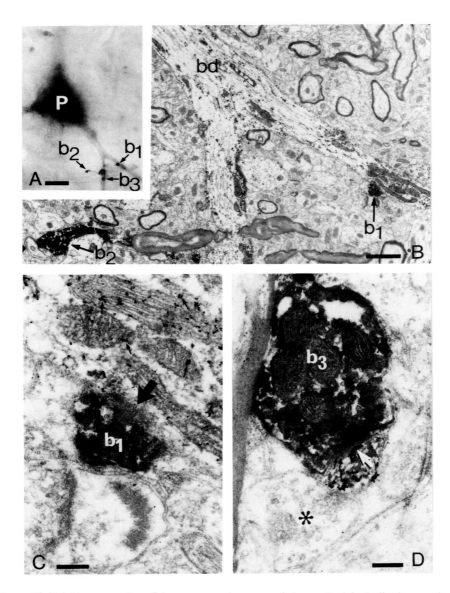

Figure 10. Golgi impregnation of the postsynaptic targets of electrophysiologically characterized and HRP-filled thalamocortical afferents in the cat striate cortex. (A) Golgi-impregnated and gold-toned pyramidal cell (P) in layer III that received contacts from eight boutons on its basal dendrites from an HRP-filled geniculocortical axon (Y type). Two HRP-filled boutons (b_1,b_2) are in focus in this micrograph, and another (b_3) is out of focus. (B) Electron micrograph of the basal dendrite (bd) of the pyramidal cell and two of the HRP-filled boutons (b_1 and b_2). (C) Enlarged view of the asymmetric synapse (arrow) established by one HRP-filled bouton (b_1) with the basal dendrite. The scattered electron-dense granules (small arrows) in the dendrite represent Golgi gold precipitate. (D) The HRP-filled bouton (b_3, slightly out of focus in A) establishes an asymmetric synaptic contact (large white arrow) with a spine originating from the basal dendrite of the pyramidal cell seen in A. The pre- and postsynaptic membranes are indicated by small arrows. The spine also receives symmetrical synaptic input from an unlabeled terminal (asterisk). Scales: A, 10 μm; B, 1 μm; C,D, 0.25 μm.

approach allowed us to establish that one axon only provides a small fraction of the geniculate afferent input to an individual cell, since the maximum number of synapses made between one axon and a single postsynaptic cell was found to be eight, although in most cases it was only one.

The same approach was used by Kisvárday and colleagues (1987) to study the synaptic connections of an electrophysiologically characterized basket cell in layer V of the kitten visual cortex (Fig. 11). Perikarya and basal and apical dendrites of layer V pyramidal cells were shown by Golgi impregnation to be the major postsynaptic sites of this neuron. The Golgi-impregnated pyramidal neuron shown as an example in Fig. 11 was contacted by 34 boutons of this basket cell.

D. Afferent and Efferent Synaptic Connections of Golgi-Impregnated Neurons as Revealed by Horseradish Peroxidase Transport

Anterograde or retrograde transport of horseradish peroxidase can be used to study the input and output relationships of identified Golgi-impregnated neurons with distant brain areas (Bolam and Izzo, 1986; Freund and Somogyi, 1983; Freund et al., 1984; Izzo and Bolam, 1986; Somogyi et al., 1979, 1981a). By using chromogens for the peroxidase reaction that produce an electron-dense reaction end product, it is possible to examine synaptic connections between HRP-labeled terminals and Golgi-impregnated neurons. The retrogradely labeled and Golgi-impregnated neurons can also be studied in both the light and the electron microscope.

This approach has been applied successfully in studies of the synaptic connections of identified striatonigral neurons (Bolam and Izzo, 1986; Freund et al., 1984; Izzo and Bolam, 1986). Following injections of HRP into the substantia nigra, the cell bodies and occasionally some of the most proximal dendrites of striatonigral neurons are labeled. The dendritic tree can then be visualized using the section–Golgi procedure (Fig. 12A), and synaptic contacts established by labeled (immunostained, HRP-labeled, or degenerating) terminals can be traced on different parts of the neuron. Tyrosine hydroxylase (Figs. 7–9; Freund et al., 1984), choline acetyltransferase (Bolam and Izzo, 1986), and substance P (Izzo and Bolam, 1986) immunoreactive synaptic inputs were localized on striatonigral neurons identified by retrograde HRP transport and Golgi impregnation. Axon terminals of the nigrostriatal projection and local collaterals of striatonigral neurons also become labeled following injections of HRP into the substantia nigra, and synaptic connections between retrogradely labeled, Golgi-impregnated neurons and terminals labeled by transported HRP can frequently be found (Fig. 12B–D). Immunoreactive boutons can easily be distinguished from terminals labeled by transported HRP. The peroxidase reaction end product is confined to dense bodies or smooth endoplasmic reticulum in the case of the latter. In the immunocytochemically stained profiles, the reaction end product surrounds the membranes of all cytoplasmic organelles (Fig. 12B–D). It has

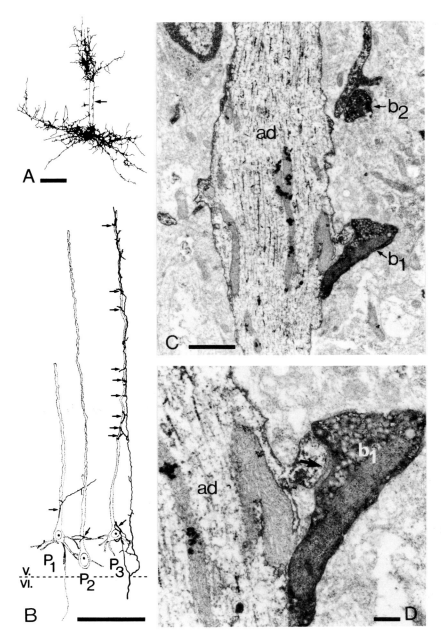

Figure 11. Golgi impregnation of the postsynaptic targets of an electrophysiologically characterized and HRP-filled basket cell in layer V of the kitten visual cortex. (A) Computer reconstruction of the basket cell axon. (B) One of the collaterals (arrow in A) that gave rise to the supragranular tuft followed the apical dendrite of a layer V pyramidal cell (P_3, contacts indicated by arrows) visualized here by Golgi impregnation. Other pyramidal cells (P_1, P_2) received fewer contacts (arrows). (C,D) Electron micrographs of two boutons (b_1, b_2) contacting spines of the Golgi-impregnated and gold-toned apical dendrite (ad) of P_3. (D) The HRP-filled bouton (b_1) is shown at higher power to establish a symmetrical synaptic contact (arrow). Data from Kisvárday *et al.* (1987). Scales: A, 200 μm; B, 100 μm; C, 1 μm; D, 0.2 μm.

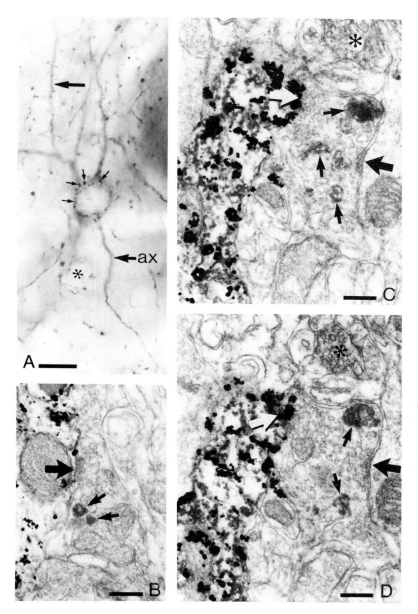

Figure 12. Combination of Golgi impregnation with HRP transport at the light and electron microscopic level. (A) Golgi-impregnated and gold-toned medium-sized spiny neuron in the rat neostriatum retrogradely labeled by HRP (granules labeled by arrows) from the substantia nigra. A spiny dendrite (large arrow), the axon initial segment (ax), and another retrogradely HRP-labeled but not Golgi-impregnated cell body (asterisk) are indicated. (B–D) Synaptic contact (large arrows, cut tangentially in case of B and C) between a Golgi-impregnated dendrite and an axon terminal labeled by transported HRP in the rat neostriatum following an HRP injection into the substantia nigra. The HRP-labeled terminal contains dense bodies and cisternae of smooth endoplasmic reticulum (small arrows) filled with HRP reaction product. The asterisk labels TH-immunostained profile. Scales: A, 10 μm; B–D, 0.2 μm.

been shown by this approach that striatonigral neurons are in contact with each other via their local axon collaterals (Freund *et al.*, 1984).

The anterograde transport of HRP in combination with Golgi impregnation can potentially be applied to study the origin of certain inputs to identified cell types. This technique is clearly superior to the anterograde degeneration–Golgi combination (Blackstad, 1965; Frotscher *et al.*, 1981; Frotscher and Zimmer, 1983; Peters *et al.*, 1979; Somogyi, 1978; White, 1979; White and Rock, 1981), since following lesions, only a proportion of the degenerating terminals can be recognized at any one survival time. A much larger percentage of the projecting axons can be labeled by anterograde HRP transport (Mesulam and Mufson, 1980; Reperant, 1975; Sotelo and Riche, 1974). In this case care should be taken to choose a sensitive chromogen that produces an electron-dense reaction end product (Carson and Mesulam, 1982). Satisfactory results have been obtained in our laboratory using the DAB method with cobalt and nickel intensification (Adams, 1977, 1981), but the TMB method with subsequent DAB stabilization and cobalt–nickel intensification is likely to be more sensitive (Rye *et al.*, 1984).

III. ADVANTAGES AND LIMITATIONS

The major advantage of the combined techniques is that several aspects of the synaptic organization of neuronal circuits can now be studied directly in the same material. Thus, the results obtained in this way can be interpreted without resort to inferential arguments. These combinations form a bridge among electrophysiological, neurochemical, and morphological approaches.

The main limitation is that the procedures are very time consuming; thus, only a limited sample of neurons can be studied. In some cases this makes the generalization of the results difficult. Another limitation is that the identification of neuronal interactions depends on the morphologically defined synaptic contact. It is not yet clear how much neuronal communication takes place at nonsynaptic sites. In places where such interactions are significant, they will not be revealed by our techniques.

In the combined procedures conflicting technical requirements have to be satisfied. For example, immunocytochemical procedures usually need pretreatment of the sections, e.g., freeze–thawing or the use of detergents, in order to increase the penetration of antibodies. Unfortunately, any treatment that disrupts the integrity of cell membranes also decreases the quality of Golgi impregnation. Frequently, even with treatments to enhance the penetration of antibodies, the preembedding methods will achieve immunoreactivity only in the superficial few micrometers depth of the sections. The degree of antibody penetration varies from area to area and also from antiserum to antiserum. This means that although the processes of Golgi-impregnated neurons will cross the entire 80- to 100-μm-thick section, only at the two surfaces of the section will immunoreactivity be present. Furthermore, as a result of limited antibody penetration the quantification of preembedding immunostaining is very difficult if at all possible. False negative staining of cell bodies and/or axon terminals can occur at any depth in the section. Further uncertainties arise when colchicine treatment is required to increase the concentration of the antigen in cell bodies. The region uniformly affected by colchicine cannot be determined.

These difficulties do not apply to the combination of postembedding immunocytochemistry and Golgi impregnation, but this latter technique can be used for only a limited range of antigens (see Section IIA and Somogyi and Freund, Chapter 9, this volume). In this case quantification of immunostained elements is possible, although the loss of antigenic sites as a result of osmium treatment and embedding should be taken into account. With antisera to GABA, the density of stained profiles in a given area appears to be the same both in osmium-treated and untreated material provided the same fixative and procedure were used for perfusion fixation. The staining intensity and the level of background nonspecific staining can vary from animal to animal.

The combination of postembedding GABA immunocytochemistry and Golgi impregnation is the easiest and most informative approach to study the synaptic connections of identified types of GABAergic cells in any brain area where neurons can be Golgi impregnated. The conventional Golgi electron microscopic techniques can be used to study the synaptic input and output of the individual identified neurons. Semithin sections can subsequently be cut from the cell body of the neuron at any stage for postembedding immunostaining.

The major limitation of demonstrating synaptic contacts between Golgi-impregnated and physiologically characterized cells is that the probability of impregnating neurons postsynaptic to the HRP-filled terminals is very low. We have tried to overcome this by recycling sections several times. Although this increases the chance of impregnating cells in the area covered by the HRP-filled neuron, the quality of impregnation becomes poorer with each cycle.

Whenever synaptic contacts are found in this combination, their interpretation requires caution. The distribution of synapses established by a single afferent axon on its target cells is likely to be uneven (Figs. 10 and 11; see Section II.C; Hamos *et al.*, 1987); therefore, the generalization of quantitative data obtained in this way is not possible. More conclusive results could be obtained by intracellular iontophoresis of a marker that is transported across synapses. In this case those targets receiving the largest number of synapses from the injected neuron could contain the highest levels of the transsynaptic label. We have seen in our material evidence for a weak transsynaptic spread of HRP in cases of heavily filled axons (Freund *et al.*, 1985a). Some markers appear to cross the synaptic membrane much more readily than HRP. The C fragment of tetanus toxin (Dumas *et al.*, 1979; Evinger and Erichsen, 1986), certain types of viruses (Kristensson *et al.*, 1982), tritiated amino acids (Grafstein, 1971), wheat germ agglutinin (Ruda and Coulter, 1982), and the complex of WGA and HRP (Gerfen *et al.*, 1982; Itaya and van Hoesen, 1982) have been used for transsynaptic labeling. However, to our knowledge, none of these markers has yet been applied in intracellular recording and marking experiments or in electron microscopic studies of the transsynaptically labeled neurons.

The procedures described in this chapter have not gained widespread application. One reason is that their use requires expertise in a diverse range of anatomic techniques rarely present in the same laboratory. The other reason is that in many parts of the nervous system it is not necessary to apply combinations of techniques for the recognition of neuronal types. For example, in the isodendritic central core of the brain, stretching from the spinal cord to the the hypothalamus, neurons differ more biochemically than in the distribution of their processes. In complex neural centers, neurons that share biochemical characteristics evolved into different forms as a result of the differences in their input, output, and functional properties. Our examples show that the converse can also be found, and morphologically similar cells can have different neurochemical characteristics. In these networks the only way to unravel the precise rules of synaptic interactions is to demonstrate the anatomic, physiological, and neurochemical properties directly in the interacting neurons.

IV. APPENDIX: METHODS

A. Preparation of the Animals: Extracellular HRP and Colchicine Injections

The combination of Golgi impregnation and the localization of endogenous or exogeneously applied substances in the brain often requires the pretreatment of animals prior to fixation. To illustrate the combined procedures, material from adult rats and cats of either sexes is used.

1. Colchicine Injections

To enhance the concentration of antigen, the cats used for glutamic acid decarboxylase (GAD) immunocytochemistry received unilateral injections of colchicine (BHD) directly into the lateral gyrus of the cortex through a glass capillary with 50-μm tip diameter (Somogyi *et al.*, 1983). The animals were sedated with ketamine hydrochloride (0.4 mg/kg Ketanest[R] i.m.) and anesthetized with xylazine hydrochloride (1 ml/kg, Rompun[R], Bayer). The injection capillary was advanced from the caudal to the rostral pole, parallel with the sagittal sulcus, 3 mm lateral, and at an angle approximately 20° to the surface of the cortex. After the capillary had been advanced 12 mm, it was gradually withdrawn, and 0.2 μl colchicine (6 μg/μl, dissolved in artificial cerebrospinal fluid) was injected at every 1.0–1.2 mm over a distance of 10 mm. Thus, altogether 2 μl of solution containing 12 μg colchicine was injected.

2. The Intracellular Iontophoresis of HRP

Iontophoresis of HRP in cats following electrophysiological characterization is described in detail by Martin and Whitteridge (1984), and all such cells used in our experiments derive from their material.

3. HRP–WGA Injections

Rats were injected with 80 nl of a conjugate of horseradish peroxidase and wheat germ agglutinin (HRP–WGA; final concentration approximately 3% HRP) in the substantia nigra under chloral hydrate (350 mg/kg i.p.) anaesthesia (Freund *et al.*, 1984). Glass capillaries attached to a gas pressure delivery system and coordinates of *A* (earbar zero), 2.2; *L*, 6.2; *V*, 6.4, at an oblique lateral angle (Somogyi *et al.*, 1979) were used.

4. Preparation of Animals for Acetylcholinesterase Histochemistry

Rats received intramuscular injections of a mixture of diisopropylphosphorofluoridate (DFP, Sigma Chemical Company, 1.8 mg/kg), and atropine sulfate (BDH Chemicals, 6 mg/kg) dissolved in saline (Bolam *et al.*, 1984a). Injection volumes were approximately 0.1 ml.

B. Preparation of Tissue Sections: Fixation, Sectioning, and Embedding

For subsequent histology, the animals were perfused with one of three fixatives, according to the type of experiment. Fixative A was used for experiments involving extracellular injection or intracellular iontophoresis of HRP (Martin and Whitteridge, 1984; Somogyi *et al.*, 1979). It consists of 0.5–1% paraformaldehyde (TAAB) and 2.5% glutaraldehyde (TAAB, Reading) dissolved in 0.1 M phosphate buffer (PB, pH 7.2–7.4). Fixative B was used in our electron microscopic and Golgi electron microscopic degeneration studies and consists of 1% each of paraformaldehyde and glutaraldehyde dissolved in 0.1 M PB at pH 7.2–7.4. Fixatives A and B give the best results for the immunocytochemical localization of GABA, whereas fixative C, containing 4% paraformaldehyde, 0.05–0.1% glutaraldehyde, and approximately 0.2% picric acid in 0.1 M PB (pH 7.1–7.4)(Somogyi and Takagi, 1982), is used for the immunocytochemical detection of various enzymes and neuropeptides and also for acetylcholinesterase histochemistry. For the latter, the use of a fixative containing 2% paraformaldehyde and 2% glutaraldehyde gives equally good results.

The colchicine-injected cats were reanesthetized after 24 hr with chloral hydrate (350 mg/kg i.p.) and perfused through the heart first with Tyrode's solution (gassed with a mixture of 95% O_2 and 5% CO_2) and then with fixative C.

The cats used for electrophysiological recordings and intracellular HRP filling were perfused at the end of the recording session (1–18 hr following the iontophoresis) in the same way: first with saline, then with fixative A.

The rats that received HRP–WGA injections were reanesthetized with chloral hydrate (350 mg/kg i.p.) after 24–36 hr survival time and perfused through the heart first with Tyrode's solution and then with fixative A. Fixative C was used for the immunohistochemical localization of proteins (Freund et al., 1984).

Rats used for acetylcholinesterase histochemistry were perfused under chloral hydrate anesthesia (350 mg/kg i.p.) in the same way 4–6 hr after the DFP injection.

Brains were removed from the skull, and the areas of interest dissected into about $6 \times 5 \times 2$ mm blocks. They were postfixed in the same fixatives for various lengths of time, usually 1–6 hr. In order to increase penetration of antibodies in preembedding immunocytochemistry, some blocks were immersed in 10% and 20% sucrose in 0.1 M PB until they sank and then frozen in liquid nitrogen and thawed. Blocks were then sectioned on a Vibratome (Oxford Instruments), usually at 80–100 μm, the thickness optimal for the section–Golgi impregnation and also for most histochemical procedures. Following washes in several changes of 0.1 M PB, the sections were processed for HRP or immunohistochemistry.

For acetylcholinesterase histochemistry (Bolam et al., 1984a), the blocks were washed and sectioned in 0.1 M sodium cacodylate buffer (pH 7.2). The sections were then washed and stored in the same buffer at 4°C for up to 12 hr before the histochemical reaction.

The thorough removal of unbound fixative from the tissue is especially important for immunocytochemistry, and we therefore wash the sections at least five times for 30 min each.

The HRP–WGA injection sites were sectioned similarly, and they were revealed by conventional light microscopic HRP histochemistry using 3,3'-diaminobenzidine tetra-HCl (DAB) as chromogen (see below for details).

C. Histochemical Staining Techniques

1. Preembedding Immunocytochemistry

The primary antisera used for the illustrations were raised in rabbits with the exception of monoclonal antibodies (rat) to substance P. Incubations were carried out in small glass vials in the following order at room temperature using phosphate-buffered saline (PBS, pH 7.3–7.4) containing 1% normal goat (or rabbit for the substance P) serum (NGS, Miles or Cappel) for all the washes and antibody dilutions unless otherwise stated:

1. One hour in 20% normal goat (or rabbit) serum diluted in PBS.
2. Wash for three times 20 min.
3. Overnight (or 6–36 hr) at 4°C in the primary antiserum (rabbit, rat) at dilutions 1 : 1000 for the anti-tyrosine-hydroxylase (van den Pol *et al.*, 1984), 1 : 500 or 1 : 1000 for the anti-glutamate-decarboxylase (Wu *et al.*, 1982), 1 : 600 for the anti-[Met]-enkephalin (Micevych and Elde, 1980), or 1 : 1000 for the anti-substance-P (Cuello *et al.*, 1979).
4. Wash for three times 30 min.
5. Six hours (occasionally 1–36 hr was used with satisfactory results) in goat antirabbit immunoglobulin (Miles) diluted 1 : 40 or rabbit antirat (Miles) diluted 1 : 50.
6. Wash for three times 30 min.
7. Overnight at 4°C in rabbit peroxidase–antiperoxidase (PAP) complex (Miles) diluted 1 : 80 or 1 : 100 or rat PAP (Sternberger, Meyer Inc.) 1 : 100 dilution.
8. Wash for three times 30 min in PBS only.
9. Wash twice for 20 min in 0.05 M Tris-HCl buffer (pH 7.4–7.6).
10. Preincubation for 20 min in dark in DAB (50 mg/100 ml) dissolved in the same Tris-HCl buffer.
11. Incubation in the same DAB solution after the addition of 1% hydrogen peroxide to a final concentration of 0.01%. The appropriate time of incubation has to be judged by visual examination of the sections as they are turning brown; this is usually 2–8 min.
12. Wash three times 20 min in 0.05 M Tris-HCl buffer (pH 7.4).

Following a few rinses in 0.1 M PB, the sections can be osmium treated and processed for Golgi impregnation (see below). The vials containing the sections were subjected to agitation in all the above steps.

2. Intra- and Extracellularly Injected HRP Enzyme Histochemistry

The histochemical reaction for intracellularly delivered HRP follows the method of Hanker *et al.* (1977), with cobalt and nickel intensification (Adams, 1981) as described earlier (Martin and Whitteridge, 1984) and also in Chapter 9 (Somogyi and Freund) in this book.

For the visualization of retrogradely or anterogradely transported HRP we use DAB as the chromogen (see above for immunoperoxidase reaction). This reaction produces an electron-dense end product. The sections are incubated for 20–30 min. If immunocytochemistry is to be carried out on the same sections at a later stage, then a shorter incubation time (5–8 min) should be used, since the immunoperoxidase reaction will add to the background. With this shorter time, however, the reaction may not be sensitive enough to visualize anterogradely labeled terminals.

The use of cobalt and nickel intensification (Adams, 1981) for the detection of anterograde labeling is advisable (not used in the illustrated material).

The density and distribution of retrogradely labeled neurons can be checked at this stage in the light microscope. The end product of retrogradely transported HRP is present in the perinuclear cytoplasm and most proximal dendrites of the labeled neurons in the form of dark brown granules.

3. Acetylcholinesterase Histochemistry

The procedure of Koelle and Friedenwald (1949) was used and modified for electron microscopy (Bolam *et al.*, 1984a; Lewis and Knight, 1977). All steps were carried out at 4°C with constant agitation unless otherwise stated.

1. Wash twice for 20 min in succinate buffer, which is made by mixing 2 ml 0.5 M succinic acid, 2 ml 0.2 M calcium acetate, and 120 ml isotonic sodium sulfate (38 g/liter), adjusting to pH 5.3 with 1 M sodium hydroxide, and then diluting to 200 ml with distilled water.
2. Incubate for 4 hr in a medium that consists of 2.5 ml 0.5 succinic acid (pH 5.3), 4.5 ml distilled water, 20 ml isotonic sodium sulfate, and 20 ml of the following supernatant solution. This is prepared on the day of incubation by dissolving 200 mg acetylthiocholine iodide (Sigma Chemical Company) in 8 ml distilled water and then adding 14 ml of 0.1 M copper sulfate. This solution has to be filtered using a Millipore™ filter (0.22-μm pore size). Glycine (124 mg) is then added to 20 ml of the filtrate to form the supernatant. In some experiments ethopropazine hydrochloride (1.75 mg) was added to the final incubation medium to inhibit nonspecific cholinesterase.
3. Wash twice in succinate buffer for 30 min.
4. Sulfide treatment twice for 30 min. The sulfide medium is prepared by mixing 10 ml 0.5 M succinic acid, 1 ml 0.2 M calcium acetate, and 60 ml isotonic sodium sulfate adjusted to pH 5.3 with freshly prepared 4% sodium sulfide (approximately 25 ml is needed). Dilute this to a final volume of 100 ml with distilled water.
5. Wash in succinate buffer four times for 15 min.
6. Postfixation in modified Dalton's osmium (Dalton, 1955) for 30 min at 4°C without shaking (pH 5.6).
7. Wash four times in distilled water for 3 min.

The sections are now ready for Golgi impregnation (see below). Note that these sections have already been osmium treated; thus, the second step (see Fig. 13) of the section–Golgi procedure will follow. At this stage, AChE-positive neurons can be seen in the sections under the light microscope with a grayish precipitate contained in their perikarya and most proximal dendrites, which often outlines the nuclear membrane and Golgi apparatus.

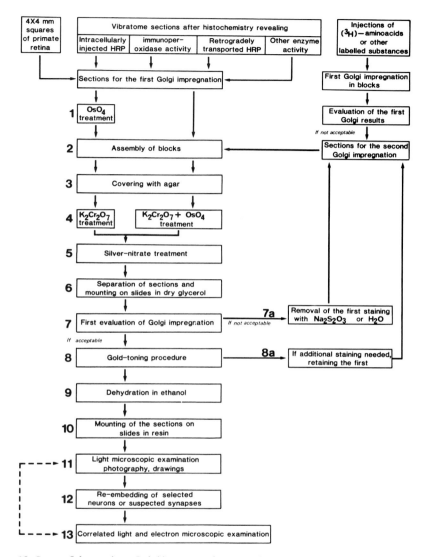

Figure 13. Steps of the section–Golgi impregnation procedure for light and electron microscopy.

D. Section–Golgi Impregnation

The Golgi impregnation procedure for sections (Freund and Somogyi, 1983) is outlined in Fig. 13, and in the description we follow the numbered steps in the scheme. Once the histochemical procedures are completed, the sections can be processed for Golgi impregnation. Unless otherwise stated, the steps are all carried out with solutions at room temperature.

1. Osmium Tetroxide Treatment

This is required both for electron microscopy and for the rapid Golgi impregnation. In the original method it was suggested that the OsO_4 treatment could be done either before the assembly of blocks or following the assembly by including OsO_4 in the potassium dichromate solution. Experience shows that it is better to treat the sections before assembly. This way the sections are much easier to handle, and their separation is also more successful. We use 0.5% OsO_4 (in 0.1 M PB at ph 7.4) for 1 hr or 1% for 40 min after incubation in Hanker–Yates reagent (intracellular HRP injections), 1% OsO_4 for 40–90 min after immunocytochemistry with DAB as chromogen, and 1% OsO_4 for 20–30 min after DAB or Hanker–Yates reagent in retrograde or anterograde HRP-transport experiments. Generally, the concentration of OsO_4 has to be decided in pilot experiments, depending on the chromogen used in peroxidase reaction and the area of the brain being studied. Although the sections turn black in the osmium, they should still remain sufficiently transparent for light microscopic examination.

In addition to the sections of interest, a few 100- to 200-μm-thick sections from the same area with the same shape are cut and treated with OsO_4 for later use as top and bottom cover sections of the block assembly.

If OsO_4 is included in the potassium dichromate solution, either 0.5% or 1% is used for 1–3 days. Osmium treatment in the $K_2Cr_2O_7$ solution results in sections with much lighter background than the same concentration given in phosphate buffer.

Following the OsO_4 treatment the sections are washed three times in 0.1 M PB for 10 min and rinsed twice in distilled water (3 min).

2. Assembly of Blocks

The sections are piled on top of each other on a silicon rubber plate using a fine brush (Fig. 14). Ideally, the sections should have matching shapes and sizes. Preferably sections cut from the same block on the Vibratome should be used, so that they can be assembled with matching edges. Uneven edges make the later separation of sections very difficult, as the agar will fill all spaces that occur between overhanging edges. The distilled water is repeatedly blotted at the bottom of the pile to get the sections tightly together, but care should be taken to prevent drying. Two osmium-treated but not incubated covering sections (100–200 μm thick) are used at the top and bottom, since these usually cannot be separated from the agar after the impregnation. Sections that have previously been processed for different histochemical reactions can be put into the same block if the edges are matching.

3. Covering with Agar

The block obtained in this way is surrounded with 5% agar in distilled water (Fig. 14). The agar should be cool enough to set as soon as it comes

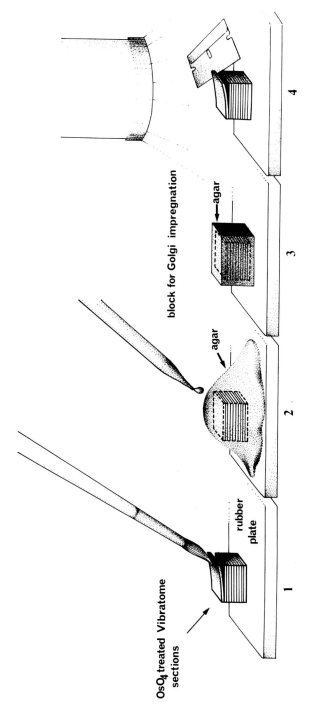

Figure 14. The main steps in the assembly of sections into blocks suitable for Golgi impregnation and their separation following impregnation. 1: The osmium-treated sections (80–100 μm thick) are placed on top of each other while the buffer is repeatedly blotted at the bottom section. 2: The pile is then covered with agar from both sides. 3: The excess agar is trimmed off, leaving an 0.5- to 1-mm-thick layer around the block. 4: Following Golgi impregnation, the sections are separated under a dissecting microscope using a blunt razor blade, forceps, and a brush.

out of the pipette, to avoid excessive heating of the block. While the agar is poured on, the sections should be kept tightly together (pressed with a spatula); otherwise silver chromate crystals will be formed in the gaps between sections. When the agar sets, the block is turned over, and the bottom face is also covered. Then the excess agar is trimmed off with a razor blade so that about 0.5–1.0 mm is left on all sides around the sections.

4. Potassium Dichromate Treatment

We use the same 3.5% potassium dichromate solution overnight for all blocks, but any concentration between 2% and 4% can give good results. The ratio between the potassium dichromate and silver nitrate concentration determines the amount of silver chromate crystals and the density of impregnated neuronal elements formed within the tissue. If osmium treatment was not carried out before the block assembly, then OsO_4 is included in the potassium dichromate solution (see also step 1 above). Here treatment is usually for 1–6 days, but for small blocks a few hours can be sufficient.

5. Silver Nitrate Treatment

Following a few seconds rinse in double-distilled water, the blocks are transferred into silver nitrate solution. The concentration and duration of $AgNO_3$ treatment depend on the size of the block, the concentration of potassium dichromate used previously, and the density of Golgi-impregnated neurons required. In general, blocks assembled from immunostained sections require higher concentrations of $AgNO_3$ than the solid tissue blocks of the same size for conventional Golgi impregnation, and even higher if the sections have been freeze–thawed for the facilitation of antibody penetration. Depending on the brain area, for a block of immunostained sections of $7 \times 6 \times 4$ mm size including the agar, 0.8–1.2% $AgNO_3$ is used, and 1.0–1.4% if they were frozen and thawed. For this size of block assembled from sections containing only HRP-injected cells or transported HRP reaction end product, a concentration 0.6–0.8% gives the best results, which is similar to that for conventional Golgi blocks. The blocks are left in this solution until the interior of the block is in equilibrium with the solution, i.e., for at least 4–8 hr or overnight if convenient. If the silver concentration is relatively low, large crystals will be present on the surface of the block and the sections, and there will be few impregnated neuronal structures in the sections.

6. Separation of Sections

This step is carried out under a dissecting microscope on a silicon rubber plate using a blunt razor blade, forceps, and a fine brush. The agar has to be removed first from each side of the block, together with the cover sections if necessary. The rest of the sections are separated by advancing the blunt razor blade horizontally between the top section and the rest of the block while the block is gently pushed toward the blade by the brush. If the blade is too sharp it can cut into the sections. Dry glycerol is repeatedly put on the block to make separation easier and to avoid breaking and drying of sections. If silver chromate crystals have formed between sections, these bind them together, but the ease of separation greatly depends on the fixative used. Immunostained sections are the most difficult to separate, because the fixative usually contains low concentrations of glutaraldehyde. Each separated section is placed on the rubber plate, and the surface crystals are removed by gentle brushing and rinsing in dry glycerol or silver nitrate solution. Thereafter they are mounted on slides in a drop of glycerol under coverslips.

The separation may be easier if small pieces of Parafilm™ are inserted between the sections during the assembly (Frotscher and Leranth, 1986).

7. First Evaluation of the Impregnation

The examination of sections in the light microscope should be as short as possible if recycling is necessary. At this stage the number and density of Golgi-impregnated structures are evaluated in areas of interest. If judged satisfactory, the sections can be stored on slides in glycerol at 4°C for several days prior to gold toning.

Recycling for Repeated Golgi Impregnation

If the first impregnation is not satisfactory but the sections are still in good condition, they can be reassembled into blocks in the same way as in step 2 and impregnated again. Before the second cycle the precipitate formed during the first impregnation can be removed from the sections by immersing them in 1% sodium thiosulfate for three times 15 min (or in distilled water for a longer period) with constant agitation, followed by washing in distilled water for three times 5 min. There can be many reasons why the first impregnation may not be satisfactory. Having too many or too few impregnated cells is the most frequent cause of failure, or the lack of the desired cell type in the desired area or position. The former can be altered by changing the concentration ratio of the dichromate and silver nitrate solutions in the appropriate direction.

8. Gold Toning

This is carried out after the method of Fairén et al. (1977) supplemented with illumination of the sections. Before gold toning the sections are illuminated on both sides for 30–45 min either on a microscope stage with a heat filter or by using a Schott Mainz KL 150B fiberoptic illuminating device containing a 15V, 150-W bulb focused into an 8-mm circle at full strength while the sections are cooled by cold air blowing from a hair dryer. If the sections turn pink or purple, the cooling was insufficient. The illumination is necessary to gold tone the thin processes in the full depth of the section; it also allows a shorter time in gold chloride, and this in turn reduces the number of heavily gold-toned yellow to brown perikarya. The subsequent steps are carried out at 0°C in an ice bath: 10–20 min in 0.05% $NaHAuCl_4 \cdot 2H_2O$ (containing 0.25% glycerol), three 2-min rinses in distilled water, 2 min in 0.2% oxalic acid, and three 2-min rinses in water. This is followed by three times 15 min in 1% sodium thiosulfate at room temperature.

Recycling after Gold Toning

This may be required if the Golgi-impregnated section contains few neurons that are preserved by gold toning. Additional neurons can be Golgi impregnated by assembling the gold-toned sections into a new block. After the second Golgi impregnation, gold toning is carried out again, and this does not affect the neurons obtained in the first cycle.

9-13. Dehydration, Mounting, and Correlated Light and Electron Microscopy

These procedures are essentially the same for each combination of techniques and are described in Section IV.F.

14. Recent Modifications

To eliminate the assembly and separation of sections (steps 2, 3, and 6), the "single section–Golgi" technique was introduced by Gabbott and Somogyi (1984) and later modified by Izzo *et al.* (1987). Individual immunostained, osmium- and $K_2Cr_2O_7$-treated (3.5% for 1–2 hr) sections are "sandwiched" between glass coverslips or microscope slides, which are held together by glue or tape. Then either the whole assembly or one end is immersed in the silver nitrate solution (1–2%) for 6–24 hr. The duration of silver nitrate treatment is determined by regular light microscopic monitoring of the course of impregnation. Sections can be recycled in the same way as above if the first impregnation is not satisfactory.

The use of this procedure is advisable if the Golgi impregnation of only a few sections is required or if the available sections are of irregular shape and size.

E. Golgi Impregnation of Tissue Blocks

Following fixation, the area of interest is dissected into blocks of roughly $5 \times 4 \times 2$ mm in size, washed in several changes of 0.1 M PB (pH 7.2–7.4), and immersed in 1% OsO_4 (in 0.1 M PB) for 6–8 hr. The osmium tetroxide solution has to be replaced with a fresh solution of the same concentration if its color changes. The blocks are transferred directly to 2–5% potassium dichromate solution for 1–3 days. If the block has not been OsO_4 treated earlier, this can also be done at this stage by including 0.5–1% OsO_4 in the dichromate solution. A large volume (20–30 ml) of this solution is required for one block in order to dilute sufficiently the phosphate ions present in the block; otherwise, silver phosphate crystals will be formed during the next step. The blocks are rinsed for a few seconds in distilled water and transferred into 0.6–0.8% silver nitrate solution, usually for 1 day, although 6–10 hr may be sufficient depending on the block size. The blocks are then most conveniently sliced with a tissue chopper (Sorvall TC-2) at 60- to 120-μm thickness using agar support. Sections are mounted on slides in a drop of dry glycerol and stored at 4°C awaiting gold toning. The gold-toning procedure is the same as following section–Golgi impregnation (see above). At the end of this procedure the sections will contain neurons visualized in detail by the gray to black Golgi gold precipitate. Their processes can be followed from section to section in contrast to neurons obtained in the section–Golgi impregnation procedure, which reveals cells only in single sections.

F. Correlated Light and Electron Microscopy

Following the gold-toning procedure the sections are dehydrated in ethanol (1% uranyl acetate is included in the 70% ethanol step for 40 min), embedded and mounted on slides in Durcupan ACM resin (Fluka) under a coverslip, and cured at 56°C for 2 days. The slides can be stored in this form permanently. Selected neurons can be drawn using a camera lucida, photographed, and reembedded in Durcupan in plastic capsules, as described earlier (Somogyi *et al.*, 1979; Somogyi and Takagi, 1982). Different parts of the selected neuron(s) can now be sectioned on an ultramicrotome for correlated electron microscopy or postembedding immunocytochemistry. The surface of the block is examined from time to time in the light microscope during sectioning in order to identify the appropriate parts of the neurons in the electron microscope. High-magnification light micrographs taken before the reembedding also help the correlation. The serial ultrathin sections are mounted on Formvar-coated single-slot grids, stained with lead citrate (Reynolds, 1963), and examined in the electron microscope.

G. Postembedding Immunocytochemistry of Golgi-Impregnated Neurons

Golgi-impregnated and gold-toned neurons are selected, drawn, photo-graphed, and reembedded as described above. Serial semithin sections (0.5–1.0 μm thick) are cut from the somata of the selected neurons and dried on a hotplate onto slides coated with gelatin or egg white. Care should be taken to have at least three sections of a perikaryon, including the nucleus of the cell, on different slides.

1. The resin is etched using ethanolic sodium hydroxide (Lane and Europa, 1965) for 20–30 min.
2. Wash three times in absolute ethanol for 5 min.
3. Wash twice in distilled water for 5 min.
4. Sodium metaperiodate (NaIO$_4$; 1% solution in H$_2$O) treatment for 7 min. The solution is freshly prepared and is used for removing the osmium from the tissue.
5. Wash twice in distilled water for 5 min.
6. Wash in Tris (10 mM) phosphate (10 mM)-buffered isotonic saline (TPBS), pH 7.4, twice for 10 min.

The same TPBS containing 1% normal goat or sheep serum is used for all the washes and antibody dilutions. The subsequent steps are carried out in a humid chamber at room temperature with the following sequence of reagents layered over the slides:

7. Heat inactivated normal sheep or goat serum, 20%, for 20 min.
8. Rinse in TPBS.
9. Two hours in primary antisera to GABA (Hodgson *et al.*, 1985)(code no. GABA-7 or GABA-9) or the same sera after solid-phase adsorption to GABA, all diluted 1 : 2000 to 1 : 5000.
10. Wash three times in TPBS for 10 min.
11. Goat antirabbit IgG (Miles or Dako) for 40–90 min, diluted 1 : 40.
12. Wash three times in TPBS for 10 min.
13. Rabbit peroxidase–antiperoxidase complex (PAP, Dako, diluted 1 : 100) for 60–90 min, followed by wash in TPBS.
14. Peroxidase enzyme reaction is carried out using DAB as the chromo-gen; preincubation for 5 min in DAB (50 mg/100 ml of 0.05 M Tris-HCl buffer) only, then incubation in the same solution for 2–6 min after the addition of 1% H$_2$O$_2$ to a final concentration of 0.01%.
15. Wash in 0.05 M Tris and then in 0.1 M PB. A few drops of 2% OsO$_4$ are added to the last wash to intensify the reaction end product.
16. The sections are dehydrated and covered with XAM neutral mounting medium (BDH).

ACKNOWLEDGMENTS. We thank Mrs. Dorothy Rhodes for typing the manu-script and Mrs. Klara Somogyi for the photographic work. We are grateful to Dr. J. P. Bolam for providing illustrations from his published material.

REFERENCES

Adams, J. C., 1977, Technical considerations on the use of horseradish peroxidase as a neuronal marker, *Neuroscience* **2:**141–145.

Adams, J. C., 1981, Heavy metal intensification of DAB-based HRP reaction product, *J. Histochem. Cytochem.* **29:**775.

Blackstad, T. W., 1965, Mapping of experimental axon degeneration by electron microscopy of Golgi preparations, *Z. Zellforsch.* **67:**819–834.

Balckstad, T. W., 1969, Studies on the hippocampus: Methods of analysis, in: *The Interneuron* (M. Brazier, ed.), UCLA Forum in Medical Sciences, Los Angeles, pp. 391–414.

Bolam, J. P., and Izzo, P. N., 1986, Cholinergic boutons in synaptic contact with striatonigral neurons in the rat neostriatum, *Neurosci. Lett. Suppl.* **26:**S312.

Bolam, J. P., Ingham, C. A., and Smith, A. D., 1984a, The section-Golgi-impregnation procedure. 3. Combination of Golgi-impregnation with enzyme histochemistry and electron microscopy to characterize acetylcholinesterase-containing neurons in the rat neostriatum, *Neuroscience* **12:**687–709.

Bolam, J. P., Wainer, B. H., and Smith, A. D., 1984b, Characterization of cholinergic neurons in the rat neostriatum. A combination of choline acetyltransferase immunocytochemistry, Golgi-impregnation and electron microscopy, *Neuroscience* **12:**711–718.

Bolam, J. P., Powell, J. F., Wu, J.-Y., and Smith, A. D., 1985, Glutamate decarboxylase-immunoreactive structures in the rat neostriatum: A correlated light and electron microscopic study including a combination of Golgi impregnation with immunocytochemistry, *J. Comp. Neurol.* **237:**1–20.

Carson, K. A., and Mesulam, M.-M., 1982, Electron microscopic tracing of neural connections with horseradish peroxidase, in: *Tracing Neural Connections with Horseradish Peroxidase, Methods in the Neurosciences* (M.-M. Mesulam, ed.), John Wiley & Sons, Chichester, pp. 153–184.

Cuello, A. C., Galfre, G., and Milstein, C., 1979, Detection of substance P in the central nervous system by a monoclonal antibody, *Proc. Natl. Acad. Sci. U.S.A.* **76:**3532–3536.

Dalton, A. J., 1955, A chrome–osmium fixative for electron microscopy, *Anat. Rec.* **121:**281.

DeFelipe, J., Hendry, S. H. C., Jones, E. G., and Schmechel, D., 1985, Variability in the terminations of GABAergic chandelier cell axons on initial segments of pyramidal cell axons in the monkey sensory–motor cortex, *J. Comp. Neurol.* **231:**364–384.

Dumas, M., Schwab, M. E., Baumann, R., and Thoenen, H., 1979, Retrograde transport of tetanus toxin through a chain of two neurons, *Brain Res.* **165:**354–357.

Evinger, C., and Erichsen, J. T., 1986, Transsynaptic retrograde transport of fragment C of tetanus toxin demonstrated by immunohistochemical localization, *Brain Res.* **380:**383–388.

Fairén, A., and Valverde, F., 1980, A specialised type of neuron in the visual cortex of cat: A Golgi and electron microscope study of chandelier cells, *J. Comp. Neurol.* **194:**761–780.

Fairén, A., Peters, A., and Saldanha, J., 1977, A new procedure for examining Golgi impregnated neurons by light and electron microscopy, *J. Neurocytol.* **6:**311–338.

Freund, T. F., and Somogyi, P., 1983, The section–Golgi impregnation procedure. 1. Description of the method and its combination with histochemistry after intracellular iontophoresis or retrograde transport of horseradish peroxidase, *Neuroscience* **9:**463–470.

Freund, T. F., Martin, K. A. C., Smith, A. D., and Somogyi, P., 1983, Glutamate decarboxylase-immunoreactive terminals of Golgi-impregnated axoaxonic cells and of presumed basket cells in synaptic contact with pyramidal neurons of the cat's visual cortex, *J. Comp. Neurol.* **221:**263–278.

Freund, T. F., Powell, J. F., and Smith, A. D., 1984, Tyrosine hydroxylase-immunoreactive boutons in synaptic contact with identified striatonigral neurons, with particular reference to dendritic spines, *Neuroscience* **13:**1189–1215.

Freund, T. F., Martin, K. A. C., and Whitteridge, D., 1985a, Innervation of cat visual areas 17 and 18 by physiologically identified X- and Y-type thalamic afferents. I. Arborization patterns and quantitative distribution of postsynaptic elements, *J. Comp. Neurol.* **242:**263–274.

Freund, T. F., Martin, K. A. C., Somogyi, P., and Whitteridge, D., 1985b, Innervation of cat visual areas 17 and 18 by physiologically identified X- and Y-type thalamic afferents. II. Identification of postsynaptic targets by GABA immunocytochemistry and Golgi impregnation, *J. Comp. Neurol.* **242:**275–291.

Frotscher, M., and Leranth, C., 1986, The cholinergic innervation of the rat fascia dentata: Identification of target structures on granule cells by combining choline acetyltransferase immunocytochemistry and Golgi impregnation, *J. Comp. Neurol.* **243:**58–70.

Frotscher, M., and Zimmer, J., 1983, Commissural fibers terminate on non-pyramidal neurons in the guinea pig hippocampus—a combined Golgi/EM degeneration study, *Brain Res.* **265:**289–293.

Frotscher, M., Rinne, U., Hassler, R., and Wagner, A., 1981, Termination of cortical afferents on identified neurons in the caudate nucleus of the cat: A combined Golgi/EM degeneration study, *Exp. Brain Res.* **41:**329–337.

Gabbott, P. L. A., and Somogyi, J., 1984, The 'single' section Golgi-impregnation procedure: Methodological description, *J. Neurosci. Methods* **11:**221–230.

Gerfen, C. R., O'Leary, D. D. M., and Cowan, W. M., 1982, A note on the transneuronal transport of wheat germ agglutinin-conjugated horseradish peroxidase in the avian and rodent visual systems, *Exp. Brain Res.* **48:**443–448.

Golgi, C., 1883, Recherches sur l'histologie des centres nerveux, *Arch. Ital. Biol.* **3:**285–317.

Grafstein, B., 1971, Transneuronal transfer of radioactivity in the central nervous system, *Science* **172:**177–179.

Hamos, J. E., Van Horn, S. C., Raczkowski, D., and Sherman, S. M., 1987, Synaptic circuits involving an individual retinogeniculate axon in the cat, *J. Comp. Neurol.* **259:**165–192.

Hanker, J. S., Yates, P. E., Metz, C. B., and Rustioni, A., 1977, A new specific, sensitive and non-carcinogenic reagent for the demonstration of horseradish peroxidase, *Histochem J.* **9:**789–792.

Hodgson, A. J., Penke, B., Erdei, A., Chubb, I. W., and Somogyi, P., 1985, Antiserum to γ-aminobutyric acid. I. Production and characterization using a new model system, *J. Histochem. Cytochem.* **33:**229–239.

Itaya, S. D., and van Hoesen, G. W., 1982, WGA–HRP as a transneuronal marker in the visual pathways of monkey and rat, *Brain Res.* **236:**199–204.

Izzo, P. N., and Bolam, J. P., 1986, The post-synaptic targets of substance P-immunoreactive boutons in the rat neostriatum, *Neurosci. Lett. Suppl.* **26:**S312.

Izzo, P. N., Graybiel, A. M., and Bolam, J. P., 1987, Characterization of substance P- and Met-enkephalin-immunoreactive neurons in the caudate nucleus of cat and ferret by a single section Golgi procedure, *Neuroscience* **20:**577–587.

Kisvárday, Z. F., Cowey, A., and Somogyi, P., 1986, Synaptic relationships of a type of GABA-immunoreactive neuron (clutch cell), spiny stellate cells and lateral geniculate nucleus afferents in layer IVC of the monkey striate cortex, *Neuroscience* **19:**741–761.

Kisvárday, Z. F., Martin, K. A. C., Friedlander, M. J., and Somogyi, P., 1987, Evidence for interlaminar inhibitory circuits in striate cortex of cat, *J. Comp. Neurol.* **260:**1–19.

Koelle, G. B., and Friedenwald, J. S., 1949, A histochemical method for localizing cholinesterase activity, *Proc. Soc. Exp. Biol. Med.* **70:**617–622.

Kristensson, K., Ninnesmo, I., Persson, L., and Lycke, E., 1982, Neuron to neuron transmission of herpes simplex virus. Transport of virus from skin to brainstem nuclei, *J. Neurol. Sci.* **54:**149–156.

Lane, B. P., and Europa, D. L., 1965, Differential staining of ultrathin sections of Epon-embedded tissues for light microscopy, *J. Histochem. Cytochem.* **13:**579–582.

Lewis, P. R., and Knight, D. P., 1977, Staining methods for sectioned material, in: *Practical Methods in Electron Microscopy*, Vol. 5 (A. M. Glauert, ed.), North-Holland, Amsterdam, pp. 1–311.

Martin, K. A. C., and Whitteridge, D., 1984, Form, function, and intracortical projections of spiny neurones in the striate visual cortex of the cat, *J. Physiol. (Lond.)* **353:**463–504.

Mesulam, M.-M., and Mufson, E. J., 1980, The rapid anterograde transport of horseradish peroxidase, *Neuroscience* **5:**1277–1286.

Micevych, P., and Elde, R., 1980, Relationship between enkephalinergic neurons and the vasopressin–oxytocin neuroendocrine system of the cat: An immunohistochemical study, *J. Comp. Neurol.* **190:**135–146.

Millhouse, O. E., 1981, The Golgi methods, in: *Neuroanatomical Tract-Tracing Methods* (L. Heimer and M. J. RoBards, eds.), Plenum Press, New York. pp. 311–344.

Peters, A., 1984, Chandelier cells, in: *Cerebral Cortex. Cellular Components of the Cerebral Cortex,* Vol. 1 (E. G. Jones and A. Peters, eds.), Plenum Press, New York, pp. 361–380.

Peters, A., Proskauer, C. C., Feldman, M. L., and Kimerer, L., 1979, The projection of the lateral geniculate nucleus to area 17 of the rat cerebral cortex. V. Degenerating axon terminals synapsing with Golgi impregnated neurons, *J. Neurocytol.* **8:**331–357.

Peters, A., Proskauer, C. C., and Ribak, C. E., 1982, Chandelier cells in rat visual cortex, *J. Comp. Neurol.* **206:**397–416.

Ramon y Cajal, S., 1891, Sur la structure de l'ecorce cerebrale de quelques mammiferes, *Cellule* **7:**3–54.

Ramon y Cajal, S., 1911, *Histologie du Systeme Nerveux de l'Homme et des Vertebres,* Maloine, Paris.

Reperant, J., 1975, The orthograde transport of horseradish peroxidase in the visual system, *Brain Res.* **85:**307–312.

Reynolds, E. S., 1963, The use of lead citrate at high pH as an electron opaque stain in electron microscopy, *J. Cell. Biol.* **17:**208–212.

Ribak, C. E., 1978, Aspinous and sparsely-spinous stellate neurons in the visual cortex of rats contain glutamic acid decarboxylase, *J. Neurocytol.* **7:**461–478.

Ruda, M., and Coulter, J. D., 1982, Axonal and transneuronal transport of wheat germ agglutinin demonstrated by immunocytochemistry, *Brain Res.* **249:**237–246.

Rye, D. B., Saper, C. B., and Wainer, B. H., 1984, Stabilization of the tetramethylbenzidine (TMB) reaction product: Application for retrograde and anterograde tracing, and combination with immunohistochemistry, *J. Histochem. Cytochem.* **32:**1145–1153.

Somogyi, P., 1977, A specific axo-axonal interneuron in the visual cortex of the rat, *Brain Res.* **136:**345–350.

Somogyi, P., 1978, The study of Golgi stained cells and of experimental degeneration under the electron microscope: A direct method for the identification in the visual cortex of three successive links in a neuron chain, *Neuroscience* **3:**167–180.

Somogyi, P., 1986, Seven distinct types of GABA-immunoreactive neuron in the visual cortex of cat, *Soc. Neurosci. Abstr.* **12:**583.

Somogyi, P., and Hodgson, A. J., 1985, Antiserum to γ-aminobutyric acid. III. Demonstration of GABA in Golgi-impregnated neurons and in conventional electron microscopic sections of cat striate cortex, *J. Histochem. Cytochem.* **33:**249–257.

Somogyi, P., and Smith, A. D., 1979, Projection of neostriatal spiny neurons to the substantia nigra. Application of a combined Golgi-staining and horseradish peroxidase transport procedure at both light and electronmicroscopic levels, *Brain Res.* **178:**3–15.

Somogyi, P., and Takagi, H., 1982, A note on the use of picric acid–paraformaldehyde–glutaraldehyde fixative for correlated light and electron microscopic immunocytochemistry, *Neuroscience* **7:**1779–1783.

Somogyi, P., Hodgson, A. J., and Smith, A. D., 1979, An approach to tracing neuron networks in the cerebral cortex and basal ganglia. Combination of Golgi-staining, retrograde transport of horseradish peroxidase and anterograde degeneration of synaptic boutons in the same material, *Neuroscience* **4:**1805–1852.

Somogyi, P., Bolam, J. P., and Smith, A. D., 1981a, Monosynaptic cortical input and local axon collaterals of identified striatonigral neurons. A light and electron microscopic study using the Golgi-peroxidase transport–degeneration procedure, *J. Comp. Neurol.* **195:**567–584.

Somogyi, P., Freund, T. F., Halász, N., and Kisvárday, Z. F., 1981b, Selectivity of neuronal ³H-GABA accumulation in the visual cortex as revealed by Golgi staining of the labelled neurons, *Brain Res.* **225:**431–436.

Somogyi, P., Freund, T. F., and Cowey, A., 1982, The axo-axonic interneuron in the cerebral cortex of the rat, cat and monkey, *Neuroscience* **7:**2577–2607.

Somogyi, P., Freund, T. F., Wu, J.-Y., and Smith, A. D., 1983, The section Golgi impregnation procedure. 2. Immunocytochemical demonstration of glutamate decarboxylase in Golgi-impregnated neurons and in their afferent synaptic boutons in the visual cortex of the cat, *Neuroscience* **9**:475–490.

Somogyi, P., Freund, T. F., Hodgson, A. J., Somogyi, J., Beroukas, D., and Chubb, I. W., 1985, Identified axo-axonic cells are immunoreactive for GABA in the hippocampus and visual cortex of the cat, *Brain Res.* **332**:143–149.

Sotelo, C., and Riche, D., 1974, The smooth endoplasmic reticulum and the retrograde and fast orthograde transport of horseradish peroxidase in the nigro-striato-nigral loop, *Anat. Embryol.* **146**:209–218.

Stell, W. K., 1965, Correlation of retinal cytoarchitecture and ultrastructure in Golgi preparations, *Anat. Rec.* **153**:389–397.

Stell, W. K., 1967, The structure and relationships of horizontal cells and photoreceptor–bipolar synaptic complexes in goldfish retina, *Am. J. Anat.* **121**:401–424.

Szentágothai, J., 1975, What the "Reazione Nera" has given to us, in: *Golgi Centennial Symposium Proceedings* (M. Santini, ed.), Raven Press, New York, pp. 1–12.

Szentágothai, J., 1978, The neuron network of the cerebral cortex: A functional interpretation. The Ferrier Lecture, 1977, *Proc. R. Soc. Lond. [Biol.]* **201**:219–248.

Szentágothai, J., and Arbib, M. A., 1974, Conceptual models of neural organization, *Neurosci. Res. Prog. Bull.* **12**:305–510.

van den Pol, A. N., Herbst, R., and Powell, J. F., 1984, Tyrosine hydroxylase-immunoreactive neurons of the hypothalamus: A light and electron microscopic study, *Neuroscience* **13**:1117–1156.

White, E. L., 1979, Thalamocortical synaptic relations: A review with emphasis on the projections of specific thalamic nuclei to the primary sensory areas of the neocortex, *Brain Res. Rev.* **1**:275–313.

White, E. L., and Rock, M. P., 1981, A comparison of thalamocortical and other synaptic inputs to dendrites of two non-spiny neurons in a single barrel of mouse SmI cortex, *J. Comp. Neurol.* **195**:265–278.

Wu, J.-Y., Lin, C.-T., Brandon, T. S., Mohler, H., and Richards, J. G., 1982, Regulation and immunocytochemical characterization of glutamic acid decarboylase, in: *Cytochemical Methods in Neuroanatomy* (V. Chan-Palay and S. L. Palay, eds.) Alan R. Liss, New York, pp. 279–296.

9

Immunocytochemistry and Synaptic Relationships of Physiologically Characterized HRP-Filled Neurons

PETER SOMOGYI and
TAMÁS F. FREUND

I. INTRODUCTION

The combination of intracellular recording and marking of neurons with horseradish peroxidase (HRP) has greatly extended the understanding of neuronal circuits. As discussed in Chapter 7 by Kitai *et al.*, this approach is suitable for the reconstruction of the axonal and dendritic arborizations of neurons over several millimeters, thus providing a more complete picture of individual cells than was possible with previous methods. In addition, the direct correlation of electrophysiological and structural data becomes possible. In most cases the interpretation of the possible role of identified neurons would benefit greatly from a knowledge of their biochemical character-

PETER SOMOGYI and TAMÁS F. FREUND • MRC Anatomical Neuropharmacology Unit, University Department of Pharmacology, Oxford OX1 3QT, United Kingdom. *Present address for T.F.F.:* First Department of Anatomy, Semmelweis University Medical School, H-1450 Budapest, Hungary.

istics, especially their transmitters. The identification of the transmitters of the postsynaptic cells would also be useful because each neuron or afferent system is likely to contact several neurochemically, morphologically, and/or physiologically distinct neuron populations.

In the vertebrate nervous system information about the transmitters of physiologically characterized cells and their postsynaptic targets has largely been predicted from separate neurochemical, pharmacological, or histochemical experiments. Among the few exceptions, dopamine has been localized in intracellularly recorded mesencephalic neurons by fluorescence microscopy following the elevation of dopamine levels by intracellular injection of drugs (Grace and Bunney, 1983). Fluorescence microscopy and intracellularly injected fluorescent dyes were also used to determine the chemical nature of intracellularly recorded noradrenergic and serotoninergic neurons (Aghajanian and Vandermaelen, 1982; Weiler and Ammermuller, 1986). The neurons characterized in these procedures, however, could not be processed for electron microscopy.

Immunocytochemistry was employed to reveal neurophysin, enkephalin, and arginine vasotocin immunoreactivity in magnocellular paraventricular neurons in the hypothalamus (Reaves *et al.*, 1983). In these studies, intracellularly injected Lucifer yellow and Procion yellow were used to locate the recorded cells. Immunofluorescence combined with intracellular recording and dye injection was also used in the peripheral nervous system to study the response properties of neurons containing different neuropeptides (Bornstein *et al.*, 1986). Reaves *et al.* (1983) were also able to study the labeled cells in the electron microscope following deposition of DAB in the fluorescent dye-filled cells. However, the marking of neurons with HRP has the advantage that cells can be reconstructed from serial sections over distances of several millimeters, and they are particularly suitable for electron microscopic analysis.

In order to provide direct information about the neurochemical characteristics of intracellularly recorded cells, we combined intracellular HRP filling with light and electron microscopic postembedding immunocytochemistry. Following intracellular recording, the tissue containing the HRP-filled cells is processed for electron microscopic analysis. Thus, the afferent and efferent synaptic connections of the physiologically characterized HRP-filled neurons can be studied at the ultrastructural level. In addition, the connections of these same neurons can also be established by stimulation of the cell's input and output pathways during the electrophysiological recording.

The application of immunocytochemistry to cells that had been processed for conventional electron microscopy is illustrated here with examples using an antiserum to γ-aminobutyric acid (GABA). The development of antisera to amino acid neurotransmitters opened up new possibilities for their immunocytochemical localization in the central nervous system (Seguela *et al.*, 1984; Somogyi *et al.*, 1984; Storm-Mathisen *et al.*, 1983). The antibodies are usually raised against amino acid–aldehyde–protein conjugates that resemble the form of the amino acid in aldehyde-fixed tissue. This could explain why epitopes (antigenic determinants) produced during fixation of amino acids in the tissue seem to be less sensitive to tissue-processing conditions than most proteins and peptides. The particular property that has proved most advantageous is that fixed amino acids, and in particular GABA, are recognized by antibodies following routine osmium tetroxide treatment, dehydration, and epoxy resin embedding for electron microscopy (Somogyi and Hodgson, 1985). The procedures, however, should not be restricted to the localization of amino acids, since there are an increasing number of other molecules that can be localized under similar conditions (Bendayan *et al.*, 1986; Graber and Kreutzberg, 1985; Hearn *et al.*, 1985; Theodosis *et al.*, 1986; van den Pol, 1985).

Two methods are illustrated. They are described in detail in the Appendix (Section IV).

Postembedding immunocytochemistry using the unlabeled antibody enzyme method is carried out on semithin sections (0.5–1 μm), which are cut from osmium-treated 80-μm-thick sections containing the physiologically characterized HRP-filled neuron (Freund *et al.*, 1985; Kisvarday *et al.*, 1985). First, the synaptic contacts between the physiologically characterized presynaptic cell and its postsynaptic target are identified by correlated light and electron microscopy. Semithin sections are then cut from parts of the postsynaptic neuron still in the thick section, and the presence or absence of the epitopes is established in the postsynaptic cell. Several antisera can be tested on consecutive sections.

Postembedding immunocytochemistry using immunogold methods is carried out on ultrathin sections cut from the 80-μm-thick osmium-treated section containing the HRP-filled neuron (Somogyi and Soltesz, 1986). Alternate ribbons of sections are studied, either conventionally for the identification of synaptic connections or after the immunogold reaction. Since it is necessary to remove the osmium from the sections prior to the immunoreaction, the HRP-filled processes are difficult to locate without studying the alternate, nonimmunoreacted grids. This method is suitable for demonstrating immunoreactivity both in the HRP-filled cells and in their postsynaptic targets. Alternate grids can be reacted for different epitopes, or the same grid can be reacted for several epitopes using different sizes of colloidal gold.

II. APPLICATIONS OF THE COMBINED TECHNIQUES

The simultaneous demonstration of physiological, structural, and biochemical properties in neuronal networks has several potential applications. The most basic situations are summarized in Fig. 1, but further combinations are clearly possible. Some of the circuits are illustrated by examples from recent results obtained in the cortex using antisera to GABA.

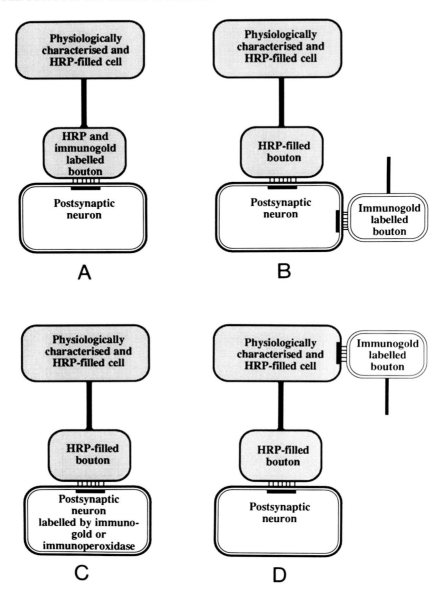

Figure 1. Summary of some basic combinations of intracellular recording and marking studies with immunocytochemistry. In all cases the illustrated synaptic connections are established by electron microscopy. Additional, especially long-range, connections can be investigated using electrical or natural stimulation of the appropriate pathways. Cases A–C are illustrated in this chapter by examples obtained using antisera to GABA in the visual cortex (see also Figs. 2–4 for A, Figs. 5 and 6 for B, Fig. 7 for C). The examination of further circuits is clearly possible.

A. Demonstration of GABA Immunoreactivity in Intracellularly Recorded Neurons

In the cerebral cortex the majority of axosomatic boutons are thought to originate from the so-called cortical basket cell (Jones, 1975; Marin-Padilla, 1969; Marin-Padilla and Stibitz, 1974; Ramon y Cajal, 1911; Szentagothai, 1973, 1983). Intracellular HRP filling studies combined with electron microscopy and the quantitative evaluation of efferent synaptic connections provided evidence for the existence of three types of basket cell in the visual cortex of the cat (Kisvarday *et al.*, 1985, 1987; Martin *et al.*, 1983; Somogyi *et al.*, 1983). All three cell types establish type II synaptic contacts (Figs. 2B,C and 4), and they make 20–30% of their synapses with the somata of other neurons (Kisvarday *et al.*, 1985, 1987; Somogyi *et al.*, 1983), the rest being with dendrites and dendritic spines.

On the basis of similarities between the identified basket cells and neurons immunoreactive for GABA (Somogyi and Hodgson, 1985; Somogyi *et al.*, 1985) or the GABA-synthetic enzyme glutamate decarboxylase (Freund *et al.*, 1983; Hendry *et al.*, 1983; Ribak, 1978), it has been proposed that these neurons may use GABA as their transmitter (Kisvarday *et al.*, 1985; Martin *et al.*, 1983; Somogyi *et al.*, 1983). This assumption, however, was based on indirect comparisons (for discussion see Somogyi and Soltesz, 1986). In order to overcome the inherent uncertainties of the inferential evidence, we tested directly for the presence of immunoreactive GABA in synaptic terminals of identified basket and clutch cells (Somogyi and Soltesz, 1986; Kisvarday *et al.*, 1987) using the electron microscopic immunogold protocol described in the Appendix (Section IV).

GABA immunoreactivity was demonstrated in the identified HRP-filled boutons, in the dendrites of three clutch cells and in the myelinated axons of both basket and clutch cells (Somogyi and Soltesz, 1986; Kisvarday*et al.*, 1987). The GABA-immunolabeled basket cell terminals made synapses with somata (Fig. 2B,C), dendritic shafts (Figs. 3C and 4A,B), and dendritic spines (Fig. 4C,D). Dendritic spines that received a synapse from a GABA-positive basket or clutch cell bouton also received a type I synaptic contact from a GABA-negative bouton (Fig. 4C,D). This indicates that selective interaction can take place on single spines between a GABAergic basket cell terminal and another input. A few of the postsynaptic dendrites were also immunoreactive for GABA (Fig. 3C), indicating synaptic interactions between GABAergic basket and other GABA-containing cells. The fine structural characteristics of the majority of postsynaptic targets suggested that they were pyramidal and spiny stellate cells.

There was great variation among the reactivities of the individual cells, just as there was variation in the general reactivity of the tissue from animal to animal. This is probably explained by differences in fixation, because in general, tissue showing poor ultrastructural preservation reacted poorly and also showed the highest background deposition of gold. In the same reaction there was little variation among the boutons of an individual cell, but those

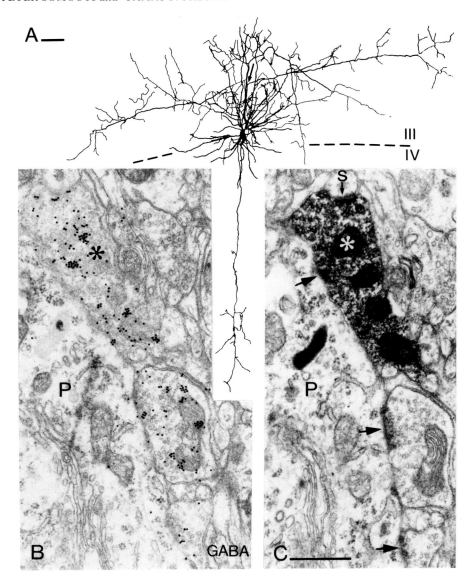

Figure 2. Immunogold demonstration of GABA in a basket cell. (A) Intracellularly recorded, HRP-filled large basket cell in the cat striate cortex that was shown to receive monosynaptic X-type thalamic and also callosal input and had a simple-type receptive field (Martin *et al.*, 1983). Arrow points to main axon. (B,C) Serial EM sections of a bouton of the basket cell (asterisk) that contacts the soma of a pyramidal cell along with two other boutons (arrows). All three are GABA-positive as seen in B from the selective accumulation of colloidal gold particles. This cell was lightly filled with HRP; thus, the bouton lost all electron density following sodium metaperiodate treatment. The HRP-filled bouton also makes a synapse with a spine (s). Data from work by Somogyi *et al.* (1983) and Somogyi and Soltesz (1986). Scales: A, 100 μm; B,C, 0.5 μm.

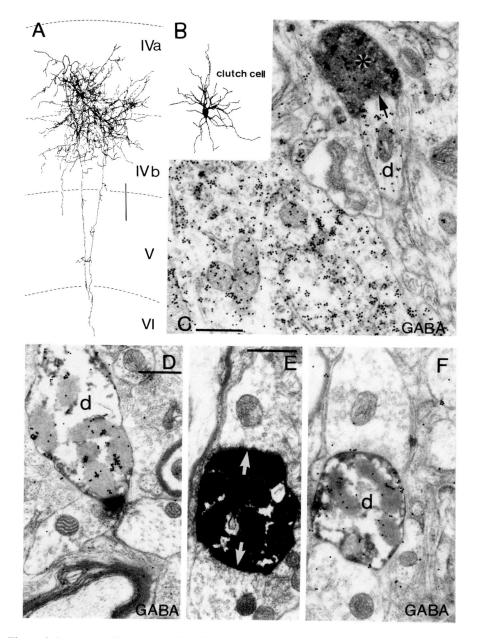

Figure 3. Immunogold demonstration of GABA in a clutch cell. (A,B) Axonal (A) and dendritic (B) arborizations of the HRP-filled cell that was shown to be monosynaptically activated by Y-type thalamic afferents and had a complex-type receptive field (Martin *et al.*, 1983). (C–F) Electron micrographs of dendrites (d in D and F) and a bouton (asterisk in C) of the clutch cell. This cell was heavily filled with HRP, and the section was treated for only a short time with sodium metaperiodate, so the bouton retained some of its electron density. The selective accumulation of gold particles demonstrates that they are immunoreactive for GABA, as is a soma (lower left in C) and the dendrite (d) contacted by the clutch cell terminal. (E) The same dendrite as in F, but this section was not immunoreacted. Arrows mark synapses. Data from work by Kisvarday *et al.* (1985) and Somogyi and Soltesz (1986). Scales: A,B, 100 μm; C–F, 0.5 μm.

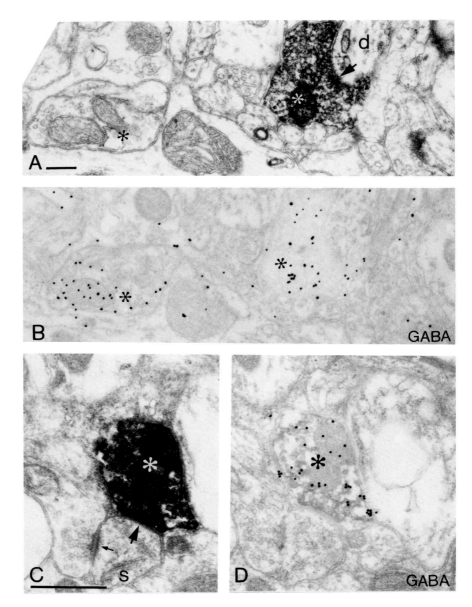

Figure 4. HRP-filled boutons revealed by 3,3'-diaminobenzidine (A) or *p*-phenylenediamine/ pyrocatechol (C) as chromogens. (A,B) Serial sections of two GABA-positive boutons (asterisk). The HRP-filled bouton of a basket cell on the right makes a synapse (arrow) with a dendrite (d). GABA immunoreactivity in B is visualized using protein-A-coated colloidal gold. (C,D) Serial sections of a GABA-positive clutch cell bouton (asterisk) making a type II synapse (large arrow) with a spine (s) that also receives a type I synapse (small arrow) from an immunonegative terminal. GABA immunoreactivity in D is visualized using IgG-coated colloidal gold. Scales: A and B, 0.2 μm; C and D, 0.5 μm.

sections of a bouton that contained many mitochondria usually exhibited higher gold density. Mitochondria usually show strong immunoreactivity for GABA, but only in those neuronal profiles whose other parts are also immunoreactive (Figs. 2B and 4B,D). This immunoreactivity may reflect the endogenous GABA content of mitochondria or could result from cytosolic GABA that was fixed to mitochondrial basic proteins. The dendrites of clutch cells were also immunoreactive for GABA (Fig. 3D,F). Both proximal and distal dendrites were GABA-positive, most of the gold being deposited over mitochondria (Fig. 3D,F). Both clutch and basket cells have myelinated axons, and these also showed immunoreactivity for GABA (Somogyi and Soltesz, 1986). Many myelinated axons were GABA-positive in the cortical neuropile, and the density of gold particles was usually very high over them.

These studies provided direct evidence for the presence of immunoreactive GABA in identified basket and clutch cells, and the results strongly suggest that GABA is a neurotransmitter at their synapses. In the electrophysiological parts of the experiment, orthodromic activation of basket cells by visual and electrical stimulation demonstrated that some of them receive mono-, others polysynaptic thalamic input, and they can be activated either by the Y or the X stream of thalamic afferents (Martin *et al.*, 1983). One of the basket cells was also shown to receive callosal input. The laminar distribution of the synaptic terminals, identified by the HRP filling, demonstrates that GABAergic basket cells that have similar target specificity segregate into different laminae and that the same GABAergic cells can take part in both horizontal and radial interactions. Since the spatial distributions of their axonal arborization are largely complementary, our findings demonstrate that in the different cortical laminae different sets of basket cells use the same transmitter, presumably for similar operations.

B. Demonstration of GABA in Postsynaptic Targets of Intracellularly Recorded Neurons: Immunogold Method

The identification of an antigen in the postsynaptic elements of intracellularly recorded cells may help to clarify hypotheses for their roles. For example, there are numerous hypotheses for the role of the local axon collaterals of pyramidal cells. Most hypotheses predict that pyramidal cells activate specific classes of postsynaptic cells. According to one hypothesis the local axon collaterals may activate inhibitory interneurons, thereby providing the structural basis of recurrent inhibition (Phillips, 1959; Stefanis and Jasper, 1964; Creutzfeldt *et al.*, 1969). The major inhibitory transmitter in cortex is GABA; thus, we were able to test the above hypothesis by testing for the presence of GABA in structures postsynaptic to pyramidal cell axon collaterals (Kisvarday *et al.*, 1986).

In the cat visual cortex two pyramidal cells in layer III were examined in the electron microscope. These cells were of special interest because of their clumped axon arborization near and also 0.4–1.0 mm from the cell body, in register in layers III and V (Fig. 5A). Of 191 synaptic contacts established by the axons, only one bouton contacted a cell body, and that was immunoreactive for GABA. The major targets were dendritic spines (84 and 87%), which probably originated from other pyramidal cells, and the remainder were dendritic shafts. Only about a third of the postsynaptic dendrites tested showed immunoreactivity for GABA (Fig. 5B,D); thus, all in all, putative inhibitory cells formed not more than 5% of the postsynaptic targets of these pyramidal cells. The primary role of both the intra- and intercolumnar collateral systems is probably the activation of other excitatory cells (Kisvarday *et al.*, 1986). The presence of a small population of GABAergic cells among the targets, however, may be significant if they receive highly convergent input from a large population of pyramidal cells. It is unclear why GABA is present in the dendrites or whether the dendrites of all neurons that use GABA as transmitter have sufficient levels for immunocytochemical demonstration. Interestingly, not only proximal dendrites, which could be expected to contain high levels of glutamate decarboxylase synthesized in the endoplasmic reticulum, were GABA-positive; many small-diameter distal dendrites also showed strong immunoreactivity. As in the case of synaptic boutons, most of the gold particles were located over the mitochondria.

In the previous discussion of basket cells we mentioned that a few of the dendrites postsynaptic to basket terminals were also immunoreactive for GABA (Fig. 3C). These two examples illustrate that the immunogold–GABA method is well suited for determining the proportion of putative GABAergic targets postsynaptic to physiologically characterized axons.

Some afferent pathways provide synapses onto the somata of their target neurons. In these situations another strategy can be used, and this is illustrated by an example from the visual system. The specific visual afferents arriving mainly from the lateral geniculate nucleus of the thalamus to the cortex terminate principally in layer IV and to a lesser extent in layer VI (Rosenquist *et al.*, 1974; LeVay and Gilbert, 1976). It has been known from degeneration studies that a small proportion of the terminals made synapses with the somata of nonpyramidal cells (Garey and Powell, 1971). This was confirmed in recent experiments (Freund *et al.*, 1985) by examining the terminations of intracellularly recorded, HRP-filled, and resin-embedded thalamic axons (Fig. 6). Furthermore, it was discovered that each thalamic axon made multiple contacts (Fig. 6B) with the somata of about seven to ten neurons that seemed similar in size and shape to a population of large GABA-positive cells demonstrated previously. Using electron microscopy of the HRP-filled axons, Freund *et al.* (1985) showed synaptic contacts between the thalamic terminals and the large somata (Fig. 6D,E). The cells postsynaptic to the intracellularly recorded axons were tested for the presence of GABA. Semithin (0.5-μm) sections were cut from the somata still in the block and reacted using the unlabeled antibody peroxidase–antiperoxidase technique described in the Appendix (Section IV). Every cell that received somatic input from the axons was GABA-positive (Fig. 6C), and their fine structural

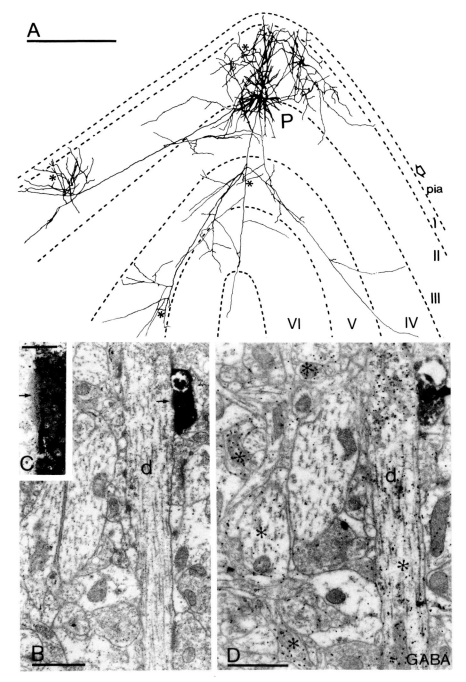

Figure 5. GABA immunoreactivity in postsynaptic targets of HRP-filled neurons. (A) Pyramidal cell (P) in layer III of cat striate cortex. The axon forms distinct clumps of terminals (asterisks). Open arrow denotes border of areas 17 and 18. (B,D) Serial sections of a bouton of the pyramidal cell in synaptic contact (arrow) with a dendrite (d). The dendrite and several neuronal processes (asterisk) are immunoreactive for GABA, as shown by the accumulation of gold particles in D. (C) The synaptic junction is shown at higher magnification. Data from the work of Kisvarday *et al.* (1986). Scales: A, 500 μm; B,D, 1 μm; C, 0.2 μm.

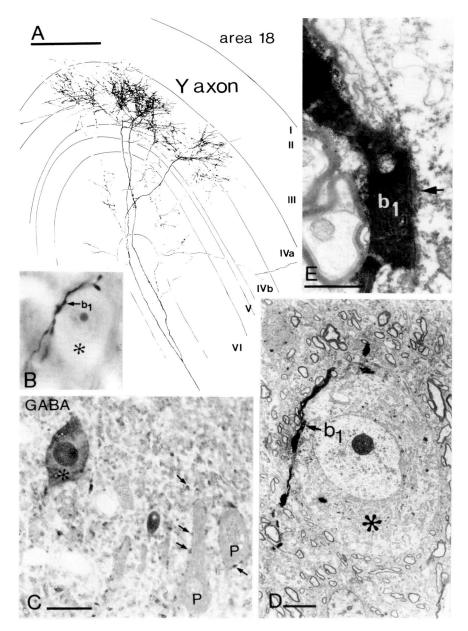

Figure 6. Immunoperoxidase demonstration of GABA in a cell postsynaptic to a thalamic Y-type axon in area 18 of the cat's visual cortex. (A) Drawing of the axon terminating predominantly in layer IV. (B) One collateral contacts a large soma (asterisk) as seen in an 80-μm-thick section. (C) The same soma is immunopositive for GABA as shown in a 0.5-μm-thick section. Immunoreactive puncta surrounding pyramidal cells (P) and also present in the neuropil (arrows) represent mainly nerve terminals. (D) Electron micrograph of the postsynaptic cell in contact with the HRP-filled collateral. The synaptic bouton (b_1) is shown at higher magnification in E, where arrow indicates synaptic junction. Data from the work of Freund *et al.* (1985). Scales: A, 500 μm; B,C, 20 μm; E, 0.5 μm.

characteristics agreed well with those of identified basket and clutch cells. Furthermore, it could be shown that X-type afferents contacted GABA-positive somata that, as a population, were significantly smaller than the ones contacted by the Y axons.

This study demonstrated that GABAergic, presumably inhibitory, neurons are activated at the first stage of cortical processing and that the cells are of a select population of GABA-containing neurons probably corresponding to basket and clutch cells. The size difference between the GABA-positive cells contacted by the two functionally distinct streams of visual afferents provides evidence for the segregation of parallel functional channels at the first step of processing in the primary visual cortex. In this example the electrophysiological recording showed the functional type of the afferents, electron microscopy identified their target cells, and immunocytochemistry revealed the putative transmitter of the later. At present only our combined methods can provide all this information in one experiment.

C. Convergence of HRP-Filled and Immunolabeled Boutons onto the Same Postsynaptic Cell

The postsynaptic targets of HRP-filled neurons received synapses from many other boutons in addition to the ones labeled by HRP (Fig. 2B,C). Some of these boutons were GABA-positive. In the case of the basket cells whose terminals were also immunopositive, this demonstrated the convergence of several GABAergic cells to the same neuron.

The terminals of pyramidal cells, however, were never immunoreactive for GABA, and all available evidence suggests that their direct effect on other cells is excitatory. The presence of GABA-containing and presumably inhibitory synapses near the synapses established by pyramidal cells suggests that their effect may be selectively reduced under certain circumstances. This would especially apply to the pyramidal terminals on dendritic spines, whose excitatory effect would be selectively reduced by appropriately timed input from the GABAergic bouton contacting the same spine (Fig. 7B). This arrangement could provide the basis for the "synaptic veto mechanism" (Koch and Poggio, 1983). These examples illustrate the potential of the immunogold method for mapping the origin and the chemistry of inputs that may influence each other's action on the postsynaptic cell.

III. ADVANTAGES AND LIMITATIONS

The retrospective localization of GABA in electrophysiologically characterized HRP-filled cells that were embedded for electron microscopy is possible because the epitopes remain recognizable by the antiserum following tissue processing. Other methods, outlined in Section I, have also been used to localize the putative transmitter of physiologically characterized neurons

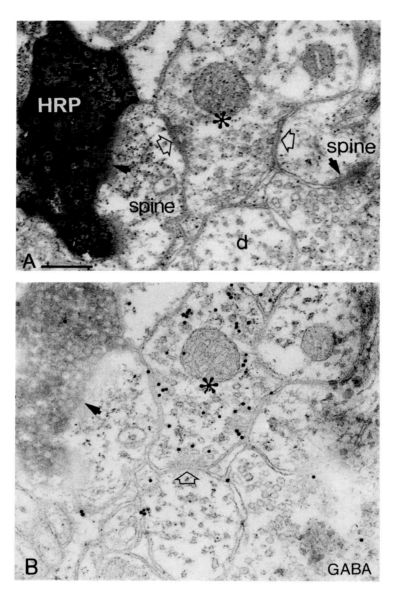

Figure 7. Convergence of synaptic input onto a dendritic spine from an HRP-filled pyramidal cell bouton and from a GABA-positive terminal (asterisk) in layer III of cat striate cortex. GABA immunoreactivity is shown in B by the accumulation of colloidal gold particles over the bouton that makes type II synapses (open arrows) with two spines and a dendrite (d). Both spines receive type I synapses (filled arrows). Small, irregularly shaped electron-dense particles, present in both pictures, are artifacts of tissue processing unrelated to the immunocytochemical reaction. Figure courtesy of Z. F. Kisvarday and K. A. C. Martin. Scale: A,B, 0.5 μm.

in the central nervous system, and the transmitters of many identified neurons in invertebrates have been established. HRP filling has the advantage that it not only gives a very detailed image of the cell but also allows the axonal arborizations to be followed over dozens of sections covering several millimeters in the brain. As a result of the high electron density of the reaction end product formed by HRP, the HRP-filled neurons are particularly suitable for electron microscopic analysis of their synaptic connections. The specimens are also permanent, and by using the postembedding methods, several antigens can be localized in serial electron microscopic sections of the same HRP-filled process.

It is not yet clear how generally applicable the demonstration of transmitter within the intracellularly recorded HRP-filled neurons will be. The impalement of the cell and the injection of HRP may cause damage that upsets the normal biochemical machinery for transmitter production. In the case of GABA, its levels are known to increase postmortem in the brain (Balcom *et al.*, 1975; Van der Heyden and Korf, 1978); thus, any damage to the cell may even increase its GABA levels. Other transmitters, however, could decrease following HRP filling. Therefore, negative results concerning the intracellularly recorded cell, as generally in immunocytochemistry, should be treated with caution.

In order to achieve electron microscopic localization of synapses, in most studies the tissue will be osmium treated and embedded in resin. A wide range of antigens has been localized in nervous tissue following embedding into epoxy and other resins, but few of these studies included osmium treatment. Of the neuroactive substances, a few peptides such as LHRH (van den Pol, 1985), oxytocin (Theodosis *et al.*, 1986), neurophysin (van den Pol, 1984, 1985), and the amino acids glutamate (Somogyi *et al.*, 1986) and GABA (Somogyi and Hodgson, 1985; van den Pol, 1985) have been localized in osmium-treated tissue. The immunoreactivity of fixed GABA is not changed by osmium treatment. Unfortunately, the immunoreactivity of many other epitopes, especially on proteins, is sensitive to osmium treatment and embedding and will be lost during processing of the tissue. Thus, the major limitation of the above procedures is that, at the moment, they can only be applied to relatively few antigens. However, from new developments along several lines it can be predicted that the localization of more and more antigens will become possible under conditions that permit the analysis of synaptic connections.

First, new resins are being introduced that preserve tissue antigenicity better. Both Lowicryl 4KM (Roth *et al.*, 1981; van den Pol, 1984) and LR White (e. g., Cohen, 1985) have great potential for immunocytochemical studies of the brain. We have used epoxy resin for the localization of GABA because the embedding into this material is simpler, and most of our cells were processed before the introduction of the new resins. Secondly, antibodies are developed to an increasing number of small neuroactive molecules that are resistant to tissue-processing conditions following their fixation. In addition to GABA, the localization of glycine (van den Pol and Görcs, 1986) and glutamate (Somogyi *et al.,* 1986) has been achieved under postembedding conditions in material similar to that used in the studies for GABA.

In this review, besides providing a detailed methodological description, we have also tried to illustrate the potential of the procedures. It should be clear that our examples, related to one transmitter and in only one area of the brain, merely mark the beginning of future applications.

IV. APPENDIX: METHODS

A flow diagram of the combined procedures is provided in Fig. 8. The steps are described below, together with technical comments on possible difficulties.

1. Preparation of animals, intracellular recording, and HRP filling; electrophysiological characterization of connections. Several reviews have described in detail the current techniques for intracellular recording and HRP filling (Brown and Fyffe 1984; Kitai and Bishop, 1981); therefore, only a brief summary is given of the electrophysiological recording carried out by Martin and Whitteridge (1984) in the visual cortex and reported earlier by them. All the cells illustrated here derive from their material. The cats were prepared under halothane–nitrous oxide–oxygen anesthesia; they were paralyzed, artificially ventilated, and maintained under anesthesia with Althesin® (Glaxo) or barbiturate. Stimulating electrodes were placed in the optic chiasm, in the optic radiation above the lateral geniculate nucleus (LGN), in the white matter of the visual cortex a few millimeters from the recording site, and in the contralateral visual cortex. Electrical stimulation of the cells through these electrodes provided the basis for determining the mono- or polysynaptic nature of their thalamic input and the presence of a callosal input. Electrical stimulation was also used to determine the type of visual afferents (X or Y) providing their predominant thalamic input (Bullier and Henry, 1979; Martin and Whitteridge, 1984). Glass electrodes filled with 4% solution of HRP (Bohringer, grade 1) dissolved in 0.2 M KCl and 0.05 M Tris (pH 7.9) were used for extracellular recording of the receptive field properties of the cells using visual stimulation. The membrane of the cell was then penetrated, the receptive field was examined again, and the cell was filled with HRP using 2-to 4nA positive current pulses, following the procedures of Friedlander *et al.* (1981).

2. Perfusion, fixation, and removal of brain. At the end of the recording experiment the animals were given a lethal dose of anesthetic; they were removed from the ventilation apparatus and were perfused through the heart with saline followed by fixative. The fixative consisted of 2.5% glutaraldehyde, 1% paraformaldehyde, and 0.1 M sodium phosphate buffer (PB, pH 7.4). Several neurons were filled in each animal; thus, 2–20 hr elapsed between filling the cell and the fixation.

In general, a high concentration of glutaraldehyde in the fixative results in good immunoreactivity for amino acids (Ottersen and Storm-Mathisen,

1. Intracellular recording and HRP-filling
   Electrophysiological characterization of connections

2. Perfusion fixation and removal of brain

3. Sectioning on Vibratome and washing of sections

4. HRP enzyme-histochemistry

5. Osmium treatment and flat-embedding in epoxy resin

6. Light microscopic analysis
   Photography, drawing and reconstruction of HRP-filled cells

7. Reembedding for electron microscopy

|

8.   IMMUNOCYTOCHEMISTRY

A. Semithin sections Immunoperoxidase method	B. Ultrathin sections Immunogold method
9A.Cut semithin sections of somata and mount on slides	9B. Cut serial EM sections onto Formvar coated gold grids
10A.Etching resin in ethanolic NaOH	10B.Periodic acid treatment and wash
11A.Wash in ethanol and distilled water	11B.Wash in distilled water
12A.Removal of osmium in sodium periodate	12B.Removal of osmium in sodium periodate
13A.Wash in water and buffered saline	13B.Wash in water and buffered saline
14A.Blocking serum	14B.Blocking protein solution
15A.Primary antiserum (to GABA) and wash	15B.Primary antiserum (to GABA) and wash
16A.Bridge antibody followed by wash	16B.Wash and polyethilene glycol treatement
17A.PAP-complex followed by wash	17B.IgG or Protein A coated colloidal gold
18A.Immunoperoxidase enzyme reaction	18B.Wash followed by uranyl acetate and lead citrate treatment for contrasting
19A.Wash, dehydration and mounting. Identification of immunopositive cells and correlation with electron micrographs	19B.Identification of immunopositive pre- and postsynaptic structures. Correlation with HRP filled profiles from non-reacted grids

Figure 8. Flow diagram of combined procedures for immunocytochemical characterization of the afferent and efferent synaptic connections of intracellularly recorded neurons.

1984; Somogyi *et al.*, 1985; Storm-Mathisen *et al.*, 1983). However, even with 2.5% glutaraldehyde, as above, considerable variation in immunoreactivity and background staining from animal to animal was produced. This indicates that for strong immunoreactivity the method of delivering the fixative to the cells is more important than the concentration of the cross-linking aldehyde. This is supported by our finding (Somogyi *et al.*, 1985) that much lower glutaraldehyde concentrations, down to 0.05%, can produce excellent immunoreactivity. Using our antiserum to GABA, we found no improvement by increasing the glutaraldehyde concentration further as recommended by others (Seguela *et al.*, 1984; Ottersen and Storm-Mathisen, 1984).

3. Sectioning. Following the perfusion, 5- to 10-mm-thick slices of the visual cortex were cut in the frontal plane and sectioned at 80 μm on a Vibratome (Oxford Instruments). The tissue was submerged in 0.1 M sodium phosphate buffer, and the sections were collected in the same buffer, serially in trays. Thereafter the sections were washed free of fixative in three changes of buffer, 30 min each.

4. HRP enzyme histochemistry. Most sections were processed according to the method of Hanker *et al.* (1977), supplemented with cobalt and nickel intensification (Adams, 1981) as described earlier (Martin and Whitteridge, 1984). The procedure is as follows:

1. The sections are washed in sodium cacodylate buffer (0.1 M, pH 5.1) twice for 10 min. All subsequent steps are carried out at 4°C.
2. They are preincubated for 15 min in a 5 : 1 mixture of intensifying solution [consisting of 0.4% $(NH_4)_2SO_4 \cdot NiSO_4 \cdot 6H_2O$ and 0.6% $CoCl_2$] and chromogen solution (consisting of 0.1% catechol and 0.05% *p*-phenylenediamine dihydrochloride dissolved in 0.1 M cacodylate buffer at pH 5.1).
3. The sections are washed for 5 min in 0.1 M PB, pH 7.4.
4. The sections are incubated, with agitation, for 15 min in the chromogen solution in the presence of 0.01% H_2O_2.
5. They are washed twice for 10 min in 0.1 m PB.

Some sections were processed in 0.1 M PB, using 3,3′-diaminobenzidine tetrahydrochloride (DAB, Sigma) as the chromogen (Graham and Karnovsky, 1966) both without and with cobalt intensification according to Adams (1977).

As far as the visualization of the intracellularly injected cells is concerned, the reaction of Hanker *et al.* (1977) is more sensitive than the DAB procedure. In the intracellularly injected cells GABA immunoreactivity remained equally detectable whether HRP was reacted with DAB or *p*-phenylenediamine/pyrocatechol (Fig. 4). The use of heavy metal intensification does not affect the immunoreactivity.

5. Osmium treatment and flat embedding. Following the enzyme reaction the sections were washed extensively in 0.1 M PB and treated for 30–40 min with 1% OsO_4 dissolved in 0.1 M PB. They were washed again in PB and dehydrated in an ascending series of ethanol, followed by propylene oxide and embedding in Durcupan (Fluka) epoxy resin. We prefer to use this resin because of its hardness, but postembedding immunostaining for GABA has been achieved using a variety of other resins, including Epon (van den Pol, 1985), Spurr (Theodosis *et al.*, 1986), and L. R. White (unpublished observation). Durcupan is made up by mixing with a spatula 10 g of component A (epoxy resin), 10 g of component B (hardener 964), 0.3 g of component C (accelerator 964, phenol derivative, harmful), and 0.3 g of component D (plasticizer). The sections are taken from propylene oxide, put into the resin contained in disposable aluminum foil wells, and kept overnight at room temperature. The following day they are placed serially onto glass microscope slides and covered with glass coverslips. Durcupan has high viscosity at room temperature, and the osmium-treated sections are very rigid and can easily break. Therefore, the transfer of the sections is carried out on a warming table in order to increase the fluidity of the resin. Neither the slides nor the coverslips were specially cleaned because during reembedding for electron microscopy the cured resin has to be separated from the glass. This may be difficult when acid-cleaned glass is used. The use of siliconized slides and coverslips or acetate foil instead of glass (Hollander, 1970; for review see Brown and Fyffe, 1984) has been recommended, but we have found the use of plain glass both convenient and satisfactory. The slides were then placed into an oven, and the resin was cured at 56°C for 2 days. These specimens can be stored permanently.

We routinely enhance contrast *en bloc* during dehydration by including 1% uranyl acetate in the 70% ethanol for 40 min. This does not interfere with immunocytochemistry for any of the antigens we have tested so far.

   6. Light microscopic analysis. The HRP-filled cells were then drawn using a drawing tube, and in addition some of them were reconstructed in three dimensions using a computerized microscope system (Capowski and Rethelyi, 1982; Zsuppan, 1984). Complete reconstructions of the neurons can be done at this stage, and any feature of the cell can be recorded on light micrographs. Those parts of the dendritic and axonal fields that were subsequently resectioned for electron microscopy were photographed in small focal steps using an X100 oil-immersion objective, and these photographs were used to correlate the light and electron microscopic images of the same neuronal process.

   7. Reembedding for electron microscopy. Selected parts of the sections were reembedded as described earlier (Somogyi *et al.*, 1979). In order to transfer the resin-embedded section from the slide to a resin block that can be fixed into the specimen arm of the ultramicrotome, first the cover slip is removed by inserting a razor blade between the coverslip and the resin. Scoring the glass with a diamond pen once the blade is under the glass makes it possible to remove only part of the coverslip so the majority of the sections remain protected. We cut out only a small part (1–3 mm^2) of the section that contains the area of interest, using a scalpel and stereomicroscope. During this operation the slide is kept on a warming plate to make the resin softer. The small piece of section is then lifted from the slide with the tip of a scalpel or a pointed razor blade. It is placed into a flat-bottom embedding capsule that is cut to about 5–8 mm height. The capsule is filled with resin, and a coverslip is placed on top of the resin, parallel to the bottom, in a way that ensures that no air bubbles remain in the capsule. After the curing of the resin and removal of the coverslip, the block is now in a cylinder that has an optically smooth, flat bottom. This cylinder can be placed on a microscope slide and examined in the light microscope with dry objectives at any time during the subsequent trimming and sectioning.

   8A. Immunocytochemistry. A series: Semithin section, postembedding immunoperoxidase method. When the axons of intracellularly HRP-injected neurons contact the cell bodies of other cells, it is possible to localize the antigens in the soma of the postsynaptic neuron at the light microscopic level. First the presumed contact is located in the 80-μm-thick section while it is still on the slide. Following reembedding the synaptic contact is confirmed or rejected by electron microscopy. Alternatively, axosomatic contacts provided by the HRP-filled cell may be located during electron microscopy. In both cases immunocytochemistry is carried out on semithin sections cut from the remaining part of the postsynaptic soma still in the block.

The immunocytochemical reaction steps are described below, expanded after Somogyi *et al.* (1984).

9A. The resin-embedded semithin sections (0.5–2 μm) are placed into gelatin- or egg-albumen-coated slides, flattened on a drop of warm water, and gently dried on a hotplate. Drying too quickly and at high temperatures should be avoided to prevent the sections sticking too tightly. The reaction is often uneven over the section, those parts that are not tightly stuck to the slide reacting much more strongly, presumably because the etching (see below) of the resin takes place from both sides. Uncoated slides can also be used, but sometimes the sections may float off. If the reaction is not carried out on the day of the sectioning, the slides are kept in a 56°C oven overnight.

10A. Etching of the resin is carried out in ethanolic sodium hydroxide (Lane and Europa, 1965) in Coplin jars. The solution is made up at least a day before it is used by adding NaOH pellets to absolute ethanol. It is stirred several times during the first day and can be used for weeks. It turns brown, but this does not diminish its effectiveness. From here on care should be taken not to allow the drying of the sections.

11A. Following etching the slides are washed in three changes of absolute ethanol and two changes of distilled water, 5 min each.

12A. Sodium periodate (NaIO$_4$, 1%, freshly made) is used to remove the osmium. Usually 7–10 min is sufficient, but if this treatment proves ineffective, the concentration of NaIO$_4$ can be increased or the duration of treatment extended. We have obtained good results using saturated NaIO$_4$ for up to 1 hr. This treatment is followed by two 5-min washes in distilled water.

13A. Two 10-min washes in Tris (10 mM) phosphate (10 mM)-buffered saline (TPBS) are applied. Other buffered salt solutions such as TBS or PBS can also be used, both here and in the subsequent steps.

14A. The slides are placed horizontally into a moist chamber, and all antibody solutions are applied to them in this way. We use a plastic box with wet tissue in the bottom. Most of the buffer is drained from the slides; only a thin layer of fluid is left over the sections. Thereafter, blocking protein solution is layered over them. Usually 10% normal serum of the species that produced the bridge antibody is used; in the case of GABA immunocytochemistry we use normal goat serum for 20 min. Then the serum is drained.

15A. Antiserum to GABA, raised in rabbit, is overlaid for 1–2 hr and diluted with 1% normal goat serum in TPBS at dilutions from 1 : 1000 to 1 : 5000. The antisera we use have been raised to GABA conjugated to bovine serum albumen by glutaraldehyde, and they have been extensively characterized for crossreactivity with a large number of related molecules, both in a nitrocellulose test system and on sections of the brain (Hodgson *et al.*, 1985; Somogyi *et al.*, 1985). In this step, control sera can be used to replace the antiserum to GABA.

16A. Slides are rinsed with TPBS from a pressure bottle and washed in Coplin jars in 1% NGS twice for 10 min. Bridge antibodies (goat antirabbit IgG, Miles) diluted 1 : 30 with 1% NGS are applied for 40 min, followed by a rinse in TPBS and two washes in 1% NGS for 10 min.

17A. Peroxidase–antiperoxidase complex (diluted 1 : 100) is applied for 1 hr, followed by two 15-min washes in TPBS and 10 min in 0.1 M PB. It should be noted that although we generally use the unlabeled antibody enzyme method (Sternberger *et al.*, 1970), other methods such as the use of peroxidase-conjugated second antibody, avidin–biotin methods, or silver-intensified gold methods produce equally good results on semithin sections.

18A. For the peroxidase enzyme method, the slides are preincubated in 0.05% DAB dissolved in 50 mM Tris buffer (pH 7.0–7.4). Five minutes later, 1% H_2O_2 is added to a final concentration of 0.01%, and the slides are incubated for a further 5–10 min. Thereafter they are washed in 0.1 M phosphate buffer for three times 5 min, and the contrast is increased by treating them for 5 min in 0.01% osmium tetroxide in 0.1 M PB.

19A. The slides are washed three times 5 min in distilled water, dehydrated in ethanol followed by xylene, and covered with a synthetic mounting medium under coverslip.

20A. The immunoreactive cells are dark brown, and immunoreactive puncta corresponding to immunoreactive dendrites, axons, and nerve terminals can clearly be recognized. Because the osmium is removed from the sections, the originally black or dark brown HRP-filled processes of the physiologically characterized cells become pale brown or ocher, and they are more difficult to locate than before the immunoreaction.

8B. Immunocytochemistry. B series: Postembedding immunogold technique for ultrathin sections; demonstration of GABA immunoreactivity. Serial ultrathin sections are used. From each series only every second grid is incubated for immunocytochemistry. The incubation in sodium metaperiodate greatly reduces the electron density of the HRP reaction end product, probably by removing the osmium. This makes the localization of the HRP-filled processes and synaptic contacts difficult. Therefore, unreacted serial sections are indispensable for the efficient collection of a reasonable sample of HRP-filled profiles. The reduction of electron density was observed in both the 3,3′-diaminobenzidine- and the p-phenylenediamine/pyrocatechol-reacted HRP-filled processes. In lightly filled cells all traces of the HRP reaction disappeared, and the processes could only be identified by their location. Therefore, the HRP-filled processes are first localized in sections on the nonincubated grids. Thereafter the same process is located in the consecutive sections that are reacted to reveal GABA, using capillaries, myelinated axons, and other conspicuous structures as fiducial marks.

9B. Serial sections are cut and picked up onto Formvar-coated single-slot gold grids. Only three to five sections are placed on each grid in order to have the same boutons represented on more than one grid. The immunocytochemical method follows procedure I of Somogyi and Hodgson (1985) with small modifications. Droplets of solutions for the immunocytochemical reaction are put on Parafilm™ in Petri dishes. The Parafilm™ is surrounded with wet paper tissue to avoid drying the grids. Unless otherwise stated, the grids are floated on the droplets at room temperature with the sections facing down. When grids are transferred from one droplet to another, the excess fluid is removed from the grids by filter paper, but the sections are never allowed to dry. All reagents and washing solutions are Millipore filtered (pore size 0.22 μm). The following steps are carried out:

10B. Pretreatment of the resin in 1% periodic acid (H_5IO_6, BDH Chemicals Ltd., freshly prepared) for 7–10 min.

11B. Three washes in double-distilled water by dipping the grids several times into vials, followed by 5 min in double-distilled water.

12B. Removal of osmium in 1% sodium periodate ($NaIO_4$, BDH Chemicals Ltd., freshly prepared) for 7 min, as recommended by Bendayan and Zollinger (1983). For some specimens a longer time may be necessary; it is worth trying a series of different times when using unfamiliar material.

13B. Washing as in step 2. The grids are blotted with filter paper on the side opposite the sections. From now on unless otherwise stated the grids are not dipped into any solution but are just floated on the droplets. Occasionally if a grid sinks in the droplet it is put into the droplets in all subsequent steps with the sections facing upward. Two 10-min periods in Tris (10 mM) phosphate (10 mM)-buffered isotonic saline (TPBS), pH 7.4.

14B. Blocking of nonspecific reaction with either a solution of 5% normal goat serum for 20 min if IgG-coated colloidal gold is to be the reagent later or with a solution of 0.5% ovalbumin if protein-A-coated colloidal gold is to be the reagent later. One to two minutes in TPBS.

15B. Antiserum to GABA for 1–2 hr produced in rabbit against a GABA–glutaraldehyde–bovine serum albumin conjugate (Hodgson *et al.*, 1985). It is diluted with 1% normal goat serum at 1 : 1000 to 1 : 3000. For control studies some grids are reacted with the same antiserum diluted 1 : 1000 and preincubated for 4 hr with GABA or other amino acids attached to polyacrylamide beads with glutaraldehyde as described elsewhere (Hodgson *et al.*, 1985).

16B. Washing in three changes of 1% goat serum diluted with TPBS, 15 min each. Three to five minutes in 0.05% solution of polyethylene glycol (mol. wt. 15,000–20,000, Sigma) dissolved in 50 mM Tris buffer, pH 7.0. This step is carried out to avoid the mixing of the TPBS with the protein-coated colloidal gold in the next step.

17B. Goat antirabbit IgG-coated colloidal gold (15 nm, Janssen Life Science Products), usually diluted to 1 : 10 to 1 : 40 depending on the batch, for 1–2 hr. It is diluted with the same solution as used in step 11. In other experiments protein-A-coated colloidal gold is used as reported earlier (Somogyi and Hodgson, 1985).

18B. Three dips in double-distilled water, followed by 10 min in double-distilled water. Staining with uranyl acetate and alkaline lead citrate to increase contrast for electron microscopy. Three dips in double-distilled water and blotting with filter paper.

19B. Immunopositive pre- and postsynaptic elements are recognized in the electron microscope on the basis of the high gold density over the intracellular organelles. If the HRP reaction end product is no longer obvious because of the decrease of its electron density, the alternate series of unreacted grids should be studied first for orientation.

ACKNOWLEDGMENT. The authors thank Mrs. Dorothy Rhodes for secretarial assistance.

REFERENCES

Adams, J. C., 1977, Technical considerations on the use of horseradish peroxidase as a neuronal marker, *Neuroscience* **2:**141–145.

Adams, J. C., 1981, Heavy metal intensification of DAB-based HRP reaction product, *J. Histochem. Cytochem.* **29:**775.

Aghajanian, G. K., and Vandermaelen, C. P., 1982, Intracellular identification of central noradrenergic and serotonergic neurons by a new double labeling procedure, *J. Neurosci.* **2:**1786–1792.

Balcom, G. J., Lenox, R. H., and Meyerhoff, J. L., 1975, Regional γ-aminobutyric acid levels in rat brain determined after microwave fixation, *J. Neurochem.* **24:**609–613.

Bendayan, M., and Zollinger, M., 1983, Ultrastructural localization of antigenic sites on osmium-fixed tissues applying the protein A–gold technique, *J. Histochem. Cytochem.* **31:**101–109.

Bendayan, M., Nanci, A., Herbener, G. H., Gregoire, S., and Duhr, M. A., 1986, A review of the study of protein secretion applying the protein A–gold immunocytochemical approach, *Am. J. Anat.* **175:**379–400.

Bornstein, J. C., Costa, M., and Furness, J. B., 1986, Synaptic inputs to immunohistochemically identified neurones in the submucous plexus of the guinea-pig small intestine, *J. Physiol. (Lond.)* **381:**465–482.

Brown, A. G., and Fyffe, R. E. W., 1984, *Intracellular Staining of Mammalian Neurones*, Academic Press, London.

Bullier, J., and Henry, G. H., 1979, Laminar distribution of first-order neurons and afferent terminals in cat striate cortex, *J. Neurophysiol.* **42:**1271–1281.

Capowski, J. J., and Rethelyi, M., 1982, Neuron reconstruction using a quantimet image analysing computer system, *Acta Morphol. Acad. Sci. Hung.* **30:**241–249.

Cohen, R. S., Chung, S. K., and Pfaff, D. W., 1985, Immunocytochemical localization of actin in dendritic spines of the cerebral cortex using colloidal gold as a probe, *Cell. Mol. Neurobiol.* **5:**271–284.

Creutzfeldt, O., Maekawa, K., and Hosli, L., 1969, Forms of spontaneous and evoked postsynaptic potentials of cortical nerve cells, *Prog. Brain Res.* **31:**265–273.

Freund, T. F., Martin, K. A. C., Smith, A. D., and Somogyi, P., 1983, Glutamate decarboxylase-immunoreactive terminals of Golgi-impregnated axoaxonic cells and of presumed basket cells in synaptic contact with pyramidal neurons of the cat's visual cortex, *J. Comp. Neurol.* **221:**263–278.

Freund, T. F., Martin, K. A. C., Somogyi, P., and Whitteridge, D., 1985, Innervation of cat visual areas 17 and 18 by physiologically identified X- and Y-type thalamic afferents. II. Identification of postsynaptic targets by GABA immunocytochemistry and Golgi impregnation, *J. Comp. Neurol.* **242:**275–291.

Friedlander, M. J., Lin, C.-S., Stanford, L. R., and Sherman, S. M., 1981, Morphology of functionally identified neurons in lateral geniculate nucleus of the cat, *J. Neurophysiol.* **46:**80–129.

Garey, L. J., and Powell, T. P. S., 1971, An experimental study of the termination of the lateral geniculo-cortical pathway in the cat and monkey, *Proc. R. Soc. Lond. [Biol.]* **179:**41–63.

Graber, M. B., and Kreutzberg, G. W., 1985, Immuno gold staining (IGS) for electron microscopical demonstration of glial fibrillary acidic (GFA) protein in LR white embedded tissue, *Histochemistry* **83:**497–500.

Grace, A. A., and Bunney, B. S., 1983, Intracellular and extracellular electrophysiology of nigral dopaminergic neurones—1. Identification and characterization, *Neuroscience* **10:**301–315.

Graham, R. C., and Karnovsky, M. J., 1966, The early stages of absorption of injected horseradish peroxidase in the proximal tubules of mouse kidney: Ultrastructural cytochemistry by a new technique, *J. Histochem. Cytochem.* **14:**291–302.

Hanker, J. S., Yates, P. E., Metz, C. B., and Rustioni, A., 1977, A new specific, sensitive and non-carcinogenic reagent for the demonstration of horseradish peroxidase, *Histochem. J.* **9:**789–792.

Hearn, S. A., Silver, M. M., and Sholdice, J. A., 1985, Immunoelectron microscopic labeling of immunoglobulin in plasma cells after osmium fixation and epoxy embedding, *J. Histochem. Cytochem.* **33:**1212–1218.

Hendry, S. H. C., Houser, C. R., Jones, E. G., and Vaughn, J. E., 1983, Synaptic organization of immunocytochemically identified GABA neurones in the monkey sensory–motor cortex, *J. Neurocytol.* **12:**639–660.

Hodgson, A. J., Penke, B., Erdei, A., Chubb, I. W., and Somogyi, P., 1985, Antiserum to γ-aminobutyric acid. I. Production and characterisation using a new model system, *J. Histochem. Cytochem.* **33:**229–239.

Hollander, H., 1970, The section embedding (SE) technique. A new method for the combined light microscopic and electron microscopic examination of central nervous tissue, *Brain Res.* **20:**39–47.

Jones, E. G., 1975, Varieties and distribution of non-pyramidal cells in the somatic sensory cortex of the squirrel monkey, *J. Comp. Neurol.* **160:**205–268.

Kisvarday, Z. F., Martin, K. A. C., Whitteridge, D., and Somogyi, P., 1985, Synaptic connections of intracellularly filled clutch cells: A type of small basket cell in the visual cortex of the cat, *J. Comp. Neurol.* **241:**111–137.

Kisvarday, Z. F., Martin, K. A. C., Freund, T. F., Magloczky, Z., Whitteridge, D., and Somogyi, P., 1986, Synaptic targets of HRP-filled layer III pyramidal cells in the cat striate cortex, *Exp. Brain Res.* **64:**541–552.

Kisvarday, Z. F., Martin, K. A. C., Friedlander, M. J., and Somogyi, P., 1981, Evidence for interlaminar inhibitory circuits in striate cortex of cat, *J. Comp. Neurol.* **260:**1–19.

Kitai, S. T., and Bishop, G. A., 1981, Horseradish peroxidase: Intracellular staining of neurons, in : *Neuroanatomical Tract-Tracing Methods*, (L. Heimer and M. J. RoBards, eds.), Plenum Press, New York, pp. 262–277.

Koch, C., and Poggio, T., 1983, A theoretical analysis of electrical properties of spines, *Proc. R. Soc. Lond. [Biol.]* **218:**455–477.

Lane, B. P., and Europa, D. L., 1965, Differential staining of ultrathin sections of Epon-embedded tissues for light microscopy, *J. Histochem. Cytochem.* **13:**579–582.

LeVay, S., and Gilbert, C. D., 1976, Laminar patterns of geniculocortical projection in the cat, *Brain Res.* **113:**1–19.

Marin-Padilla, M., 1969, Origin of the pericellular baskets of the pyramidal cells of the human motor cortex: A Golgi study, *Brain Res.* **14:**633–646.

Marin-Padilla, M., and Stibitz, G. R., 1974, Three-dimensional reconstruction of the basket cell of the human motor cortex, *Brain Res.* **70:**511–514.

Martin, K. A. C., and Whitteridge, D., 1984, Form, function, and intracortical projections of spiny neurones in the striate visual cortex of the cat, *J. Physiol. (Lond.)* **353:**463–504.

Martin, K. A. C., Somogyi, P., and Whitteridge, D., 1983, Physiological and morphological properties of identified basket cells in the cat's visual cortex, *Exp. Brain Res.* **50:**193–200.

Ottersen, O. P., and Storm-Mathisen, J., 1984, Glutamate- and GABA-containing neurons in the mouse and rat brain, as demonstrated with a new immunocytochemical technique, *J. Comp. Neurol.* **229**:374–392.

Phillips, C. G. 1959, Actions of antidromic pyramidal volleys on single Betz cells in the cat, *Q. J. Exp. Physiol.* **44**:1–25.

Ramon y Cajal, S., 1911, *Histologie du Systeme Nerveux de l'Homme et des Vertebres*, Vol. II, Maloine, Paris.

Reaves, T. A., Cumming, R., Libber, M. T., and Hayward, J. N., 1983, Immunocytochemical identification of intracellularly dye-marked neurons: A double-labelling technique for light and electron microscopic analysis, in: *Techniques in Immunocytochemistry*, Vol. 2 (G. R. Bullock, and P. Petrusz, eds.), Academic Press, London, pp. 71–84.

Ribak, C. E., 1978, Aspinous and sparsely-spinous stellate neurons in the visual cortex of rats contain glutamic acid decarboxylase, *J. Neurocytol.* **7**:461–478.

Rosenquist, A. C., Edwards, S. B., and Palmer, L. A., 1974, An autoradiographic study of the projections of the dorsal lateral geniculate nucleus and the posterior nucleus in the cat, *Brain Res.* **80**:71–93.

Roth, J., Bendayan, M., Carlemalm, E., Villiger, W., and Garavito, M., 1981, Enhancement of structural preservation and immunocytochemical staining in low temperature embedded pancreatic tissue, *J. Histochem. Cytochem.* **29**:663–671.

Seguela, P., Geffard, M., Buijs, R. M., and Le Moal, M., 1984, Antibodies against γ-aminobutyric acid: Specificity studies and immunocytochemical results, *Proc. Natl. Acad. Sci. U. S. A.* **81**:3888–3892.

Somogyi, P., and Hodgson, A. J., 1985, Antiserum to γ-aminobutyric acid. III. Demonstration of GABA in Golgi-impregnated neurons and in conventional electron microscopic sections of cat striate cortex. *J. Histochem. Cytochem.* **33**:249–257.

Somogyi, P., and Soltesz, I., 1986, Immunogold demonstration of GABA in synaptic terminals of intracellularly recorded, horseradish peroxidase-filled basket cells and clutch cells in the cat's visual cortex, *Neuroscience* **19**:1051–1065.

Somogyi, P., Hodgson, A. J., and Smith, A. D., 1979, An approach to tracing neuron networks in the cerebral cortex and basal ganglia. Combination of Golgi-staining, retrograde transport of horseradish peroxidase and anterograde degeneration of synaptic boutons in the same material, *Neuroscience* **4**:1805–1852.

Somogyi, P., Kisvarday, Z. F., Martin, K. A. C., and Whitteridge, D., 1983, Synaptic connections of morphologically identified and physiologically characterized large basket cells in the striate cortex of cat, *Neuroscience* **10**:261–294.

Somogyi, P., Hodgson, A. J., Smith, A. D., Nunzi, M. G., Gorio, A., and Wu, J.-Y., 1984, Different populations of GABAergic neurons in the visual cortex and hippocampus of cat contain somatostatin- or cholecystokinin-immunoreactive material, *J. Neurosci.* **4**:2590–2603.

Somogyi, P., Hodgson, A. J., Chubb, I. W., Penke, B., and Erdei, A., 1985, Antiserum to γ-aminobutyric acid. II. Immunocytochemical application to the central nervous system, *J. Histochem. Cytochem.* **33**:240–248.

Somogyi, P., Halasy, K., Somogyi, J., Storm-Mathisen, J., and Ottersen, O. P., 1986, Quantification of immunogold labeling reveals enrichment of glutamate in mossy and parallel fibre terminals in cat cerebellum, *Neuroscience* **19**:1045–1050.

Stefanis, C., and Jasper, H. H., 1964, Recurrent collateral inhibition in pyramidal tract neurons, *J. Neurophysiol.* **27**:855–877.

Sternberger, L. A., Hardy, P. H., Jr., Cuculis, J. J., and Meyer, H. G., 1970, The unlabelled antibody enzyme method of immunohistochemistry. Preparation and properties of soluble antigen–antibody complex (horseradish peroxidase–antihorseradish peroxidase) and its use in identification of spirochetes, *J. Histochem. Cytochem.* **18**:315–333.

Storm-Mathisen, J., Leknes, A. K., Bore, A. T., Vaaland, J. L., Edminson, P., Haug, F.-M. S., and Ottersen, O. P., 1983, First visualization of glutamate and GABA in neurones by immunocytochemistry, *Nature* **301**:517–520.

Szentagothai, J., 1973, Synaptology of the visual cortex, in: *Handbook of Sensory Physiology* (R. Jung, H. Autrum, W. R. Loewenstein, D. M. McKay, and H. L. Tenber, eds.), Springer-Verlag, Berlin, pp. 270–321.

Szentagothai, J., 1983, The modular architectonic principle of neural centers, *Rev. Physiol. Biochem. Pharmacol.* **98:**11–61.

Theodosis, D. T., Chapman, D. B., Montagnese, C., Poulain, D. A., and Morris, J. F., 1986, Structural plasticity in the hypothalamic supraoptic nucleus at lactation affects oxytocin-, but not vasopressin-secreting neurones, *Neuroscience* **17:**661–678.

van den Pol, A. N., 1984, Colloidal gold and biotin–avidin conjugates as ultrastructural markers for neural antigens, *Q. J. Exp. Physiol.* **69:**1–33.

van den Pol, A., 1985, Dual ultrastructural localization of two neurotransmitter-related antigens: Colloidal gold-labeled neurophysin-immunoreactive supraoptic neurons receive peroxidase-labeled glutamate decarboxylase- or gold-labeled GABA-immunoreactive synapses, *J. Neurosci.* **5:**2940–2954.

van den Pol, A. N., and Görcs, T., 1986, Glycine immunoreactive neurons and presynaptic boutons in the spinal cord, *Soc. Neurosci. Abstr.* **12:**771.

van der Heyden, J. A. M., and Korf, J., 1978, Regional levels of GABA in the brain: Rapid semiautomated assay and prevention of postmortem increase by 3-mercapto-propionic acid, *J. Neurochem.* **31:**197–203.

Weiler, R., and Ammermuller, J., 1986, Immunocytochemical localization of serotonin in intracellularly analyzed and dye-injected ganglion cells of the turtle retina, *Neurosci. Lett.* **72:**147–152.

Zsuppan, F., 1984, A new approach to merging neuronal tree segments traced from serial sections, *J. Neurosci. Methods* **10:**199–204.

10

In Situ Hybridization Combined with Retrograde Fluorescent Tract Tracing

BIBIE M. CHRONWALL,
MICHAEL E. LEWIS,
JAMES S. SCHWABER,
and THOMAS L. O'DONOHUE

I. INTRODUCTION

In situ hybridization histochemistry is one of the most recent additions to neurobiological methods. In this method, a labeled DNA or RNA sequence is hybridized to its specific complementary messenger RNA (mRNA) in his-

The authors wish to dedicate this chapter to the memory of T. L. O'Donohue.

BIBIE M. CHRONWALL • School of Basic Life Sciences, Division of Structure and Systems Biology, University of Missouri, Kansas City, Missouri 64108. MICHAEL E. LEWIS • Cephalon Inc., West Chester, Pennsylvania 19380. JAMES S. SCHWABER • Neurobiology Group, E. I. DuPont de Nemours and Co., Inc., Wilmington, Delaware 19858. THOMAS L. O'DONOHUE • J. D. Searle & Co., CNS Research, St. Louis, Missouri.

tological sections and visualized by autoradiography or histochemistry. The method originated in the field of molecular genetics and was originally used for localization of specific DNAs in metaphase chromosomes (Gall and Pardue, 1969; Jones and Robertson, 1970; Jacob *et al.*, 1971). Later, globin mRNA was detected in dispersed mammalian cells (Harrison *et al.*, 1973). The early studies are good sources for information on techniques and their application to the analysis of invertebrate development (Capco and Jeffery, 1978; Angerer and Angerer, 1981; McAllister *et al.*, 1983; Cox *et al.*, 1984). This chapter focuses on the mammalian CNS. Most commonly, probes are radioactively labeled, but biotinylated probes have also been tried (Singer and Ward, 1982; Varndell *et al.*, 1984; Binder *et al.*, 1986). An advantage of using radioactively labeled probes is that grain counting will give a relative quantification of mRNA levels in specific cells (Szabo *et al.*, 1977; Brahic and Haase, 1978; Griffin *et al.*, 1985; Uhl and Sasek, 1986; Wilcox *et al.*, 1986a,b; Young *et al.*, 1986b; Chronwall *et al.*, 1987). Compared to immunohistochemistry, *in situ* hybridization offers the advantage of localizing the anatomic site for protein synthesis, not merely detecting the presence of the protein. *In situ* hybridization may also have a higher degree of specificity. *In situ* hybridization is technically more complicated than immunohistochemistry and should be reserved for studies in which mRNA presence or levels are of interest. However, it enables the histologist to address a new set of questions concerning the presence of or changes in the amount of a certain mRNA, to manipulate this biosynthetic potential, and to get an answer at the cellular level. One of the most exciting concepts to emerge from this work is that changes in neuropeptide-related mRNAs are specifically coupled to altered utilization of the neuropeptides in brain and neuroendocrine tissue.

Tissues as heterogeneous as the mammalian brain (Siegel and Young, 1986; Whittemore *et al.*, 1986; Nojiri *et al.*, 1985; Gee *et al.*, 1983; Bloch *et al.*, 1986; Lewis *et al.*, 1986a; Uhl and Sasek, 1986; Young *et al.*, 1986a; Gehlert *et al.*, 1987) and pituitary (Pochet *et al.*, 1981; Gee *et al.*, 1983; Bloch *et al.*, 1985, 1986; Lewis *et al.*, 1986c) have been analyzed for different mRNAs at the cellular level. In experiments in which gene expression has been pharmacologically manipulated, *in situ* hybridization has become an invaluable tool (Wolfson *et al.*, 1985; Angulo *et al.*, 1986; Lewis *et al.*, 1986c; Kelsey *et al.*,1986; Baldino and Davis, 1986; Sherman *et al.*, 1986; Davis *et al.*, 1986a; Yamamoto *et al.*, 1986; Young *et al.*, 1986a; Chronwall *et al.*, 1987). Changes in mRNA levels during brain development (Griffin *et al.*, 1985) as well as changes in mRNA levels in neurological disease states (Griffin *et al.*, 1982; Uhl *et al.*, 1985; Fuller *et al.*, 1985) have also been elucidated with *in situ* hybridization.

Various combinations of axonal tracing and other histochemical methods, most notably immunohistochemistry (reviews: Hökfelt *et al.*, 1983; Skirboll *et al.*, 1984), link one or more transmitters to a neuron with known projections. Very recently the combination of axonal tracing and *in situ* hybridization has been applied to study the mRNA levels of different neuronal populations with known projections (Chronwall, 1985; Wilcox *et al.*, 1985, 1986b;

Schalling *et al.*, 1986; Schwaber *et al.*, 1989), and the present chapter presents variations of such combinations.

In such a combination, the axonal tracing is performed first, and after a suitable survival time, the tissue is prepared and hybridized to a probe. The choice of the tract-tracing method is limited by the specific requirements for the retention and unmasking of mRNAs and optimal hybridization conditions. Different aspects of the *in situ* hybridization technique have been reviewed recently (Gee and Roberts, 1983; Coghlan *et al.*, 1985; Griffin and Morrison, 1985; Lewis *et al.*, 1985b, 1986b; Bloch *et al.*, 1986). Here, we give a step-by-step discussion of the technique. It is important to establish this technique by itself first, before attempting to combine it with any axonal tracing method.

In considering the ways of combining the two techniques, one must decide to what extent various markers are mutually distinguishable and what methodological compromises have to be made. A section on how to examine and document the results and an appendix with detailed protocols conclude the chapter.

II. AXONAL TRACING METHODS

The past decade has seen an explosive growth in the field of neuroanatomy, largely driven by the development of new tract-tracing methods based on the active axonal transport of various markers. Several generations of such markers have rapidly superseded one another, each offering improvements, such that the ease of use, resolving power, and sensitivity of these methods are now quite good.

Retrograde axonal transport tracers have also recently come to include several fluorescent dyes, many of them originally introduced by Kuypers and his associates (reviewed by Hökfelt *et al.*, 1983; Skirboll *et al.*, 1984). The dyes offer numerous advantages, including ease of double staining, which permits study of axonal collateralization or combination with other techniques. The dyes initially available suffered disadvantages, however, including rapid fading, uptake by fibers of passage, diffuse, undefined injection locations, and leakage from labeled neurons. The search for improved dyes has led to the continual, rapid introduction of new fluorescent markers. The most recent in this series are fluorescent latex microspheres or beads (Katz *et al.*, 1984) and fluorogold (Schmued and Fallon, 1986), which appear to have overcome most of the earlier problems. These markers can be combined with other methods such as immunohistochemistry and *in situ* hybridization.

III. *IN SITU* HYBRIDIZATION

In situ hybridization subsumes a wide diversity of procedures for localizing specific nucleic acid sequences within cells. All of these procedures require

(1) a probe, which is a nucleic acid sequence partially or fully complementary to the sequence to be detected, (2) an incubation step in which the probe is hybridized to the endogenous nucleic acid, and (3) a method for detecting the location of the probe in a tissue preparation. As with any histochemical procedure, demonstration of the specificity of cellular labeling is critical. The following discussion describes several types of probes, how they are labeled for detection, the conditions under which hybridization occurs, and how to determine the specificity of hybridization. We emphasize the simplicity of using synthetic oligonucleotide probes. Thus, readers who wish to avoid "cloning jargon" may safely pass over the following sections on cDNA and cRNA probes.

A. Types of Probes

1. cDNA Probes

Hybridization probes have traditionally been obtained from cloned pieces of DNA that are complementary to a particular mRNA species. The complementary DNA (cDNA) clones must be isolated from cDNA libraries (a collection of clones derived from a total tissue mRNA population) of clones, which are prepared by reverse transcribing mRNAs into cDNA copies and are then made double-stranded and inserted into appropriate cDNA cloning vectors (for methods, see Maniatis *et al.*, 1982; Davis *et al.*, 1986b). Few histochemists will take the considerable trouble to prepare a new cDNA library; most anatomists who want a cDNA library will obtain one from a sympathetic molecular biologist, but it is also possible to purchase such libraries from Clontech Laboratories, Inc. (Palo Alto, CA).

Histochemists may find the commercially available cDNA libraries containing λ-gt 11 recombinant phage (bacteriophage vector) to be of particular interest, since these libraries can be screened with antisera, and positive clones detected by familiar antibody localization techniques (Huynh *et al.*, 1985). However, the majority of histochemists who use cloned cDNAs will obtain the purified clone from a molecular biologist who has already screened a library to isolate the clone of interest (Maniatis *et al.*, 1982; Davis *et al.*,1986b). Having obtained the clone generally as a stab of *E. coli* containing the recombinant plasmid,* the histochemist will then have to grow the cells, purify the plasmid, excise the cloned DNA from the plasmid with an appropriate restriction endonuclease, purify the DNA fragment by electrophoresis, elute the fragment from the gel, and perhaps further purify the fragment by column chromatography. The DNA fragment is then labeled by nick translation, i.e., using DNase I to generate random nicks and DNA polymerase I to initiate DNA synthesis with radioactive nucleotide triphosphates at the nick sites (Fig. 1). The radioactive DNA fragments are then purified by phenol–chloroform extraction or column chromatography (see Maniatis *et*

---

*A plasmid is a small independently replicating bacterial DNA molecule not linked to the main chromosome with a cDNA copy of the relevant mRNA.

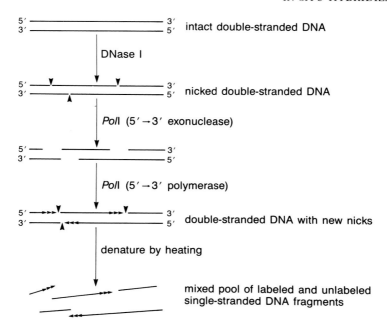

Figure 1. Preparation of cDNA hybridization probes by nick translation. The nick translation reaction is used to incorporate radioactive nucleotide phosphates into unlabeled double-stranded DNA. This DNA is nicked by DNase I (large arrowheads), and the exonuclease and polymerase activities of *E. coli* DNA polymerase I (Pol I) then remove parts of the DNA at the nick sites and replace them by introducing radioactive nucleotide phosphates (small arrowheads). The now double-stranded radioactive DNA must be denatured by heating to generate a mixed pool of labeled and unlabeled single-stranded DNA fragments. Those fragments from the strand that are complementary to the mRNA can now hybridize to the mRNA *in situ*.

al., 1982, or Davis *et al.*, 1986b, for details). This route to obtaining hybridization probes obviously requires the establishment of microbiological and molecular biological techniques, which is a disadvantage for the non-molecular-biologist who simply wishes to obtain probes for histochemical studies. Nick-translated cDNA probes have further disadvantages (Lewis *et al.*, 1985b), such as their long and variable lengths as well as their tendency to reassociate during the hybridization procedure.

2. cRNA Probes

An alternative, increasingly popular method for obtaining hybridization probes is the use of recently constructed plasmids containing promotor sequences (e.g., Sp6 and T7, that are recognized by RNA polymerase to start RNA synthesis) for transcription *in vitro* by DNA-dependent RNA polymerases (Green *et al.*, 1983; Cox *et al.*, 1984; Johnson and Johnson, 1984; Melton *et al.*, 1984). When a cDNA fragment is appropriately cloned into this

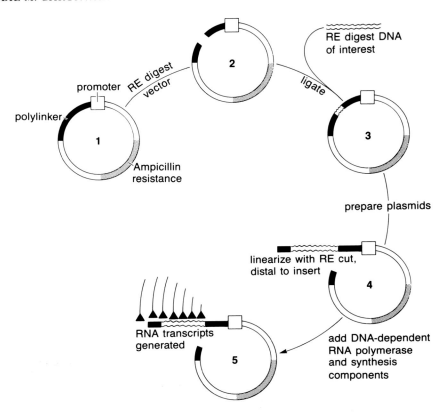

Figure 2. Preparation of hybridization probes by RNA transcript synthesis. The transcription reaction uses plasmids with a DNA-dependent RNA polymerase promoter such as Sp6. The appropriate cloned DNA is ligated into the plasmid, which has been opened by the action of a restriction endonuclease (RE). Bacterial cells are made permeable to the plasmid and are grown on an agar plate containing an antibiotic (e.g., ampicillin) that will kill cells not containing the plasmid (which confers resistance to the antibiotic.) A large quantity of cells is then grown, the plasmids are purified from them, and linearized plasmid is used as a template to direct the synthesis of a radioactive complementary RNA, which will then be purified and used as a hybridization probe.

type of plasmid, the RNA polymerase will repeatedly transcribe the cloned sequence (in the presence of radiolabeled precursor), resulting in the generation of large quantities of single-stranded RNA probes of very high specific activity (Fig. 2) (see Davis *et al.*, 1986b, for methods). These cRNA probes are up to eight times more sensitive than cDNA probes (Cox *et al.*, 1984), and hybridization background can be markedly reduced by the use of (1) posthybridization RNase treatment to digest unhybridized cRNA and mRNA and (2) elevated washing temperatures, which are permitted by the greater thermal stability of RNA–RNA duplexes compared to DNA–RNA hybrids (Angerer *et al.*, 1985). Despite these clear advantages, molecular biological expertise is still needed in order to obtain RNA probes, which may require hydrolysis into smaller fragments for effective tissue penetration (Cox *et al.,* 1984).

3. Synthetic Oligonucleotide Probes

A third route to obtaining hybridization probes, which is presently the simplest for the non-molecular-biologist, is to have synthetic oligonucleotides prepared in a sequence complementary to the mRNA of interest (see Lewis *et al.,* 1985b, 1988 for reviews). These probes are short (e.g., 20–50 nucleotides) single-stranded segments of DNA that are readily synthesized by automated apparatus, e.g., the Applied Biosystems Model 380A or the Vega Coder 300 DNA Synthesizer (Matteucci and Caruthers, 1981), and then HPLC purified (Fritz *et al.,* 1978) for subsequent radiolabeling. Nucleotide or amino acid sequence information is needed to design the probe, and different design strategies are required, depending on the information available (Lathe, 1985; Lewis *et al.,* 1985b; Davis *et al.,* 1986b). Fortunately, many research institutions and universities now have oligonucleotide synthesis facilities, and a number of companies will undertake the custom synthesis and purification of a specified DNA sequence on a cost-effective basis (see Section VI.G). Furthermore, synthetic oligonucleotide probes for several neuronal and nonneuronal mRNAs are now commercially available (see Section VI.G), and more should become available as increasing numbers of histochemists add *in situ* hybridization to their technical repertoire. The following discussion of probe labeling is based on the use of synthetic oligonucleotides for *in situ* hybridization studies.

B. Probe Labeling

Once the oligonucleotide probe is obtained, several labeling options must be considered. Nonradioisotopic methods such as biotinylation (Singer and Ward, 1982) are appealing, particularly to histochemists who are accustomed to using biotinylated antibodies for immunocytochemistry. Unfortunately, a number of investigators, including ourselves, have generally been unsuccessful in obtaining reliable, sensitive detection of hybridization in tissue sections with such probes. An advantage of using radioisotopic labeling is the ease of quantitating the signal through grain counting (Rogers, 1979). Thus, radioisotopic methods of labeling are in general use, and the investigator is faced with a choice of three radiolabeling methods: (1) 5′-end labeling, (2) primer extension, or (3) 3′-end labeling.

The first method, 5′-end labeling, is the standard method used by molecular biologists to label synthetic oligonucleotides for screening cDNA libraries (Maniatis *et al.,* 1982; Davis *et al.,* 1986b). With this procedure, the enzyme T4 polynucleotide kinase is used to transfer a ^{32}P from $[\gamma\text{-}^{32}P]$-ATP to a free 5' OH group; this reaction can also be carried out using $[\gamma\text{-}^{35}\text{S-}$ thio]-ATP (Johnson and Johnson, 1984) to label the probe with a less energetic isotope. The method is simple (see Davis *et al.*, 1986b,c, for details) but has the disadvantage of adding only one molecule of radioisotope per molecule of probe, thus limiting the specific activity.

The second method, primer extension labeling, was introduced by Studencki and Wallace (1984) as a means for incorporating multiple labeled nucleotides into an oligonucleotide probe, using a message-sense oligonucleotide (i.e., DNA equivalent of part of mRNA sequence) as a template and the large (Klenow) fragment of *E. coli* DNA polymerase I to catalyze the extension across the template. This method has been successfully used for *in situ* hybridization studies (Uhl *et al.*, 1985; Lewis *et al.*, 1986a; Morris *et al.*, 1986) but has the disadvantages of requiring preparation of both template and primer oligonucleotides as well as electrophoretic separation of the template from the extended labeled primer after the reaction.

The third method, 3'-end labeling, is based on the ability of terminal deoxynucleotidyl transferase to catalyze the sequential addition of radioactive bases to the 3' end of oligonucleotides (Bollum, 1974), resulting in the formation of a radioactive "tail" on the probe (Fig. 3). This method was used by Lewis *et al.* (1984, 1985a,b, 1986a–c) to detect proopiomelanocortin and vasopressin mRNA by *in situ* hybridization. Collins and Hunsaker (1985) have also used this procedure to label probes for genomic blotting studies. The primer extension and 3'-end labeling methods share the advantage of being able to label probes with multiple, lower-energy radioisotopes to enhance anatomic resolution. Although both ^{3}H- and ^{125}I-labeled probes have been useful, the former requires long exposure times, and the latter can lead to high background labeling with some probes. Labeling of oligonucleotides by 3' tailing, using $[^{35}\text{S}]$-dATP as substrate in the reaction, followed by a simple chromatographic purification step, has yielded probes that give excellent anatomic (i.e., cellular) resolution after short exposure times. Thus, this method was used to prepare probes for the double-labeling studies described in this chapter and is detailed in the Appendix (Section VII.E).

C. Hybridization

1. Procedure

Once a labeled probe has been obtained, the investigator can carry out hybridization studies on appropriately prepared tissue sections (see Section IV.B and Appendix for details). Prior to hybridization, the tissue can be gently digested ("permeabilized") with proteinase K to facilitate penetration of the probe into the cells. Hybridization conditions are designed to facilitate the interaction of the labeled probe with the appropriate mRNA in the tissue while suppressing nonspecific interactions of the probe with other molecules. Before the probe is added to the tissue, the section is incubated with the

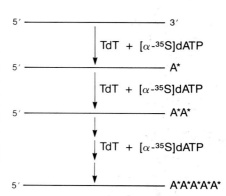

Figure 3. 3′ labeling of synthetic oligonucleotide hybridization probes. The synthesized and purified oligonucleotide is labeled by sequential addition of radioactive nucleotides to the 3′ end by terminal deoxynucleotidyl transferase. Prolonged incubation results in the addition of more nucleotides, increasing the specific activity of the probe, which is purified by chromatography as described in the Appendix (Section VII.E).

hybridization buffer, which contains (1) formamide, which facilitates hybrid formation at lower temperatures, (2) dextran sulfate, an inert polymer that appears to accelerate the rate of hybridization by exclusion of DNA from the volume taken up by the polymer, (3) $3\times$ SSC (450 mM NaCl, 45mM trisodium citrate, pH 7.0), which maintains an ionic strength consistent with a rapid rate of hybrid formation, (4) Denhardt's solution, consisting of Ficoll, polyvinylpyrrolidone, and bovine serum albumin, originally designed to saturate nonspecific binding sites on nitrocellulose, and (5) yeast tRNA and denatured salmon sperm DNA, which may occupy nonspecific binding sites and serve as "decoy" substrates for endogenous or contaminating nucleases (for further discussion, see Anderson and Young, 1985; Young and Anderson, 1985). The probe is then added to the tissue in this buffer at a temperature about 20°C below the T_m (the temperature at which half of the duplexes dissociate; see Anderson and Young, 1985; Lewis *et al.*, 1985b; Davis *et al.*, 1986b) for a period of about 16 hr. The sections are then washed at decreasing concentrations of SSC (standard sodium citrate buffer; see above) and/or at a high temperature to destabilize nonspecific hybrids, thus reducing the background. The sections are then air dried and processed for autoradiography according to standard procedures (Rogers, 1979; Edwards and Hendrickson, 1981) as outlined in Section IV.C and in the Appendix.

2. Specificity of Hybridization

Just as it is essential in immunohistochemistry to carry out certain control procedures to avoid misinterpretation of false-positive staining, so too does the correct interpretation of *in situ* hybridization studies depend on rigorous evaluation of the specificity of detected hybrids. We and other investigators have employed a number of control procedures, which are summarized below (see Lewis *et al.*, 1985a,b).

a. Peptide mRNA Localization. With appropriate fixation conditions (e.g., 4% formaldehyde perfusion, as described in the Appendix), immunohistochemical and *in situ* colocalization studies can be carried out using adjacent sections (Gee *et al.*, 1983) or sequentially on the same section (Griffin *et al.*,1983; Wolfson *et al.*, 1985; Davis *et al.*, 1986a). Strong evidence for specificity would be provided by demonstration of colocalization using multiple antisera directed against different regions of the precursor encoded by the mRNA target (i.e., three sections incubated successively with antiserum 1, DNA probe, and antiserum 2, with the same cells positive for all three markers). However, discrepancies in localization could arise for technical reasons as well as from characteristics of the cell system under investigation. This is discussed further in Section V.

b. Competition Studies. Because there is a small concentration of the target mRNA relative to potential "nonspecific hybridization" sites, only the specific hybridization signal from the labeled probe should be diminished by addition of increasing concentrations of unlabeled probe. For example, preincubation of rat pituitary sections with increasing concentrations of unlabeled oligonucleotide complementary to part of the proopiomelanocortin mRNA results in a decrease in hybridization signal from the intermediate lobe but not from the posterior lobe (Lewis *et al.*, 1986b,c). These results are consistent with the known localization of proopiomelanocortin peptides in the intermediate but not posterior lobe of rat pituitary and indicate that only the specific hybridization signal is affected by prehybridization with unlabeled probe. However, this type of study only indicates that the labeled and unlabeled probes share the same, apparently saturable target; the actual identity of this target is not demonstrated.

A second type of competition study, analogous to the preabsorption control for immunohistochemistry, can be carried out by preincubating the labeled probe with an unlabeled message-sense probe (i.e., having the mRNA sequence) prior to *in situ* hybridization. However, when these probes are hybridized together in solution before being added to the tissue, all that is being tested is whether a double-stranded probe can somehow "hybridize" nonspecifically. When such an experiment was carried out using proopiomelanocortin probes that were complementary to each other, the radioactive hybrid failed to label pituitary at all; even normal background labeling was absent (Lewis *et al.*, 1985b, 1986c). Beyond revealing that unpaired bases are necessary for nonspecific interactions, this type of study is clearly useless as a control procedure.

c. Colocalization of Related Hybrids. Probes complementary to different regions of the same mRNA should hybridize to the same cells in a series of sections. With an autoradiographic double-labeling technique (Haase *et al.*, 1985) or a recently developed nonradioactive bicolor method (Hopman *et al.*, 1986), it appears to be possible to carry out such studies on a single section. Multiple, labeled probes should be useful for enhancing hybridization signals and also confirming the effects of treatments on mRNA levels (Lewis *et al.*, 1986c)

d. Thermal Analysis of Hybrids. A powerful and sensitive index of hybridization specificity is provided by the thermal denaturation temperature (T_m) of nucleic acid hybrids. The value of T_m is determined primarily by G–C (guanine–cytosine bases) content, length, number of base-pair mismatches, and salt concentration (Bonner *et al.*, 1973; Britten *et al.*, 1974; Cantor and Schimmel, 1980). For oligonucleotides T_m can be calculated as follows:

$$T_m = 81.5 + 16.6(\log[\text{Na}^+]) + 0.41(\%\text{G} + \text{C}) - 675/(\text{probe length}) - 1.0(\%\text{mismatch}) - 0.65(\%\text{formamide})$$

where the molar concentration of Na^+ is a maximum of 0.5 (e.g., $1 \times \text{SSC}$ contains 0.165 M Na^+), the percentage of G + C bases is between 30 and 70, and the probe length is expressed as the number of bases, not exceeding 100 (Davis *et al.*, 1986b). For *in situ* hybridization, such studies may be carried out by exposing a similar series of hybridized sections to x-ray film, incubating the sections at different temperatures (e.g., 30–80°C) in a suitable buffer (e.g. 0.5 × SSC) for 1 hr, reexposing the sections to film for the same length of time, and then calculating and plotting percentage melted as a function of temperature. The interpolated "50% melted" point should compare closely to the calculated T_m, which has been found to be the case for proopiomelanocortin (Lewis *et al.*, 1985b, 1986c; Kelsey *et al.*, 1986) and vasopressin (Baldino and Davis, 1986) probes. An additional benefit of such studies is the determination of the optimal hybridization temperature, which is often considered to be about 20°C lower than the T_m value (e.g., Davis *et al.*,1986b). If the investigator is using a probe based on the sequence from one species to carry out studies on the homologous mRNA of another species, base-pair mismatches are possible and will lower the obtained T_m in relation to the calculated value (assuming no mismatches). In this case, the optimal hybridization temperature will also be lower and should be adjusted appropriately.

e. RNase Pretreatment. Treatment of sections with RNase A prior to hybridization of mRNA has invariably been found to eliminate hybridization signals (e.g., Shivers *et al.*, 1986; Uhl and Sasek, 1986), consistent with the probe target being an RNA molecule. This control procedure does not in any way establish the identity of the RNA, and it is certain that spurious hybridization, e.g., to ribosomal RNA, would also be eliminated by digestion.

f. Anticomplementary Probes. With the advent of Sp6 vectors, which can be transcribed in opposite directions to yield either complementary or anticomplementary (i.e., message-sense) probes in radioactive form, some investigators have begun to use the latter as control probes, showing generally that they hybridize poorly if at all. Logically, this procedure cannot demonstrate that hybridization of the former probes is therefore specific; all that has been shown is that the message-sense probe does not itself have a complementary target in the cell.

g. RNA Blot Analysis. To characterize further the *in situ* target of the labeled probe, RNA can be isolated from the tissue of interest (ideally, a micropunch containing the molecules under study), run through a denaturing gel, transferred to nitrocellulose, and hybridized with the probe (see Lewis *et al.*, 1985b; Davis *et al.*, 1986b; Sherman *et al.*, 1986, for details). Although this procedure is uniquely valuable in demonstrating hybridization of the probe to RNA of a particular size (consistent with the known sequence), it cannot prove that this same RNA is necessarily the target *in situ*, particularly if different hybridization conditions are used. One way to gain more confidence in RNA blot (i.e., "Northern") analysis as a control for *in situ* hybridization specificity is to demonstrate treatment effects that are detected similarly by both procedures (Sherman *et al.*, 1986).

It should be apparent from the above discussion that no one of the control procedures alone is completely sufficient to demonstrate hybridization specificity *in situ*. Instead, the careful investigator, like a good detective, will prefer to obtain several lines of evidence that consistently lead to the conclusion that the object of study is indeed what it appears to be.

IV. COMBINATION OF RETROGRADE FLUORESCENT TRACT TRACING AND *IN SITU* HYBRIDIZATION

Several considerations should be kept in mind when trying to combine axonal tract-tracing techniques with *in situ* hybridization. First, gene expression is a dynamic process that can change very rapidly with the metabolic state of the neuron. Second, the *in situ* hybridization technique requires special tissue treatment, which can not be compromised by the axonal tracing. Third, the markers have to be easily differentiated. Each of these considerations influences and limits the choice of the tract-tracing method. Of the methods available, the retrograde transport of fluorescent particles or dyes, appears to be the least disruptive to normal cellular metabolism, and there are no additional histological procedures involved apart from the hybridization. The disadvantages of this combination are that the preparations are not permanent and a fluorescence microscope is required to visualize the tracer.

A. Choice of Fluorescent Tract Tracer

We have successfully used the following tracers: fast blue, rhodamine-labeled latex microspheres, and fluorogold. Our main considerations were to choose the least toxic or least disruptive substance that showed minimal leakage and fading. Several reviews on the use of fluorescent tracers appeared recently (Hökfelt *et al.*, 1983; Skirboll *et al.*, 1984). Desirable characteristics of an optimal fluorescent marker include the following: chemically stable; brightly fluorescent; resistant to fading; can be stored and viewed repeatedly for months; low background, high signal-to-noise ratio, permitting clear photographs and unambiguous data analysis; nondisruptive of normal cellular metabolism; no processing required; nonselective; not harmed by processing requirements of *in situ* hybridization; compatible with the fixation used in present *in situ* hybridization methodologies; injection sites that remain consistent in appearance over various postinjection times; nontransient, retained after transport within the neuron; remain active after brains or sections are stored; transported from terminals and cut axons but not axons of passage; does not leak from cell, causing false-positive labeling of surrounding elements; transported in fast transport, consistent with short postinjection survival times.

1. Fast Blue

Fast blue is transported well and does not leak excessively, nor is it strikingly toxic. Though it fades in aqueous solutions, expecially during UV exposure, it is easily visualized and photographed.

2. Rhodamine-Labeled Acrylic Microspheres

The "rhodamine beads" are 0.02–0.2 μm in diameter, and their small size and hydrophobic surface, i.e., their tendency to stick to cell membranes, probably facilitate their uptake. Bead-filled neurons show no degeneration and have normal action potentials as shown by intracellular recording (Katz *et al.*, 1984). Our pilot experiments show no apparent effect on hybridization patterns; i.e., the number and distribution of labeled, mRNA-hybridized neurons in a certain area are the same in brains containing this axonal tracer as in control brains. The amount of tracer appears to be the same in double-labeled cells as in cells labeled with beads only (Fig. 4).

3. Fluorogold

Chemically, fluorogold is a "stilbene" derivative. It is easily separated to near purity and gives very reliable labeling, filling out the soma and much of the primary dendrites. The mechanisms of retrograde transport are unknown, but the tracer seems to be transported in pinocytotic vesicles (Schmued and Fallon, 1986). With fluorogold, vesicular label within the soma is visualized initially within 24 hr. If postinjection times are allowed to extend beyond 48 hr, increasing filling of the soma and the dendrites occurs. As noted above for the beads, there is no apparent difference in hybridization patterns between fluorogold-labeled and nonlabeled neurons. However, neurons double-labeled with fluorogold and silver grains were often relatively dim for the fluor. This suggests the possibility of some interference between the two markers, a problem that is undergoing further study.

B. Preparatory Steps to Combine Retrograde Fluorescent Tracing with *in Situ* Hybridization

1. Tracer Injection

If given a choice, use as low a tracer concentration as possible, avoid additives (DMSO, etc.) that can influence the target cells, and use ribonuclease-free solutions. Although colchicine injections are often used to enhance the results of immunohistochemistry, they are not necessary for *in situ* hybridization and cause unnecessary stress to experimental animals. Furthermore, colchicine is a cell toxin, and its effects on mRNA levels are not clear (Gee and Roberts, 1983; Wolfson *et al.*, 1985).

Since fluorogold and rhodamine beads have become our preference among tracers and the literature on them is scant, we would like to add some comments on their use (see also Skirboll *et al.*, Chapter 2, this volume). Fluorogold is supplied lyophilized and can be stored dry at 4°C for several months. The dye can be dissolved in water, physiological saline, or 0.2 M neutral phosphate buffer. Concentrations of 4% and 2% have been successful for use with *in situ* hybridization processing; lower concentrations produce somewhat smaller injection sites and somewhat reduced labeling. We have used dye dissolved in buffer and stored in the refrigerator for several months with good results. Rhodamine beads are supplied in an aqueous solution. This solution may be injected undiluted or diluted up to 1 : 4 in distilled H_2O or saline. We have used 1 : 4 dilutions in combination with *in situ* hybridization processing. The beads can be stored for at least 1 year in the refrigerator in a humidified container.

Pressure injections via glass pipettes in volumes of 50–75 nl have been used successfully for both tracers. Fluorogold can be iontophoresed by 5 mA positive current. Since the beads have a tendency to clump and block the glass pipette, tip sizes of 35–50 μm should be used, whereas 20 μm works well for fluorogold pressure injections. Since bead injection sites remain highly confined, several injections may be required to fill a projection field. Survival times of 24 hr are adequate for both dyes in the rat, but longer times, up to 48 hr for the beads and up to 7 days for fluorogold, lead to increased labeling. Survival time, dilution, and injection amount all interact to produce a given apparent injection site and amount of retrograde filling. Survival times up to 3 weeks have produced no diminution of label or leakage from filled cells, but long survival times do appear gradually to decrease the apparent size of the injection site. Longer survival times may be desirable if the possible effect of surgical stress on mRNA level is an important consideration. Each tracer has its pros and cons: fluorogold gives consistent success in injections, a relatively diffuse injection site, fills cells and dendrites completely,

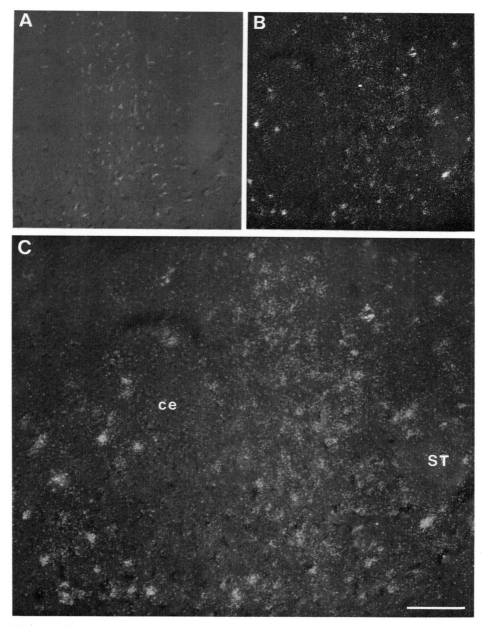

Figure 4. Photomicrographs of the same microscopic field in the left central amygdaloid nucleus under three conditions to illustrate simultaneous label for mRNA and for tract-tracing. Panel A shows neurons labeled with rhodamine latex beads from an injection into the ipsilateral nucleus of the solitary tract (NTS). Panel B is a darkfield micrograph of emulsion autoradiography for *in situ* hybridization in which labeled probes have been used to hybridize somatostatin mRNA. Panel C is a double exposure of both A and B. Bar, 100 μm.

and yields good double exposures with autoradiography. The beads some-times bind together and clog the pipette tip, causing failure to inject, but the injection site is confined, well defined, and can be seen when sectioning. Double exposures can be somewhat hard to print.

2. Anesthesia

Use conventional methods, taking into account that different types of anesthesia may involve different kinds of stress that could influence mRNA levels.

3. Fixation

Perfuse with phosphate-buffered saline (PBS) until the perfusate clears of erythrocytes, followed by 350–400 ml of 4% formaldehyde in PBS (see Appendix). For some probes a lower concentration (1%) of formaldehyde might be tried (Bloch *et al.*, 1986). Bouin's solution has been used successfully (Griffin and Morrison, 1985), and 0.05–0.1% glutaraldehyde can be added if resectioning for electron microscopy is desired. Following the perfusion the brain is removed from the skull and fixed for an additional 2 hr. The tissue can also be fixed by immersion in the fixative. Most commonly, the brain is infiltrated overnight with 30% sucrose in ribonuclease-free PBS and frozen for cryostat sectioning. Tissue containing fluorogold can be paraffin embedded (Schmued and Fallon, 1986) and *in situ* hybridization has been performed on paraffin sections (Griffin *et al.*, 1985; Chronwall *et al.*, 1987). The authors have not tried this particular combination, but it seems promising for obtaining optimal tissue preservation. The rhodamine beads should, however, not be exposed to alcohols or xylenes for more than 2 min altogether; therefore, paraffin embedding is not recommended for this tracer.

4. Preparation of Microscope Slides

In situ hybridization involves somewhat harsh tissue treatments and lengthy incubations and washes. Therefore, it is imperative to clean carefully and sub (see Section VII.B) the microscope slides to ensure tissue adherence (Griffin and Morrison, 1985).

5. Sectioning

Touch the sections only with heat-sterilized (RNase-free) tools while transferring sections to slides. Let sections fully dry onto slides to adhere well. Although thorough deparaffination is an important step prior to hybridization, paraffin sections should not be overheated when the paraffin is melted off.

6. Storage of Tissue

Store brains, preferably unsectioned, at $-30°C$ or $-70°C$. Sections mounted on slides and stored dry, dark, and cold ($-20°C$ or $4°C$) will retain their fluorescence for quite some time. The rhodamine of latex spheres lasts 1 year (Katz *et al.*, 1984), fast blue at least as long (B. M. Chronwall, unpublished observation), and tissues sectioned several months (and stored as above) prior to probe application have been successfully hybridized (B. M. Chronwall, unpublished observation).

7. Hybridization

Perform the steps discussed in Section III and in the Appendix. The permeabilization (proteinase K) step may impinge on tracer retention and should not be done for more than 10 min. In fact, this step damages tissue fixed with 1% formaldehyde and has been found unnecessary; it may even increase background labeling with several 30-base probes (R. G. Krause II and M. E. Lewis, unpublished data). The washing steps will enhance leakage of the tracer and should be kept to the absolute minimum, which allows successful hybridization with low nonspecific hybridization background. Cover containers of slides with aluminum foil in order to reduce photobleaching of a sensitive tracer.

8. Autoradiography

To visualize the radioisotope-labeled hybrids, the slides are dipped in liquid photographic emulsion under safelight, exposed in light-tight boxes at $4°C$, developed, and fixed. Autoradiography is theoretically simple and a very elegant method, but it requires some technical knowledge and carries its own set of artifacts. Rogers (1979) gives background information as well as a detailed protocol, and Edwards and Hendrickson (1981) discuss each step in detail; both sources are highly recommended. A simple protocol has been included in the Appendix (Section VII.H). In addition, we would like to give some practical hints. The use of the Thomas Duplex-Super Safelight (Thomas Instrument Company, Charlottesville VA 22901) has revolutionized emulsion dipping. Use this safe light with the red-taped filters in the vanes and the yellow-taped filters in the lamp and let the lamp warm up (30 min) before emulsion is exposed to it. The sodium light emitted by this safelight provides an astonishingly bright, easy-to-work-in darkroom.

For easy handling and economical use of the emulsion we recommend melting the bulk emulsion in the jar in a 42°C waterbath and aliquoting it into plastic slide mailers that have been prelabeled with heavy black felt pen at half and full levels.

Fill to the half mark with the liquid emulsion and store in a light-tight box in the refrigerator. Before use, fill up with distilled water (42°C) containing 1 mg/ml Dreft® detergent (dissolved in a sonicator bath), place in a waterbath (42°C), and mix well before use. Dip the slides into the emulsion in the slide mailer. Even, slow dipping consistent across slides will produce an even emulsion coat free of artifacts caused by the emulsion. Even emulsion coating also enhances quantitative comparisons across slides. The slide mailer can be capped, stored, and the emulsion reused several times before it develops too much background.

After the slides have dried in a vertical position (empty scintillation vial boxes lined with paper towels, or histology slide racks can be used) for 3 hr, they are packed in black plastic boxes (without any lining or other nonplastic material) with desiccant for exposure. Reusable desiccant capsules (Ted Pella Inc., Tustin, CA) are easy to handle and produce little dust. The slides can then be developed in the black box: remove the desiccant and simply immerse the box (keeping a finger over the slides to keep them in place) into a suitable container (such as a staining dish) with the developer. This procedure avoids reloading the slides in the darkness, which often results in scratches in the emulsion.

9. Mounting of the Preparations

The following mounting media are nonfluorescent, retain fluorescence in the tissue, and in addition give a semipermanent preparation: Entellan (Merck, Darmstadt, FRG), Fluoromount (Southern Biotechnology Associates Inc., Birmingham, AL 35226), Immumount (Accurate Chemicals), and Permafluor (Immumon, Troy, MI 48087). Polyvinyl alcohols in glycerol have proven to be very good mounting media (Lillie, 1954; Feder, 1959; Thomason and Cowart, 1966) that retain fluorescence well and harden, which prevents the coverslip from sliding around. A receipt for an inexpensive, easy to prepare medium is included in the Appendix. A polyvinylglycerol medium can also be obtained commercially (Aqua-Mount, Lerner Lab, New Haven, CT 06513).

V. EXAMINATION AND DOCUMENTATION OF PREPARATIONS

Once the technical aspects of *in situ* hybridization have been established in the laboratory, one can begin to interpret the results. The first step will be to discriminate among autoradiographic background, possible nonspecific hybridization, and specific hybridization. This will be best performed at medium magnification for overall grain distribution and relatively high magnification for individual or clusters of grains in brightfield as well as darkfield illumination. Silver grains distributed over both tissue and slide probably indicate an aged emulsion or exposure of the photographic emulsion or dipped slide to inappropriate light or heat. Clusters of grains around the edges of sections or inside blood vessels, holes, or tears in the tissue could be mechanical-stress grains in the emulsion. On the other hand, heavy labeling over white matter is most likely nonspecific hybridization, the probe adhering to myelin. Silver grains that appear over the cytoplasm of the neurons of a certain population have to be evaluated for specificity as outlined in Section III.C.2. The most commonly used control procedure is colocalization of the mRNA for a transmitter/neuropeptide (*in situ* hybridization) and the presence of the neuroactive substance that is coded for by the message (immunohistochemistry), either in the same or in serial sections. However, discrepancies in localization could arise for purely technical reasons in either method (e.g., a poor antiserum, insufficient colchicine, an insensitive immunohistochemical technique, poor labeling of the probe, or high autoradiographic background).

If technical reasons for discrepancies in localization can be ruled out, several other explanations are possible. When more numerous neurons are labeled by *in situ* hybridization than by immunohistochemistry, this could imply detection of untranslated mRNA. One reported example of such a discrepancy is the finding that many more striatal neurons are positive for apparent proenkephalin mRNA than for enkephalin immunoreactivity (Shivers *et al.*, 1986). In the reverse case of more immunoreactive neurons containing the mRNA, the peptide could have been accumulated by uptake from the surrounding tissue, or the mRNA level could be below the detection limit, given the specific activity of the probe and the length of the exposure to the emulsion. Prolonged exposure times may be necessary to detect low mRNA expression, although this approach may be unsuccessful if the signal-to-noise ratio is too low.

In situ hybridization results can be quantitated through counting of autoradiographic grains as long as certain technical precautions are taken. Only tissues that have been processed identically and that have been hybridized and emulsion dipped in the same batch should be compared, and enough material has to be analyzed to compensate for variability in results. Probe labeling as well as hybridization and exposure times have to be adapted to give neither too low nor too high grain counts to ensure that the counting is being performed in the range where grain density can be considered directly proportional to radioactivity (Rogers 1979; Szabo *et al.*, 1977). The counting can be done by eye, using a hand-held counter, or by means of a suitable image analysis system (Young *et al.*, 1986b; Wilcox *et al.*, 1986a,b; McCabe *et al.*, 1986; Chronwall *et al.*, 1987; Rogers *et al.*, 1987). Most quantitation studies are relative; i.e., mRNA levels are compared in sections from control and drug-treated animals. Recently, investigators have attempted to estimate absolute numbers of mRNA copies (Young *et al.*, 1986b; Cash and Brahic, 1986).

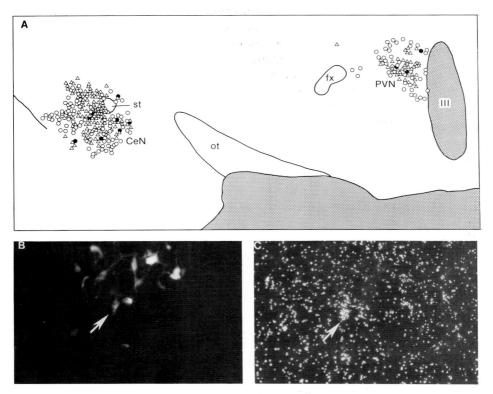

Figure 5. A is a schematic mapping of a coronal section showing the distribution of single- and double-labeled neurons. Triangles indicate cells retrogradely labeled by rhodamine beads injected into the NTS; circles indicate cells with *in situ* label for somatostatin mRNA; filled circles indicate cells with both labels. CeN, central nucleus of the amygdala; PVN, paraventricular nucleus; fx, fornix; ot, optic tract; st, stria terminalis; III, third ventricle. B and C show the same field from the CeN with retrogradely labeled cells in B and mRNA visualization in C. Arrow points to a double-labeled neuron.

Investigators with access to appropriate image analysis equipment should also be able to obtain quantitative information from preparations where *in situ* hybridization has been combined with fluorescent tract tracers, e.g., comparing cells that have been labeled by one marker but not by the other (Fig. 5A) or with varying grain counts within a neuronal population with a known projection (Wilcox *et al.*, 1986b).

Standard fluorescence microscopy is used to examine the fluorescent tracers. Fast blue is commonly viewed at 360 nm excitation wavelength. The beads require any rhodamine filter set, such as 510–560 excitation, 580 dichroic mirror, and 590 barrier filter (Fig. 4A). For fluorogold the filter requirements are 323 nm excitation (UV) and 408 nm emission at neutral pH. The *in situ* hybridization label can be viewed simultaneously using epifluorescence for the dyes and darkfield transmission microscopy for the autoradiographic grains (Fig. 4C). By dodging a hand through the subcondenser light path, the field can be rapidly scanned for double-labeled cells using ×10 or ×20 objectives. This is an important precaution to avoid misjudgment of single- versus double-labeled cells. To photograph double-labeled cells, the same field can be photographed under each condition separately without moving the stage. At least ×20 and usually ×40 objectives (×400–800 final magnification on the prints) are typically required, and "landmarks" should be included when possible to confirm the relative positions of the cells in photomicrographs (Fig. 4C). When photographing under darkfield conditions, remember to remove fluorescent filters from the light path to the camera. To show double labeling convincingly, double exposures are very valuable (Fig 4C). For these exposures, it is important to reduce the time for the darkfield exposure by approximately 1–1.5 *f*-stops to keep the brightness of each marker proportional. Documentation is most informative on color film (Fig. 4), but results can also be shown with black-and-white photomicrographs (Fig. 5B,C).

VI. SUMMARY OF ADVANTAGES AND LIMITATIONS OF *IN SITU* HYBRIDIZATION AS COMPARED TO IMMUNOHISTOCHEMISTRY

When performing *in situ* hybridization and immunohistochemistry, some procedures, like the many incubations and washes, are similar. The techniques are also similar in that both visualize the presence of specific molecules within cells. *In situ* hybridization is a relatively new technique and, like some others, is adapted from a discipline with a vocabulary of its own that sometimes seems hard to penetrate. A good solution might be to perform a hybridization together with a colleague "who knows how to" and try to understand the different steps retroactively. Here the different steps of the two techniques are compared to elucidate when to use one or the other. Probes are not yet as commercially available as antisera, but they will soon be. The probes are highly specific, can be custom made quickly, and are easy to label using commercially available kits. So far, radioactive labeling has been the most successful, which means a radiation hazard but also the advantages of a permanent signal that is easy to detect in any microscope and that, above all, is possible to quantitate. A distinct drawback of the *in situ* approach is the lack of clear-cut controls. *In situ* hybridization labels only the biosynthetic site, which means that it is limited to the detection of neuronal perikarya. On the other hand, it does not require colchicine treatment, which means that animal suffering can be avoided and also that perikarya can be labeled in human material. With *in situ* hybridization, gene expression in complex neuronal tissues such as the mammalian brain can be studied. In combination with immunohistochemistry, it can address sophisticated questions regarding posttranslational processing and in combination with tract-tracing techniques it can study the levels and regulation of mRNA in a neuron with known projections. There are many reasons why the study of specific neuronal mRNA might be of interest, but one of the most compelling is the growing evidence that couples changes in neuropeptide utilization with adjustments in the mRNA level.

VII. APPENDIX

A. Commercial Sources of Fluorescent Markers

Fluorogold:
>Fluorochrome, Inc.
>P.O. Box 4983
>Englewood, CO 80155

Rhodamine Latex Microspheres:
>Tracer Technology
>Box 7
>Bardonia, NY 10954

B. Subbing of Slides

1. Place slides in racks and wash in hot soapy water.
2. Rinse in water.
3. Soak in 8% nitric acid for 20 min.
4. Rinse well in double-distilled water.
5. Let dry in a dust-free area.
6. Prepare the subbing solution: heat 750 ml double-distilled water to 55°C; add 1.87 g gelatin (Fisher, G-8; 275 Bloom); stir without creating foam until dissolved; let cool to room temperature; add 0.187 g chromium potassium sulfate. The subbing solution can be stored up to a week in a refrigerator.
7. Dip slides slowly several times, again taking care not to cause foam.
8. Let slides dry in a dust-free area and, using gloves, put them back into their boxes.

C. Perfusion

1. Deeply anesthetize the rat and put it on ice on a tray in the sink.
2. Open the chest cavity, exposing the heart.
3. Inject 0.5 cc heparin into left ventricle (26-G needle).
4. Insert catheter into left ventricle.
5. Puncture the right atrium of the heart.
6. Using Masterflex pump set at 2, or using gravity feed, begin pumping cold saline through the rat. Pump until perfusate clears of red blood cells.

7. Begin pumping cold paraformaldehyde; to ensure that no air is introduced into the line when switching, use a T junction and tubing (solution-filled from the start) to each container and clamp off the tube not in use.
8. Continue perfusion with 4% paraformaldehyde for 20 min (300–400 ml).
9. Remove the brain and postfix for 1 hr in the same fixative, then 1 hr each in 10% and 20% sucrose in PBS at 4°C, then overnight in 30% sucrose at 4°C for cryoprotection.

D. *In Situ* Hybridization

This protocol has been adapted from methods described by Lewis *et al.* (1985b, 1986a,b) and Watson *et al.* (1987). RNase-free conditions should be maintained by the use of sterile solutions and by wearing gloves to prevent contamination with "finger nucleases."

1. Tissue Preparation

1. Perfuse animal and remove and cryoprotect its brain (Section VII.C).
2. Freeze tissue on powdered dry ice.
3. Section tissue in a cryostat at −20°C and thaw-mount tissue onto subbed slides (Section VII.B) at room temperature (RT). Wrinkles in the sections can be smoothed by careful application of an autoclaved camel's hair brush wetted with sterile PBS. Permit sections to dry (RT) for 3–16 hr and store slides at −20°C.

2. Prehybridization

1. Tissue sections are warmed to RT for at least 30 min.
2. Incubate sections with 50 μl proteinase K, 1μg/ml, for 10 min at 37° C. This step can frequently be omitted with short (e.g., 30-base) synthetic oligonucleotides.
3. Incubate for 10 min in 2× SSC at RT.
4. Excess 2× SSC is removed, and slides are placed in a Nunc culture dish lined with wetted filter paper backing.
5. Pipette 500 μl of prehybridization buffer onto each slide, covering the sections. The culture dish lid is replaced, and the slides are carefully placed into an incubator at 37–45°C for at least 1 hr.

3. Hybridization

1. The radioactive probes are diluted with prehybridization buffer, allowing 500 μl of buffer per slide with 9 × 10^5 cpm of activity per slide.

This hybridization solution is heated to incubation temperature (37–45°C).

2. Excess prehybridization buffer is removed from the slides (by decanting onto the filter paper backing), and the radioactive probe is applied at 500 μl per slide. The culture dish is carefully placed in the incubator for an overnight incubation at 37–45°C.

4. Posthybridization

1. The slides are washed as follows:

   a. 2× SSC for 2 hr at RT.
   b. 1× SSC for 2 hr at RT.
   c. 0.5× SSC for 1 hr at RT.
   d. 0.5× SSC for 0.5 hr at 37–45°C.
   e. 0.5× SSC for 0.5 hr at 37–45°C.
   f. 0.5× SSC for 0.5 hr at RT.

2. The slides are rapidly dried by blowing a gentle stream of dried compressed air over them (through a Drierite® column).

3. The dried slides are placed into an x-ray cassette with Kodak XAR-5 film and stored at RT. After developing the films (3 days of exposure is a good starting point), the slides can be dipped in liquid emulsion.

E. 3′-End Labeling of Oligonucleotides

1. In a sterile 1.5-ml Eppendorf tube add:

   5.0 μl DNA tailing buffer (International Biotechnologies Inc.)
   11.5 μl RNase-free water
   1.0 μl Oligonucleotide probe (0.005 OD)
   6.0 μl [^{35}S]-dATP (Du Pont NEN Products #NEG-034H)
   1.5 μl Terminal transferase (25 U, Boehringer Mannheim)

   Note: 3′-end labeling kits are now available: Du Pont NEN products, #NEP-100, or Boehringer Mannheim #1028 715.

2. Mix gently by flicking tube several times with finger; do not vortex. Briefly microcentrifuge tube and incubate at 37°C for 1.5 hr.

3. Near the end of the reaction, prepare NENSORB™20 (Du Pont NEN Products) #NLP-022 column as follows:

   a. Settle each column (one per reaction) by tapping side until all column matrix is at the bottom.
   b. Remove cap and attach column to ring stand over disposable beaker.
   c. Fill with 3 ml absolute methanol (HPLC grade if possible), and force through column with 10 ml syringe attached to column adaptor.
   d. Fill with 3 ml 0.1 M Tris-HCl (pH 7.5), force through with syringe.

4. At the end of the reaction:
   a. Add 500 μl Tris to reaction mixture; mix by pipetting and add to column.
   b. Apply gentle pressure to the syringe (1 drop/ 2 sec) until solution is through.
   c. Wash column with 1.5 ml Tris, forced through with syringe.
   d. Elute oligonucleotide by adding 0.5 ml of 20% ethanol (in RNase-free water); apply gentle pressure to syringe and slowly collect 10 drops in a sterile Eppendorf tube.
5. Count 3-μl aliquot by liquid scintillation counting; should get $1-2 \times 10^6$ cpm. Measure volume of eluted probe with micropipette, and add one tenth of the total volume with freshly prepared 100 mM dithiothreitol. Store at 4°C.

F. Materials for *in Situ* Hybridization and Probe Labeling

1. Equipment and Supplies

Quantity	Item	Cat. No.	Vendor
As needed	1-cc syringe with 26-G needle		
As needed	16-G 2-inch catheter		
1	Masterflex pump	7553-20	ColeParmer
1	Masterflex pumphead	7014-21	ColeParmer
As needed	Cell counter vials	14310-640	VWR
As needed	Microscope slides	48311-600	VWR
As needed	Coverslips #1, 24 mm × 50 mm	48393-081	VWR
As needed	Micro slide box	48444-003	VWR
As needed	Dricaps	19953	Ted Pella
Minimum of 2	Wheaton staining dish	25461-003	VWR
As needed	Tissue culture dish	166-508	Gibco
As needed	BioRad filter paper backing	165-0921	BioRad
1	Ice storage pail, plastic	35751-203	VWR
1	Drierite column	26668-007	VWR
As needed	X-ray cassette (Wolf 10 × 12 inches)		
As needed	Kodak XAR 5 film		
1	150-ml beaker with weights attached to bottom		
1	Porcelain spatula		
1	Glass stirring rod		
As needed	Aluminum foil		
1	Scintillation vial box		
As needed	Paper towels		

2. Solutions

In general, solutions should be prepared using sterile, double-distilled H_2O and stored in autoclaved containers.

1. Saline, physiological, 0.85 percent, cool to 4°C (Fisher SO-S-442).
2. 4 percent paraformaldehyde (made on day of use) in $2 \times$ PO_4 solution

H_2O	1 liter
NaOH (VWR VW6720-1)	7.7 g
$NaH_2PO_4H_2O$ (VWR EMSX0710-1)	33.66 g

Dissolve with stirring and heat ($2 \times$ PO_4 solution) to 75°C on a hot plate. Add 40 g paraformaldehyde (Kodak) (VWR EX-00421-7). Stir until dissolved (15–20 min). Filter through Whatman #2 paper; cool to 4°C.

3. 12 mM phosphate-buffered saline (PBS)

$2 \times$ PO_4 solution	50 ml
NaCl	9 g
H_2O	to 1 liter

4. 10 percent sucrose in PBS (2.5 g sucrose in 25 ml of PBS).
   20 percent sucrose in PBS (5.0 g sucrose in 25 ml of PBS).
   30 percent sucrose (7.5 g sucrose in 25 ml of PBS).
5. $20 \times$ SSC

NaCl	175.32 g
Na-citrate	88.23 g
H_2O	1 liter

Stir to dissolve, then autoclave. Alternatively, obtain premixed $20 \times$ concentrate (Sigma S-6639).

6. $50 \times$ Denhardts

Ficoll (Sigma F-9378)	1 g
Polyvinyl pyrrolidone (Sigma PVP260)	1 g
BSA fraction V (Sigma A70906)	1 g
H_2O	100 ml

Stir until dissolved; then sterile filter. Alternatively, obtain premixed $50 \times$ concentrate (Sigma D-2532).

7. Deionized formamide (BRL 5515UB). Mixed-bed ion-exchange resin (BioRad AG501-X8), 20–40 mesh. Stir 30 min with resin at room temperature. Filter through Whatman #1 filter paper. Aliquot and store at -20°C.
8. Salmon sperm DNA (Sigma D-1626). Dissolve DNA (Sigma type III sodium salt) in sterile H_2O, 10 mg/ml. Stir 2–4 hr at RT. Shear DNA by passing it through a sterile 18-G hypodermic needle several times. Boil 10 min, aliquot, and store at -20°C. Alternatively, obtain pre-

mixed (10 mg/ml) sonicated, denatured salmon sperm DNA (Sigma D-9156).

9. Yeast tRNA (BRL 54015A). Dissolve tRNA at 10 mg/ml, aliquot, and freeze at −20°C.

10. Alcohols: start with 200 proof punctilious alcohol.

%	Alcohol (ml)	H_2O
95	238	12
80	200	50
70	175	75

11. Proteinase K (BRL 5530UA).

12. 2× SSC (25 ml 20× SSC + 225 ml H_2O). 1× SSC (12.5 ml 20× SSC + 237.5 ml H_2O). 0.5× SSC (6.25 ml 20× SSC + 243.75 ml H_2O).

13. Prehybridization buffer (can be stored at −20°C)

Deionized formamide	5 ml
20× SSC	2.0 ml
50× Denhardts	200 μl
Salmon sperm DNA	500 μl
Yeast tRNA	250 μl
Dextran sulfate, probe grade,	2 ml
50% soln (Cat. no. 54030 Oncor, Inc.	
Gaithersburg, MD)	
Dithiothreitol	15 mg

14. Kodak D-19 developer.

15. Kodak fixer.

16. Kodak NTB2 emulsion.

17. Dithiothreitol (BRL 508UA). As probe-labeling reaction is finishing, add 7.7 mg to 500 μl sterile water, yielding a 100 mM solution.

G. Commercial Sources of Hybridization Probes

The following is a partial listing of companies that will prepare synthetic oligonucleotides to customer specification. Inclusion within this list does not constitute endorsement by the authors and is provided solely to enable the interested reader to begin to "shop" for an appropriate supplier.

Amersham Corporation, 2636 South Clearbrook Dr., Arlington Heights, IL 60005.

New England Biolabs, 32 Tozer Road, Beverly, MA 01915.

OCS Laboratories, Inc., DNA Synthesis Division, P.O. Box 2868, Denton, TX 76202.

Peninsula Laboratories, Inc., 611 Taylor Way, Belmont, CA 94002.

The Midland Certified Reagent Co., 1500 Murray St., Midland TX 79701.

Synthetic Genetics, 10457 Roselle St., Suite E, San Diego, CA 92121.

Kits are also available for investigators who wish manually to synthesize their oligonucleotides.

DNA Synthesis Kit II; New England Biolabs, 32 Tozer Road, Beverly, MA 01915.

Nucleolink Manual DNA Synthesis Kit; Pierce Chemical Co., P.O. Box 117, Rockford, IL 61105.

Some companies are beginning to offer labeled and/or unlabeled probes:

Amersham Corporation, 2636 South Clearbrook Dr., Arlington Heights, IL 60005.

Dupont NEN Research Products, 549 Albany St., Boston, MA 02118.

Oncor, P.O. Box 870, Gaithersburg, MD 20877 (also supplies other *in situ* hybridization reagents).

Pharmacia, Inc., Molecular Biology Division, 800 Centennial Ave., Piscataway, NJ 08854.

H. Autoradiography

1. In a very clean darkroom, turn on sodium vapor safelight and let warm up for 30 min.
2. Put bulk emulsion jar into a 42°C waterbath in the darkroom (if your darkroom is not equipped with revolving door or the equivalent, in light-tight cabinet in the darkroom).
3. When the emulsion is molten (30 min), bring with you into the darkroom: slide mailers (marked with felt pen at 1/2 and full levels), forceps to hold slides while dipping into mailer, glass stirring rod, slide racks, black plastic slide boxes (labeled with box content and date for development on detachable tape), desiccant capsules, aluminum foil, experimental as well as blank slides, and distilled water containing 1 mg Dreft detergent per milliliter (dissolved in a sonicator bath) and warmed to 42°C to dilute the emulsion.
4. Gently stir with clean glass rod to mix bulk emulsion without forming bubbles, aliquot 5 ml into each slide mailer, fill up to 10-ml mark with distilled water containing Dreft, cap mailers, and invert gently to mix. Store mailers in the light-tight box in refrigerator, preferably in the darkroom.
5. Dip a clean blank slide into emulsion and hold it up to safelight to check for streaks or bubbles. Dip several such slides until emulsion coat appears homogeneous and bubble-free.
6. Hold experimental slides with forceps and dip with an even up-and-down stroke. Place slides vertically in rack to dry for 20 min.
7. Pack slides into black plastic slide boxes; leave space separated by blank slide for desiccant capsules. Let continue to dry for 2 hr in safe space in the darkroom.

8. Close tops on slide boxes, detach marking tape, wrap boxes in foil, put label on again, and place in refrigerator at 4°C away from any stored radioisotopes.
9. After an appropriate exposure time, as determined with duplicate test slides, allow slides to come to room temperature.
10. Under safelight conditions, develop the slides (using the black plastic box as a rack) as follows:

    a. Kodak D-19, 16°C, for 2 min; agitate gently (rock the box) every 20 sec.
    b. Stop the development process with a rinse in water with a few drops of glacial acetic acid.
    c. Kodak fixer, 5 min (or Rapidfix 3 min), gentle agitation every 30 seconds.
    d. Water rinse in gentle stream for 30 minutes

11. Let slides dry and then coverslip using water-soluble medium. Store slides horizontally (covered slide trays) in the refrigerator.

I. Mounting Medium

Mix 20 g Vinol 205 (Air Products, P.O. Box 2662, Allentown, PA 18001, will send a l-lb free sample, which will last a lifetime) with 40 ml glycerol in 80 ml 0.05 M Tris, pH 9.0–9.5, and stir over gentle heat (50–60°C) until most Vinol is dissolved (2–3 hr); centrifuge and decant supernatant, aliquot into scintillation vials, and confirm pH before use.

ACKNOWLEDGMENTS. The authors wish to thank Rudy Krause and Joan Dubin for their invaluable technical assistance.

REFERENCES

Anderson, M. L. M., and Young, B. D., 1985, Quantitative filter hybridization, in: *Nucleic Acid Hybridisation* (B. D. Hames and S. J. Higgins, eds.), IRL Press, Oxford, pp. 73–112.

Angerer, L. M., and Angerer, R. C., 1981, Detection of poly A$^+$ RNA in sea urchin eggs and embryos by quantitative *in situ* hybridization, *Nucleic Acids Res.* **9:**2819–2840.

Angerer, R. C., Cox, K. H., and Angerer, L. M., 1985, *In situ* hybridization to cellular RNAs, in: *Genetic Engineering*, Vol. 7 (J. K. Setlow and A. Hollaender, eds.), Plenum Press, New York, pp. 43–65.

Angulo, J. A., Davis, L. G., Burkhart, B. A., and Christoph, G. R., 1986, Reduction of striatal dopaminergic neurotransmission elevates striatal proenkephalin mRNA, *Eur. J. Pharmacol.* **130:**341–343.

Baldino, F., Jr., and Davis, L. G., 1986, Glucocorticoid regulation of vasopressin messenger RNA, in: *In Situ Hybridization in Brain* (G. R. Uhl, ed.), Plenum Press, New York, pp. 97–116.

Binder, M., Tourmente, S., Roth, J., Renaud, M., and Gehring, W. J., 1986, *In situ* hybridization at the electron microscope level: Localization of transcripts on ultrathin sections of lowicryl

K4M-embedded tissue using biotinylated probes and protein A–gold complexes, *J. Cell Biol.* **102:**1646–1653.

Bloch, B., Le Guellec, D., and De Keyzer, Y., 1985, Detection of the messenger RNAs coding for the opioid peptide precursors in pituitary and adrenal by '*in situ*' hybridization: Study in several mammal species, *Neurosci. Lett.* **53:**141–148.

Bloch, B., Popovici, T., Le Guellec, D., Normand, E., Chouham, S., Guitteny, A. F., and Bohlen, P., 1986, *In situ* hybridization histochemistry for the analysis of gene expression in the endocrine and central nervous system tissues: A 3-year experience, *J. Neurosci. Res.* **16:**183–200.

Bollum, F. J., 1974, Terminal deoxynucleotidyl transferase, in: *The Enzymes*, Vol. 10 (P. D. Boyer, ed.), Academic Press, New York, pp. 145–171.

Bonner, T. I., Brenner, D. J., Neufeld, B. R., and Britten, R. J., 1973, Reduction in the rate of DNA reassociation by sequence divergence, *J. Mol. Biol.* **81:**123–135.

Brahic, M., and Haase, T., 1978, Detection of viral sequences of low reiteration frequency in *in situ* hybridization, *Proc. Natl. Acad. Sci. U.S.A.* **75:**6125–6129.

Britten, R. J., Graham, D. E., and Neufeld, B. R., 1974, DNA sequence analysis by reassociation, in: *Methods in Enzymology*, Vol. 29 (L. Grossman and K. Moldave, eds.), Academic Press, New York, pp. 363–418.

Cantor, C. R., and Schimmel, P. R., 1980, *Biophysical Chemistry*, Part III, W. H. Freeman, San Francisco.

Capco, D. G., and Jeffery, W. R., 1978, Differential distribution of poly(A)-containing RNA in the embryonic cells of *Oncopeltus fasciatus*, *Dev. Biol.* **67:**137–151.

Cash, E., and Brahic, M., 1986, Quantitative *in situ* hybridization using initial velocity measurements, *Anal. Biochem.* **157:**236–240.

Chronwall, B. M., 1985, Anatomy and physiology of the neuroendocrine arcuate nucleus, *Peptides* **6**(Suppl.2):1–11.

Chronwall, B. M., Millington, W. R., Griffin, S. W. T., Unnerstall, J. R., and O'Donohue, T. L., 1987, Histological evaluation of the dopaminergic regulation of pro-opiomelanocortin gene expression in the intermediate lobe of the rat pituitary using *in situ* hybridization and ^{3}H-thymidine uptake, *Endocrinology (N.Y.)* **120:**1201–1211.

Coghlan, J. P., Aldred, P., Haralambidis, J., Niall, H. D., Penschow, J. D., and Tregear, G. W., 1985, Review: Hybridization histochemistry, *Anal. Biochem.* **149:**1–28.

Collins, M. L., and Hunsaker, W. R., 1985, Improved hybridization assays employing tailed oligonucleotide probes: A direct comparison with 5′-end-labeled oligonucleotide probes and nick-translated plasmid probes, *Anal. Biochem.* **151:**211–224.

Cox, K. H., DeLeon, D. V., Angerer, L. M., and Angerer, R. C., 1984, Detection of mRNAs in sea urchin embryos by *in situ* hybridization using asymmetric RNA probes, *Dev. Biol.* **101:**485–502.

Davis, L. G., Arentzen, R., Reid, J. M., Manning, R. W., Wolfson, B., Lawrence, K. L., and Baldino, Jr., F., 1986a, Glucocorticoid sensitivity of vasopressin mRNA levels in the paraventricular nucleus of the rat, *Proc. Natl. Acad. Sci. U.S.A.* **83:**1145–1149.

Davis, L. G., Dibner, M. D., and Battey, J. F., 1986b, *Methods in Molecular Biology*, Elsevier, New York.

Davis, L. G., Lewis, M. E., and Baldino, F., Jr., 1986c, Synthetic oligodeoxyribonucleotide probe radiolabelling and *in situ* hybridization methodologies, in: *In Situ Hybridization in Brain* (G. Uhl, ed), Plenum Press, Oxford, pp. 230–232.

Edwards, S. T., and Hendrickson, A., 1981, The autoradiographic tracing of axonal connections in the central nervous system, in: *Neuroanatomical Tract-Tracing Methods* (L. Heimer and M. J. Robards, eds.), Plenum Press, New York, pp. 171–205.

Feder, N., 1959, Polyvinyl alcohol as an embedding medium for lipid and enzyme histochemistry, *J. Histochem. Cytochem.* **7:**292–293.

Fritz, H. J., Belagaje, R., Brown, E. L., Friz, R. H., Jones, R. A., Lees, R. G., and Khorana, H. G., 1978, High performance liquid chromatography in polynucleotide synthesis, *Biochemistry* **17:**1257–1267.

Fuller, P. J., Clements, J. A., and Funder, J. W., 1985, Localization of arginine vasopressin-neurophysin II messenger ribonucleic acid in the hypothalamus of control and Brattleboro rats by hybridization histochemistry with a synthetic pentadecamer oligonucleotide probe, *Endocrinology* **116:**2366–2368.

Gall, J. G., and Pardue, M. L., 1969, Formation and detection of RNA–DNA hybrid molecules in cytological preparations, *Proc. Natl. Acad. Sci. U.S.A.* **63:**378–383.

Gee, C. E., and Roberts, J. L., 1983, *In situ* hybridization histochemistry: A technique for the study of gene expression in single cells, *DNA* **2:**157–163.

Gee, C. E., Chen, C.-L. C., Roberts, J. L., Thompson, R., and Watson, S. J., 1983, Identification of proopiomelanocortin neurones in rat hypothalamus by *in situ* cDNA–mRNA hybridization, *Nature* **306:**374–376.

Gehlert, D. R., Chronwall, B. M., Schafer, M. P., and O'Donohue, T. L., 1987, Localization of neuropeptide Y messenger ribonucleic acid in rat and mouse brain by *in situ* hybridization, *Synapse* **1:**25–31.

Green, M., Maniatis, T., and Melton, D., 1983, Human beta-globin pre-mRNA synthesized *in vitro* is accurately spliced in *Xenopus* oocyte nuclei, *Cell* **32:**681–694.

Griffin, W. S. T., and Morrison, M. R., 1985, *In situ* hybridization—visualization and quantitation of genetic expression in mammalian brain, *Peptides* **6**(Suppl.2):89–96.

Griffin, W. S. T., Crom, E. N., and Head, J. R., 1982, Manipulation of brain DNA synthesis is achieved by using a systemic immunological disease, *Proc. Natl. Acad. Sci. U.S.A.* **79:**4783–4785.

Griffin, W. S. T., Alejos, M., Nilaver, G., and Morrison, M. R., 1983, Brain protein and messenger RNA identification in the same cell, *Brain Res. Bul.* **10:**597–601.

Griffin, W. S. T., Alejos, M. A., Cox, E. J., and Morrison, M. R., 1985, The differential distribution of beta tubulin mRNAs in individual mammalian brain cells, *J. Cell. Biochem.* **27:**205–214.

Haase, A. T., Walker, D., Stowring, L., Ventura, P., Geballe, A., Blum, H., Brahic, M., Goldberg, R., and O'Brien, K., 1985, Detection of two viral genomes in single cells by double-label hybridization *in situ* and color microautoradiography, *Science* **227:**189–192.

Harrison, P. R., Conkie, D., Paul, J., and Jones, K., 1973, Localisation of cellular globin messenger RNA by *in situ* hybridisation to complementary DNA, *FEBS Lett.* **32:**109–112.

Higgins, G. A., and Schwaber, J. S., 1983, Somatostatinergic projections from the central nucleus of the amygdala to the vagal nuclei, *Peptides* **4:**657–662.

Hökfelt, T., Skagerberg, G., Skirboll, L., and Bjorklund, A., 1983, Combination of retrograde tracing and neurotransmitter histochemistry, in: *Methods in Chemical Neuroanatomy* (A. Bjorklund and T. Hokfelt, eds.), Elsevier, Amsterdam, New York, pp. 228–285.

Hopman, A. H. N., Wiegant, J., Raap, A. K., Landegent, J. E., van der Ploeg, M., and van Duijn, P., 1986, Bi-color detection of two target DNAs by nonradioactive *in situ* hybridization, *Histochemistry* **85:**1–4.

Huynh, T. V., Young, R. A., and Davis, R. W., 1985, Constructing and screening DNA libraries in λgt10 and λgt11, in: *DNA Cloning*, Vol. 1 (D. M. Glover, ed.), IRL Press, Oxford, pp. 49–78.

Jacob, J., Todd, K., Birnstiel, M. L., and Bird, A., 1971, Molecular hybridization of ³H-labelled ribosomal RNA with DNA in ultrathin sections prepared for electron microscopy, *Biochim. Biophys. Acta* **228:**761–766.

Johnson, M. T., and Johnson, B. A., 1984, Efficient synthesis of high specific activity ³⁵S-labeled human beta-globin pre-mRNA, *Biotechniques* **2:**156–162.

Jones, K. W., and Robertson, F. W., 1970, Localisation of reiterated nucleotide sequences in *Drosophila* and mouse by *in situ* hybridisation of complementary RNA, *Chromosoma* **31:**331–345.

Katz, L. C., Burkhalter, A., and Dreyer, W. J., 1984, Fluorescent latex microspheres as a retrograde neuronal marker for *in vivo* and *in vitro* studies of visual cortex, *Nature* **310:**498–500.

Kelsey, J. E., Watson, S. J., Burke, S., Akil, H., and Roberts, J. L., 1986, Characterization of propiomelanocortin mRNA detected by *in situ* hybridization, *J. Neurosci.* **6:**38–42.

Lathe, R., 1985, Synthetic oligonucleotide probes deduced from amino acid sequence data. Theoretical and practical considerations, *J. Mol. Biol.* **183:**1–12.

Lewis, M. E., Burke, S., Sherman, T. G., Arentzen, R., and Watson, S. J., 1984, *In situ* hybridization using a 3' terminal transferase-labeled synthetic oligonucleotide probe complementary to the alpha-MSH coding region of proopiomelanocortin mRNA, *Soc. Neurosci. Abstr.* **10:**358.

Lewis, M. E., Burke, S., and Sherman, T. G., 1985a, Evaluating specificity in *in situ* hybridization histochemistry, *Soc. Neurosci. Abstr.* **11:**141.

Lewis, M. E., Sherman, T. G., and Watson, S. J., 1985b, *In situ* hybridization histochemistry with synthetic oligonucleotides: Strategies and methods, *Peptides* **6**(Suppl.2):75–87.

Lewis, M. E., Arentzen, R., and Baldino, Jr., F., 1986a, Rapid, high resolution *in situ* hybridization histochemistry with radioiodinated synthetic oligonucleotides, *J. Neurosci. Res.* **16:**117–124.

Lewis, M. E., Khachaturian, H., Schafer, M. K.-H., Watson, S. J., 1986b, Anatomical approaches to the study of neuropeptides and related mRNA in CNS, in: *Neuropeptides in Neurological Disease* (J. B. Martin and J. Barchas, eds.), Raven Press, New York, pp. 79–109.

Lewis, M. E., Sherman, T. G., Burke, S., Akil, H., Davis, L. G., Arentzen, R., and Watson, S. J., 1986c, Detection of proopiomelanocortin mRNA by *in situ* hybridization with an oligonucleotide probe, *Proc. Natl. Acad. Sci. U.S.A.* **83:**5419–5423.

Lewis, M. E., Krause, R. G., II, and Roberts-Lewis, J. M., 1988, Recent developments in the use of synthetic oligonucleotides for *in situ* hybridization histochemistry, *Synapse* **2:**308–316.

Lillie, R. D., 1954, *Histopathologic Technic and Practical Histochemistry*, Blakiston, New York, p. 105.

Maniatis, T., Fritsch, E. F., and Sambrook, J., 1982, *Molecular Cloning*, Cold Spring Harbor Laboratory Press, New York.

Matteucci, M. D., and Caruthers, M. H., 1981, Synthesis of deoxynucleotides on a polymer support, *J. Am. Chem. Soc.* **103:**3185–3191.

McAllister, L. B., Scheller, R. H., Kandel, E. R., and Axel, R., 1983, *In situ* hybridization to study the origin and fate of identified neurons, *Science* **229:**800–808.

McCabe, J. T., Morell, J. I., and Pfaff, D. W., 1986, *In situ* hybridization as a quantitative autoradiographic method: Vasopressin and oxytocin gene transcription in the Brattleboro rat, in: *In Situ Hybridization in Brain* (G. R. Uhl, ed.), Plenum Press, New York, pp. 73–95.

Melton, D. A., Krieg, P. A., Rebagliati, M. R., Maniatis, T., Zinn, K., and Green, M. R., 1984, Efficient *in vitro* synthesis of biologically active RNA and RNA hybridization probes from plasmids containing a bacteriophage SP6 promotor, *Nucleic Acids Res.* **12:**7035–7056.

Morris, B. J., Haarmann, I., Kempter, B., Hollt, V., and Herz, A., 1986, Localization of prodynorphin messenger RNA in rat brain by *in situ* hybridization using a synthetic oligonucleotide probe, *Neurosci. Lett.* **69:**104–108.

Nojiri, H., Sato, M., and Urano, A., 1985, *In situ* hybridization of the vasopressin mRNA in the rat hypothalamus by use of a synthetic oligonucleotide probe, *Neurosci. Lett.* **58:**101–105.

Pochet, R., Brocas, H., Vassart, G., Toubeau, G., Seo, H., Refetoff, S., Dumont, J. E., and Pasteels, J. L., 1981, Radioautographic localization of prolactin messenger RNA on histological sections by *in situ* hybridization, *Brain Res.* **211:**433–438.

Rogers, A. W., 1979, *Techniques of Autoradiography*, 2nd ed., Elsevier/North Holland, New York.

Rogers, W. T., Schwaber, J. S., and Lewis, M. E., 1987, Quantitation of cellular resolution *in situ* hybridization histochemistry in brain by image analysis, *Neurosci. Lett.* **82:**315–320.

Schalling, M., Hökfelt, T., Wallace, B., Goldstein, M., Filer, D., Yamin, C., Schlesinger, D. H., and Mallet, J., 1986, Tyrosine 3-hydroxylase in rat brain and adrenal medulla: Hybridization histochemistry and immunohistochemistry combined with retrograde tracing, *Proc. Natl. Acad. Sci. U.S.A.* **83:**6208–6212.

Schmued, L. C., and Fallon, J. H., 1986, Fluoro-Gold: A new fluorescent retrograde axonal tracer with numerous unique properties, *Brain Res.* **377:**147–154.

Schwaber, J. S., Chronwall, B. M., and Lewis, M. E., 1989, *In situ* hybridization histochemistry combined with markers of neuronal connectivity, *Methods Enzymol.* **168:**778–791.

Sherman, T. G., McKelvy, J. F., and Watson, S. J., 1986, Vasopressin mRNA regulation in individual hypothalamic nuclei: A northern and *in situ* hybridization analysis, *J. Neurosci.* **6:**1685–1694.

Shivers, B. D., Harlan, R. E., Romano, G. J., Howells, R. D., and Pfaff, D. W., 1986, Cellular localization of proenkephalin mRNA in rat brain: Gene expression in the caudate–putamen and cerebellar cortex, *Proc. Natl. Acad. Sci. U.S.A.* **83:**6221–6225.

Siegel, R. E., and Young, W. S., 1986, Detection of preprocholecystokinin and preproenkephalin A mRNAs in rat brain by hybridization histochemistry using complementary RNA probes, *Neuropeptides* **6:**573–580.

Singer, R. H., and Ward, D. C., 1982, Actin gene expression visualized in chicken muscle tissue culture by using *in situ* hybridization with a biotinated nucleotide analog, *Proc. Natl. Acad. Sci. U.S.A.* **79:**7331–7335.

Skirboll, L., Hokfelt, T., Norell, G., Phillipson, O., Kuypers, H. G. J. M., Bentivoglio, M., Catsman-Berrevoets, C. E., Visser, T. J., Steinbusch, H., Verhofstad, A., Cuello, A. C., Goldstein, M., and Brownstein, M., 1984, A method for specific transmitter identification of retrogradely labeled neurons: Immunofluorescence combined with fluorescence tracing, *Brain Res. Rev.* **8:**99–127.

Studencki, A. B., and Wallace, R. B., 1984, Allele-specific hybridization using oligonucleotide probes of very high specificity: Discrimination of the human beta^A and beta^S-globin genes, *DNA* **32:**7–15.

Szabo, P., Elde, R., Steffensen, D. M., and Uhlenbeck, O. C., 1977, Quantitative *in situ* hybridization of ribosomal RNA species to polytene chromosomes of *Drosophila melanogaster*, *J. Mol. Biol.* **115:**539–563.

Thomason, B. M., and Cowart, G. W., 1966, Evaluation of polyvinyl alcohols as semipermanent mountants for fluorescent-antibody studies, *J. Bacteriol.* **93:**678–769.

Uhl, G. R., and Sasek, C. A., 1986, Somatostatin mRNA: Regional variation in hybridization densities in individual neurons, *J. Neurosci.* **6:**3258–3264.

Uhl, G. R., Zingg, H. H., and Habener, J. F., 1985, Vasopressin mRNA *in situ* histochemistry: Localization and regulation studied with oligonucleotide cDNA probes in normal and Brattleboro rat hypothalamus, *Proc. Natl. Acad. Sci. U.S.A.* **82:**5555–5559.

Varndell, J. M., Polak, J. M., Minth,, C. D., Bloom, S. R., and Dixon, J. E., 1984, Visualization of messenger RNA directing peptide synthesis by *in situ* hybridisation using a novel singlestranded cDNA probe. Potential for the investigation of gene expression and endocrine cell activity, *Histochemistry* **81:**597–601.

Watson, S. J., Sherman, T. G., Kelsey, J. E., Burke, S., and Akil, H., 1987, Anatomical localization of mRNA: *In situ* hybridization of neuropeptide systems, in: *In Situ Hybridization in Neurobiology* (K. Valentino, J. Eberwine, and J. Barchas, eds.), Oxford University Press, Oxford, pp. 126–145.

Whittemore, S. R., Ebendal, T., Larkfors, L., Olson, L., Seiger, A., Stromberg, I., and Persson, H., 1986, Developmental and regional expression of β nerve growth factor messenger RNA and protein in the rat central nervous system, *Proc. Natl. Acad. Sci. U.S.A.* **83:**817–821.

Wilcox, J. N., Chronwall, B. M., O'Donohue, T. L., and Roberts, J. L., 1985, Localization of POMC mRNA in neurons functionally defined by their axonal tracing combining *in situ* hybridization with fluorescent axonal tracing, *Soc. Neurosci. Abstr.* **11:**143.

Wilcox, J. N., Gee, C. E., and Roberts, J. L., 1986a, *In situ* cDNA–mRNA hybridization: Development of a technique to measure mRNA levels in individual cells, *Methods Enzymol.* **124:**510–533.

Wilcox, J. N., Roberts, J. L., Chronwall, B. M., Bishop, J. F., and O'Donohue, T. L., 1986b, Localization of proopiomelanocortin mRNA in functional subsets of neurons defined by their axonal projections, *J. Neurosci. Res.* **16:**89–96.

Wolfson, B., Manning, R. W., Davis, L. G., Arentzen, R., and Baldino, F., Jr., 1985, Co-localization of corticotropin releasing factor and vasopressin mRNA in neurones after adrenalectomy, *Nature* **315:**59–61.

Yamamoto, N., Seo, H., Suganuma, N., Matsui, N., Nakane, T., Kuwayama, A., and Kageyama, N., 1986, Effect of estrogen on prolactin mRNA in the rat pituitary, Analysis by *in situ* hybridization and immunohistochemistry, *Neuroendocrinology* **43:**494–497.

Young, B. D. and Anderson, M. L. M., 1985, Quantitative analysis of solution hybridisation, in:

Nucleic Acid Hybridisation (B. D. Hames and S. J. Higgins, eds.), IRL Press, Oxford, pp. 47–72.

Young III, W. S., Bonner, T. I., and Brann, M. R., 1986a, Mesencephalic dopamine neurons regulate the expression of neuropeptide mRNA's in the rat forebrain, *Proc. Natl. Acad. Sci. U.S.A.* **83:**9827–9831.

Young III, W. S., Mezey, E., and Siegel, R. E., 1986b, Quantitative *in situ* hybridization histochemistry reveals increased levels of corticotrophin-releasing factor mRNA after adrenalectomy in rats, *Neurosci. Lett.* **70:**198–203.

11

Microdissection in Combination with Biochemical Microassays as a Tool in Tract Tracing

MIKLÓS PALKOVITS

I. INTRODUCTION

During the last 15 years several brain microdissection techniques have been developed (see Cuello and Carson, 1983; Palkovits and Brownstein, 1983, 1988) and applied for a number of purposes, including (1) biochemical mapping for the distribution of various substances (neurotransmitters, hormones, enzymes, receptors, amino acids, etc.) in discrete brain nuclei, (2) measuring the concentrations of above substances in brain nuclei of animals following various treatments, experimental manipulations, or pathological conditions, (3) quantitative measurements to reveal the chemical specificity of neuronal interconnections or interactions between brain regions, (4) measuring the synthesis of various substances in individual brain nuclei following precursor injections into the brain, and (5) sampling of discrete brain

MIKLÓS PALKOVITS • First Department of Anatomy, Semmelweis University Medical School, H-1450 Budapest, Hungary, and Laboratory of Cell Biology, National Institute of Mental Health, Bethesda, Maryland 20892.

nuclei for primary tissue cultures, subcellular analysis (synaptosomes), or for *in vitro* studies.

The combination of brain microdissection and neurochemical microassays is a useful adjunct to tract-tracing techniques. Thus, concentrations of various substances can be measured in individual brain nuclei following lesions (mechanical, electrolytic, or chemical) of certain brain areas or transections of neuronal pathways to determine the projection pattern of neuronal cell groups in the brain. Several reports demonstrate the feasibility and usefulness of this type of technical combination, which provides quantitative verification of immunohistochemical observations and chemical characterization of pathways revealed by classical tract-tracing techniques (e.g., Zaborszky *et al.*, 1985). In this chapter the main principles and basic technical information are reviewed with special reference to the application of microdissection techniques in tract-tracing studies. The various steps of the "micropunch" procedure are described in the Appendix (Section V.C). Detailed maps and guides are available for microdissection of rat brain nuclei (e.g., Cuello and Carson, 1983; Palkovits and Brownstein, 1983, 1988). Microdissection of brain nuclei from other mammals may be performed by the aid of stereotaxic maps listed in Table I.

II. BASIC STRATEGIES

It is well known that after transection of an axon or lesion of its parent cell body, the related nerve terminals undergo degeneration with almost total disappearance of substances synthesized by the cell. On the other hand, following axotomy a dramatic increase of these substances can occur in the proximal stump of the axon as well as in the perikaryon. The accumulation of substances in the cell body regions, as well as their depletion or disappearance in the terminal regions, can be quantitated with a high degree of sensitivity by biochemical microassays in microdissected brain nuclei.

If one assumes that the substance measured is localized in terminals, and there is a decrease of the substance following the lesion, two possibilities come to mind: (1) there is a direct connection, and the measured substance is localized in the pathway under study, or (2) no direct connection exists between the transection and the removed tissue, but the changes are induced through transynaptic effects. In general, it is difficult to identify transneuronal effects with the aid of conventional tract-tracing techniques, but *in situ* hybridization methods could give a direct answer to this problem. If the measured substance is unchanged, there are also two possibilities: (1) although the appropriate pathway has been transected, the terminals of that pathway may contain a transmitter that is unrelated to the one being measured, or (2) the pathway does use the transmitter measured, but because of rapid reinnervation (see for example Scott and Knigge, 1981), the amount of the substance does not change or may even show a slight increase. An-

Table I. Stereotaxic Atlases of Mammalian and Human Brains

Species	Authors
Opossum	Oswaldo-Cruz and Rocha-Miranda (1968)
Mouse	Sidman *et al.* (1971)
Rat	Palkovits (1980); Paxinos and Watson (1982); Palkovits and Brownstein (1988)
Cat	Snider and Niemer (1961); Verhaart (1964)
Rabbit	Monier and Gangloff (1961)
Dog	Lim *et al.* (1960); Dua-Sharma *et al.* (1970)
Farm animals	
Goat	Yoshikawa (1968)
Sheep	Yoshikawa (1968)
Cattle	Yoshikawa (1968)
Horse	Yoshikawa (1968)
Pig	Yoshikawa (1968)
Primates	
Squirrel monkey	Gergen and MacLean (1962); Emmers and Akert (1963)
Macaca	Snider and Lee (1961); Shantha *et al.* (1968)
Cebus monkey	Manocha *et al.* (1968)
Chimpanzee	Lucchi *et al.* (1965)
Baboon	Davis and Huffman (1968)
Human	Schaltenbrand and Wahren (1977)

other experimental situation is encountered when levels of substances are determined in regions of cell bodies containing the substance being studied. In this case, substances determined may be depleted secondarily to the removal of their inputs through the surgical manipulations.

In order to interpret the results, it is necessary to have complementary information about the neurons involved and their projections. For instance, immunohistochemical techniques can be applied following similar lesions to visualize pathways and terminal fields by the demonstration of disappearance of a substance from certain fibers and terminals and its accumulation in cells proximal to the lesion. Thus, the results obtained with these two procedures, i.e., immunohistochemical techniques and biochemical microassay procedures, can be used to complement each other (Zaborszky *et al.*, 1985).

III. EXPERIMENTAL CONDITIONS

To gain valuable information concerning neuronal interconnections by the aid of microdissection–microassay techniques, well-organized experimental protocols should be created. The major points of such protocols are as follows.

The optimal survival time is important. It is well known that within a few hours after transection of nerve fibers, substances transported by the axonal flow accumulate in both the proximal and distal parts of the axon close to the transection. After 2–7 days, there is a significant accumulation of substances in the proximal segments as well as in the parent cell bodies. Therefore, in order to determine the increase of substances in the perikarya following surgical manipulation, microdissections should be performed 4–7 days after lesioning. On the other hand, as a result of an axotomy, the distal part of the axon undergoes degeneration and is gradually being removed by glial cells. If the cell body was lesioned, the whole axon degenerates. Consequently, after lesions or transections, substances gradually diminish in the innervated brain area and have usually disappeared by the tenth to 14th postoperative day. The appropriate postoperative survival time for detecting the disappearance of the substance, therefore, is about 2 weeks. Ideally, it would be desirable to design experiments with different survival times in order to demonstrate dynamic changes rather than making static steady-state determinations.

Several other considerations are relevant to the use of biochemical microassays in the investigation of neuronal interconnections: (1) the sensitivity of the assays should be high enough to demonstrate depletions of the substances investigated, (2) the specificity of the assay should be tested, (3) accidental brain damage (ischemic damage, hemorrhage, abscesses following surgery) should be avoided, (4) the microdissected brain areas should be suitable for the use intended, and (5) microdissection may be performed on fresh brains for *in vivo* studies, but frozen or microwave-irradiated brains are needed to avoid postmortem alterations.

Brain lesions, including knife cuts and transections of pathways, as well as injections into the brain should be precisely localized. The surgical interventions and their side effects may be mapped on a stereotaxic atlas or characterized by three-dimnensional coordinates. Without any previous information about the chemical specificity of neuronal interconnections between certain brain areas, lesioning of large brain regions or complete surgical isolation of brain areas, such as hypothalamic deafferentation or brainstem or spinal cord hemisections, may be worthwhile. Bilateral, ipsi- or contralateral connections between brain areas can be demonstrated after appropriate brain lesions or transections. In order to obtain more detailed information, specific chemical lesions or small circumscribed electrolytic or mechanical lesions should be applied.

Control brain samples should be dissected. Samples from brain areas presumably not the targets of the experimental surgery should be removed as additional controls along with those of sham-operated animals. Demonstration of postoperative alterations only in certain brain areas but not generally in the whole brain may indicate the reliability and usefulness of the technique applied to demonstrate specific interconnections between brain areas.

IV. SUMMARY OF ADVANTAGES AND LIMITATIONS

A. Advantages

The microdissection–microassay technique provides quantitative estimates of the amount of substances in a particular brain region. With this technique, the participation and relative importance of certain chemically specified cell groups in the innervation of a brain area can be indicated by exact, comparable, and reproducible numerical data.

Measurements provided by biochemical assays are, in general, more sensitive than the changes seen in histofluorescence or in immunohistochemical staining after lesions (Kopin *et al.*, 1974; Zaborszky *et al.*, 1985). Indeed, biochemical measurements including radioimmunoassays, radioenzymatic assays, high-performance liquid chromatography, amino acid analysis, and liquid hybridization assay on discrete microdissected brain regions have reached in the past few years a degree of sensitivity that permits measuring changes in the femtogram range. Consequently, small alterations in concentrations of substances or in enzyme activities, which can not be revealed by histochemical techniques, are still detectable by biochemical measurements.

Some of the microdissection techniques, e.g., the "micropunch" method, are fast, thereby offering the possibility of investigating hundreds of brain samples within a relatively short period of time.

The sensitivity of microassays permits precise measurement of several substances in the same tissue sample. Since data are obtained from the same experimental animals, such studies provide objective comparisons and quantitative estimates of the influence of brain lesions or pathway transections on various substances in a particular region of the brain.

B. Limitations

Many brain nuclei are heterogeneous, and experimentally induced alterations measured by microassays using the punch technique or dissection of the whole nucleus may therefore be misleading or at least of restricted value. For instance, if a substance is concentrated in a small part of the nucleus (or the microdissected samples are not discrete enough), even significant changes in this small compartment may remain undetected. This problem can to some extent be resolved by the use of a grid microdissection technique (Miyata and Otsuka, 1972; Kanazawa, 1983; Godfrey and Matschinsky, 1976; Hellendal *et al.*, 1986), in which small samples are taken from the whole extent of the nucleus or area in a systematic fashion.

The microdissection technique does not provide information about the structure in which a substance resides, i.e., cell body, axon, terminal, nonneuronal elements. The spatial resolution of the technique is also limited to the size of the tissue sample. However, immunohistochemical technique can be applied following the same lesions used to visualize pathways and terminal fields by the demonstration of disappearance of a substance from certain fibers and terminals and its accumulation in cells proximal to the lesion. Thus, the results obtained with these two procedures can complement each other (Zaborszky *et al.*, 1985).

V. APPENDIX

The micropunch technique (Palkovits, 1973) is widely used and can be applied to frozen, fixed, or even living brain tissue with some modification (Palkovits and Brownstein, 1983, 1988). In the rat brain, tissue from 265 individual brain nuclei, cell groups, or cell layers can be separately removed. The lower limit is about 10 μg brain tissue (wet weight), which corresponds to a tissue pellet of 100-μm radius from a 300-μm-thick brain section. After a rather short period of training, a large number of samples (50–80) can be microdissected per hour. The reliability of the micropunch method is dependent primarily on the neuroanatomical orientations rather than on the technical procedure itself. The microdissection technique is composed of two procedures: (1) brain sectioning and (2) micropunch. The instruments needed are related to these two procedures.

A. Instrumentation

1. Instruments for Brain Sectioning

Fresh, frozen, or fixed brains can be sliced. Templates, tissue choppers, or Vibratomes are used for cutting fresh brains. Frozen brains are sliced with a cryostat or other freezing microtomes. Fixed brains can be easily cut with above instruments or even free-hand under a dissecting microscope with knives or razor blades (Palkovits and Brownstein, 1983, 1988).

2. Instruments for Microdissection

Any kind of dissecting microscope (stereomicroscope) can be used. The requirements are 6- to 20-fold magnification, upper illumination (if possible, with cool light), and a minimum of 5 inches free space under the microscope tube. A cold stage is used for microdissection from frozen sections. It can be a box or dish filled with dry ice or with a circulating cooling solution. The top of the stage should be metal, which provides good heat conductivity. Microdissection from fresh brain is performed on a rubber or other elastic stage. Microdissection needles (Fig. 1) are constructed of hard stainless steel tubing mounted in an about 2-inch-long thicker handle (Palkovits, 1973, 1980; Palkovits and Brownstein, 1983). A complete set comprises six needles with

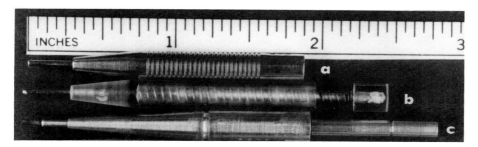

Figure 1. Microdissection needles. a, common hollow stainless steel needle; b, stainless steel tubing mounted in a plastic brass shaft with spring-loaded stylet; c, stainless steel needle equipped with a stylet.

different inside diameters, i.e., 0.2, 0.3, 0.5, 1.0, 1.5, and 2.0 mm. The needles can be equipped with a stylet (Palkovits and Brownstein, 1983, 1988).

B. Microdissection Procedure

The microdissection may be applied to fresh, frozen, or fixed brain tissue. Removal of the brain without prior fixation or freezing can be employed only if rapid (minutes) postmortem changes are not expected. In order to minimize postmortem changes, microdissection can be performed on microwave-irradiated brains or after rapid freezing in liquid nitrogen.

The major steps of the procedure are as follows.

1. Sectioning the Brain

Fresh brain slices may be made manually with a knife or razor blade on a black hard rubber plate or with the aid of mechanical devices such as templates or tissue choppers. Sectioning of frozen brains may be performed either with a freezing microtome or in a cryostat (Palkovits and Brownstein, 1983). The brains are frozen onto the specimen holder with dry ice. In general, 300-μm-thick coronal sections are cut. Several landmarks in various parts of the brain can serve to facilitate the appropriate positioning of the brain on the stage (Palkovits, 1980; Palkovits and Brownstein, 1983, 1988; Cuello and Carson, 1983). Sections are transferred and mounted on a glass microscope slide and dissected immediately or stored on dry ice or in a deep freeze.

2. Punch Technique

Nuclei from fresh brain slices can be removed by microdissection (Zigmond and Ben-Ari, 1976; Cuello and Carson, 1983) or micropunch (Palkovits, 1973; Jacobowitz, 1974; Palkovits and Brownstein, 1983) techniques. In fresh brain sections, the white matter and the ventricles serve as landmarks. By using upper illumination and black plates, myelinated structures can be easily recognized under a stereomicroscope. By using transillumination of tissue slides (Cuello and Carson, 1983), the white matter appears dark, and the nuclei transparent. Vital staining of the sections with methylene blue before microdissection may facilitate the orientation (Zigmond and Ben-Ari, 1976). Micropunch from frozen sections cut in a cryostat (Palkovits, 1973) has become the most used microdissection technique. In order to keep the slides cold during the microdissection procedure, they are placed on a cold stage under the microscope (Palkovits, 1980; Palkovits and Brownstein, 1983, 1988).

Special hollow micropunch needles of varying inner diameter (Fig. 1) are used. The proper needle should be smaller than the smallest diameter of the brain area to be removed; i.e., the tissue pellet need not contain the entire nucleus but as large a part of it as possible.

Micropunching proceeds as follows. In the first step of the punch procedure the tip of the needle is positioned exactly over the nucleus to be removed (Fig. 2a). Then, the needle is brought into a vertical position and pressed into the tissue, slightly rotated, and then quickly withdrawn. The dissected tissue pellet is then blown out of the needle or, if a needle with a stylet is used, pushed out of the needle. After a tissue sample is successfully microdissected a sharp hole remains in the section (Fig. 2b).

3. Preparation of Microdissected Brain Samples

For further biochemical studies the tissue sample must be homogenized with microhomogenizers or by sonication (Palkovits and Brownstein, 1983). When biochemical measurements are made on tissue extracts, the sample size may be determined. If there are milligram amounts of brain tissue, the samples may be weighed. The microdissected samples are usually less than 1 mg wet weight, and pellets are too small for direct weighing; therefore, their protein contents are measured. An aliquot (5–10 μl) of the well-suspended tissue homogenate is removed for protein determination, which may be carried out with the Folin phenol reagent (Lowry *et al.*, 1951; Peterson, 1977). The amount of protein in brain extract is proportional to its tissue content (about 9–13% of the wet weight of the brain is protein).

4. Validating the Microdissection Method

There are several ways to validate the microdissections. Immediately after the micropunch, sections are allowed to thaw and can be transilluminated or illuminated from above on a black background. An excellent identification of brain areas can be achieved even with lower-power magnification based

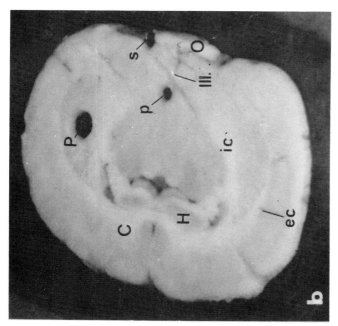

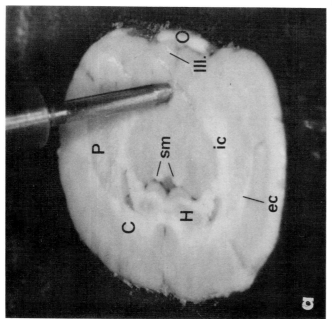

Figure 2. Micropunch technique. Coronal section of the rat forebrain 1.5 mm caudal to the bregma level. (a) The needle is positioned over the brain nucleus (paraventricular nucleus) to be dissected. (b) After punching, sharp-edged holes remain in the section. C, corpus callosum; ec, external capsule; H, hippocampus; ic, internal capsule; O, optic chiasm; P, putamen; p, paraventricular nucleus; s, supraoptic nucleus; sm, stria medullaris; III, third ventricle.

on the differential optical density of myelinated fiber bundles versus poorly myelinated areas. These sections, however, desiccate rapidly and therefore cannot be stored.

When 300-μm-thick sections yield insufficient detail, thinner sections have to be prepared by (1) alternate sectioning or (2) postsectioning. (1) After each 300-μm section a 10- to 20-μm section is cut, stained, and examined for topographical details. On the basis of the analysis of the thin section the microdissection can be validated on the adjacent thick section. (2) After the micropunching is completed, the 300-μm-thick sections should be fixed, embedded, and further cut into 10- to 20-μm-thick sections and stained. Frozen 300-μm sections can be refrozen on a gelatin block, cut into thin sections, stained, and examined under the microscope.

C. Protocol for the Micropunch

1. Determine the number of animals and the number of brain regions to be removed. When fresh brains are dissected, the number of brain areas sampled should be limited to ensure that the dissection of nuclei per brain can be finished in 2 or 3 min, otherwise the sections will be desiccated. When working with frozen sections the number of experimental animals and the number of brain regions to be punched are practically unlimited. After sectioning, the slides can be stored in a box filled with dry ice powder for weeks.
2. Prepare a dissection protocol. One should take into account the order of brain nuclei to be removed in rostrocaudal or caudorostral order (according to the serial sections), the size of the punch used, as well as the number of pellets taken from the nucleus.
3. Twice as many tubes as samples must be made ready: one for the material to be assayed and one for protein determination. The homogenizing solution is pipetted into the homogenizing vessels. The volume of the liquid required for homogenization depends on the size of the tissue samples. The solution in which the samples are homogenized is determined by the assay to be performed.
4. Decapitate the animals and remove the brains. When punching frozen sections, brains should be frozen onto the specimen holders on dry ice (Palkovits and Brownstein, 1983). The entire process should take about 1 min per animal.
5. Section the brains. Collect the sections on numbered glass slides and microdissect immediately or store them on dry ice.
6. Micropunch under a stereomicroscope.
7. Homogenize the tissue samples. Set up a schedule for mechanical homogenization or sonication. (Washing and drying of the microhomogenizers are time consuming.)
8. Remove aliquots for protein determination and then centrifuge.
9. Assay or lyophilize the samples.

REFERENCES

Cuello, A. C. (ed.), 1983, *Brain Microdissection Techniques,* John Wiley & Sons, Chichester.

Cuello, A. C., and Carson S., 1983, Microdissection of fresh rat brain tissue slices, in: *Brain Microdissection Techniques* (A. C. Cuello, ed.), John Wiley & Sons, Chichester, pp. 37–125.

Davis, R., and Huffman, R. D. 1968, *A Stereotaxic Atlas of the Brain of the Baboon (Papio papio),* University of Texas Press, Austin, London.

Dua-Sharma, S., Sharma, S., and Jacobs, H. L., 1970, *The Canine Brain in Stereotaxic Coordinates,* MIT Press, Cambridge, MA.

Emmers, R., and Akert, K., 1963, *A Stereotaxic Atlas of the Brain of the Squirrel Monkey (Saimire sciureus),* University of Wisconsin Press, Madison, WI.

Gergen, J. A., and MacLean, P. D., 1962, *A Stereotaxic Atlas of the Squirrel Monkey's Brain (Saimire sciureus),* University of Wisconsin Press, Madison, WI.

Godfrey, D. A., and Matschinsky, F. M., 1976, Approach to three-dimensional mapping of quantitative histochemical measurements applied to studies of the cochlear nucleus, *J. Histochem. Cytochem.* **24:**697–712.

Hellendall, R. P., Godfrey, D. A., Ross, C. D., Armstrong, D. M., and Price, J. L., 1986, The distribution of choline acetyltransferase in the rat amygdaloid complex and adjacent cortical areas, as determined by quantitative microassay and immunohistochemistry, *J. Comp. Neurol.* **249:**486–498.

Jacobowitz, D. M., 1974, Removal of discrete fresh regions of the rat brain, *Brain Res.* **90:**111–115.

Kanazawa, I., 1983, Grid microdissection of human brain areas, in: *Brain Microdissection Techniques* (A. C. Cuello, ed.), John Wiley & Sons, Chichester, pp. 127–153.

Kopin, I. Y., Palkovits, M., Kobayashi, R. M., and Jacobowitz, D. M., 1974, Quantitative relationship of catecholamine content and histofluorescence in brain of rats, *Brain Res.* **80:**229–235.

Lim, R. K. S., Lui, C., and Moffitt, R., 1960, *A Stereotaxic Atlas of the Dog's Brain,* Charles C. Thomas, Springfield, IL.

Lowry, O. H., Rosebrough, N. Y., Farr, A. L., and Randall, R. J., 1951, Protein measurement with the Folin phenol reagent, *J. Biol. Chem.* **193:**265–275.

Lucchi, M. R. de, Dennis, B. J., and Adey, W. R., 1965, *A Stereotaxic Atlas of the Chimpanzee Brain (Pan satyrus),* University of California Press, Berkeley, Los Angeles.

Manocha, S. L., Shantha, T. R., and Bourne, G. H., 1968, *A Stereotaxic Atlas of the Brain of the Cebus (Debus apella) Monkey,* Oxford University Press, Oxford.

Miyata, Y., and Otsuka, M., 1972, Distribution of γ-aminobutyric acid in cat spinal cord and the alteration produced by local ischemia, *J. Neurochem.* **19:**1833–1834.

Monnier, M., and Gangloff, H., 1961, *Atlas for Stereotaxic Brain Research on the Conscious Rabbit,* Elsevier, Amsterdam.

Oswaldo-Cruz, E., and Rocha-Miranda, C. E., 1968, *The Brain of the Opossum (Didelphis marsupialis). A Cytoarchitectonic Atlas in Stereotaxic Coordinates,* Instituto Biofisica Universidad Federale do Rio de Janeiro, Rio de Janeiro.

Palkovits, M., 1973, Isolated removal of hypothalamic or other brain nuclei of the rat, *Brain Res.* **59:**449–450.

Palkovits, M., 1980, *Guide and Map for the Isolated Removal of Individual Cell Groups from the Rat Brain* [Hungarian text], Akadémiai Kiadó, Budapest.

Palkovits, M., and Brownstein, M. J., 1983, Microdissection of brain areas by the punch technique, in: *Brain Microdissection Techniques* (A. C. Cuello, ed.), John Wiley & Sons, Chichester, pp. 1–36.

Palkovits, M., and Brownstein, M. J., 1988, *Maps and Guide to Microdissection of the Rat Brain,* Elsevier, New York, Amsterdam.

Paxinos, G., and Watson, C. 1982, *The Rat Brain in Stereotaxic Coordinates,* Academic Press, Sydney, New York.

Peterson, G. L., 1977, A simplification of the protein method of Lowry *et al.* which is generally more applicable, *Anal. Biochem.* **83:**346–356.

Schaltenbrand, G., and Wahren, W., 1977, *Atlas for Stereotaxy of the Human Brain*, Georg Thieme, Stuttgart.

Scott, P. M., and Knigge, K. M., 1981, Immunocytochemistry of luteinizing hormone-releasing hormone, vasopressin, and corticotropin following deafferentation of the basal hypothalamus of the male rat brain, *Cell Tissue Res.* **219:**393–402.

Shantha, T. R., Manocha, S. L., and Bourne, G. H., 1968, *A Stereotaxic Atlas of the Jawa Monkey Brains (Macaca irus)*, Williams & Wilkins, Baltimore.

Sidman, R. L., Angevine, J. B., Jr., and Taber Pierce, E., 1971, *Atlas of the Mouse Brain and Spinal Cord*, Harvard University Press, Cambridge.

Snider, R. S., and Lee, J. C., 1961, *A Stereotaxic Atlas of the Monkey Brain (Macaca mulatta)*, University of Chicago Press, Chicago.

Snider, R. S., and Niemer, W. T., 1961, *A Stereotaxic Atlas of the Cat Brain*, University Chicago Press, Chicago.

Verhaart, W. J. C., 1964, *A Stereotaxic Atlas of the Brain of the Cat*, Van Gorcum, Assen.

Yoshikawa, T., 1968, *Atlas of the Brains of Domestic Animals*, Pennsylvania State University Press, University Park.

Zaborszky, L., Alheid, G. H., Beinfeld, M. C., Eiden, L. E., Heimer, L., and Palkovits, M., 1985, Cholecystokinin innervation of the ventral striatum: A morphological and radioimmunological study, *Neuroscience* **14:**427–453.

Zigmond, R. E., and Ben-Ari, Y., 1976, A simple method for the serial sectioning of fresh brain and the removal of identifiable nuclei from stained sections for biochemical analysis, *J. Neurochem.* **26:**1285–1287.

12

Receptor Autoradiography

WILLIAM A. GEARY II and G. FREDERICK WOOTEN

I. INTRODUCTION

Receptor autoradiography involves the identification of receptors in tissue fragments or sections with the use of pharmacological binding methods. The earliest binding studies utilized high-specific-activity radiolabeled receptor ligands and crude membrane preparations. The compound or ligand was bound selectively to a receptor site, and the membranes were then separated from the radiolabeled drug solution. Under appropriate conditions, the quantity of radiolabeled drug that bound to the membranes represented the quantity of receptors in the tissue. In order to apply binding methods to the study of receptors in a tissue as complex as the brain, modifications have been made in binding methods to allow for autoradiographic localization of specifically bound radiolabeled compounds.

The principles of tissue section autoradiography have been well described by Stumpf and Roth (1966). Early autoradiographic receptor studies in frozen sections of brain were carried out in Kuhar's laboratory using *in vivo* administration of radiolabeled receptor ligands (Kuhar and Yamamura, 1975). Unnerstall *et al.* (1982) performed quantitative studies of silver grains on x-ray film for single concentrations of radioligands, employing *in vitro* labeling

WILLIAM A. GEARY II and G. FREDERICK WOOTEN • Department of Neurology, University of Virginia Medical Center, Charlottesville, Virginia 22908.

techniques. Quantitative studies of tissue tritium concentration by film autoradiography using tritium-impregnated, calibrated, plastic standards were performed by Alexander *et al.* (1981). Quantitative film autoradiography of the kinetic features of the binding of a tritium-labeled radioligand was first described by Penney *et al.* (1981). Palacios *et al.* (1981) suggested the use of computerized densitometry in the analysis of film autoradiographs of radioligands. Now, several investigators have presented well-validated methods for quantitative autoradiography of tritium-labeled receptor ligands using a variety of tritium-impregnated standards (Alexander *et al.*, 1981; Unnerstall *et al.*, 1982; Geary and Wooten, 1983, 1985a). Such methods have been used to localize and quantify numerous neurotransmitter and drug receptors in brain. Data obtained from receptor autoradiographic studies have greatly supplemented the vast information already available on brain functional anatomy from tract tracing, immunocytochemistry, and 2-deoxyglucose autoradiographic studies.

In this chapter we review the conditions for performing pharmacologically valid binding assays on brain sections and the principles involved in generating and quantifying the autoradiographic images produced by specifically bound radiolabeled ligands.

II. QUANTITATIVE RECEPTOR AUTORADIOGRAPHY

The experimental animal is sacrificed, and its brain is rapidly removed and frozen. The frozen brain is then immersed in embedding matrix and mounted on a chuck for cryostat sectioning. Frozen sections are cut at 6 to 20-μm thickness, thaw-mounted onto coverslips, and refrozen. Prior to the labeling procedure, sections are brought to room temperature and then preincubated in buffer for 30 min. Following preincubation, sections are immersed in buffer containing tritium-labeled ligands. After incubation, sections are rinsed twice in buffer and once in distilled water. The sections are then air dried and glued to an 8 × 10 inch sheet of cardboard. In the darkroom, 8 × 10 inch sheets of LKB-Ultrofilm are placed in apposition to the sections and stored in light-tight x-ray cassettes. The x-ray films are exposed for the appropriate amount of time and then removed and developed. Densitometric measurements are made over regions of the autoradiographs as well as the appropriate coexposed calibrated standards. The data are then expressed as binding site density per unit weight of tissue.

A. Tissue Preparation

1. Freezing of Brain Tissue and Preparation of Frozen Sections

The animal is anesthetized with sodium pentobarbital and decapitated. The whole brain is rapidly removed, blotted, placed in a Parafilm^{TM} sling, and immersed in liquid Freon® that is packed in dry ice for 2 min to ensure uniform freezing. If perfusion and fixation are performed, appropriate controls must be carried out to ensure that receptor number and affinity are not affected by fixation. We do not routinely use fixation procedures. The frozen brain is then immersed in embedding matrix, mounted on a brass chuck, and stored at −70°C for up to 2 weeks. Serial 6 to 20-μm sections are cut in a cryostat at −18° to −22°C, thaw-mounted onto coated coverslips, and immediately refrozen.

2. Preparation of Coverslips and Storage Conditions

Prior to use, the coverslips are coated with poly-D-lysine polymer (mol. wt. 100,000–150,000) by immersing them in a 10 mg/100 ml solution of poly-D-lysine in distilled water for 5 sec. This coating minimizes tissue loss or distortion in subsequent incubation procedures. After the tissue sections are mounted onto the coated coverslips and refrozen, they are stored over desiccant at −20°C. The length of time the sections may be stored for subsequent binding assays should be empirically determined for each ligand.

B. Choice of Conditions for Assay

1. Choice of Buffers and Temperatures

The most appropriate buffer for a particular ligand-binding study can only be determined empirically. A large number of different buffer systems have been employed in ligand-binding assays. With many ligands, the use of different buffers leads to trivial differences in specific binding, yet with some ligands, e.g., opiates, hemicholinium, and ouabain, different buffers may result in large differences in specific binding.

In general, any departure from physiological conditions in the binding assay should be validated by comparison with physiological conditions. Many investigators prefer to perform opiate radioreceptor assays in the absence of sodium in the buffer to improve the signal-to-noise ratio for agonist binding. Such departures from physiological conditions could, in theory, lead to artifactual results. Other radioreceptor assay buffer systems often contain supraphysiological concentrations of certain anions and cations, again raising questions about the physiological significance of the binding results.

The choice of temperature for binding assays is usually one of convenience. A high temperature, e.g., 37°C, increases the rate of association of ligands with receptors and minimizes tissue incubation time; however, tissue integrity on the slides or coverslips is most likely to be compromised by high-temperature incubations. Incubations carried out at a low temperature, e.g., 4°C, markedly reduce both association and dissociation rates of ligands with tissue receptors. Nevertheless, low-temperature incubations are often chosen with polypeptide ligands, for example, to minimize the effects of tissue degradative enzymes on the peptide ligands.

The choice of buffers and temperatures for binding studies is based on optimizing the binding assay without compromising the physiological significance of the results. Thus, the buffer and temperature conditions for each binding assay must be determined empirically.

2. Role of Buffer Volumes for Assays: Effects of Changes in Ligand Concentrations

Ideally, the amount of radiolabeled ligand bound to tissue at equilibrium should constitute a very small percentage of the free ligand concentration in the buffer at steady state. Thus, binding assays should be performed under conditions where the ratio of buffer volume to tissue weight is high. By meeting this condition, the effects of the loss of bound ligand from the buffer on the free ligand's true concentration are minimized when steady-state conditions are reached. This condition is difficult to achieve in two circumstances: (1) when large tissue sections, e.g., human brain sections, are being labeled, large incubation volumes are required, and (2) when on-slide incubations using small buffer volumes result in small absolute ligand availability relative to receptor density. We routinely measure tritium concentration in our buffers before and after each tissue incubation to correct for any reduction in free ligand concentration in the buffer resulting from binding to tissue. Thereby, one may determine directly that true free ligand concentration at steady state is not changed relative to the initial incubation conditions.

3. Indications for and Effects of Preincubation

Endogenous ligands may compete with radiolabeled ligands in binding studies. To minimize these effects, we routinely preincubate tissue sections in ligand-free buffer prior to exposure of the sections to buffer containing radiolabeled ligand. Serial preincubations in large buffer volumes may reduce endogenous ligand concentration of 10^{-9}- to 10^{-12}-fold. However, a potential consequence of this preincubation is the removal of cofactors, e.g., guanosine triphosphate (GTP), that might affect ligand binding affinity, unlike the *in vivo* physiological state. Such possibilities should be considered when interpreting quantitative binding data.

C. Establishing an Assay for a Specific Ligand

1. Binding Kinetics

The first step in establishing a binding assay is to determine the rate of association of a given ligand with its binding site. It is important to study the

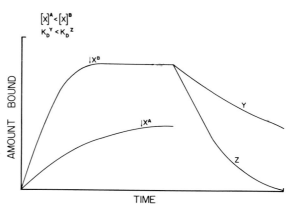

Figure 1. Theoretical "on" and "off" rates. The two theoretical "on" rates (plotted on the left side) are for a single ligand *(X)* at two different concentrations *(A* and *B)* where $[X]^A < [X]^B$. See text for discussion. The two theoretical "off" rates (plotted on the right side) reflect two different ligands *(Y* and *Z)* for the same receptor. Ligand *Z* has a lower affinity (higher K_d) than ligand *Y* for this theoretical receptor.

association rate at several different ligand concentrations. In Fig. 1, using ligand concentration X^B, it is clear that steady-state conditions are approximated because at some time point there is no further net binding; concentration X^A achieves steady-state conditions later. If the concentration X^A were employed, steady-state conditions would not be achieved in a reasonable time frame, and thus one of the critical conditions for binding assays would not be met. Such data permit the selection of a ligand concentration sufficiently high to allow steady-state conditions to be achieved in a reasonable time (i.e., 30–45 min) without wasting radiolabeled ligand.

To determine ligand–receptor affinity, knowledge of both "on" and "off" rates is required. *Y* and *Z* in Fig. 1 represent "off" rates for different ligands from the same receptor. The slower "off" rate for ligand–receptor interaction *Y* indicates a higher affinity (lower K_d) for the ligand–receptor interaction *Y* than for *Z*.

Specific binding is the difference between total binding and nonspecific binding. Nonspecific binding is the amount of binding that occurs in the presence of an excess of cold, unlabeled ligand (specific for the same binding site as the radiolabeled ligand). When the finite number of specific binding sites is saturated with unlabeled ligand, bound radioligand is an estimate of the nonspecific binding compartments. Total binding thus represents binding to the specific receptor and all other tissue compartments. Ideally, the proper concentration of unlabeled, competing ligand should be determined experimentally as illustrated in Fig. 2. In the condition on the left side of Fig. 2, the competing drug is capable of competing for up to 90% of total binding; in the condition on the right side, only 60% of the total binding is "displaced" by the inhibitor. Concentrations of inhibitor or competing ligand should be chosen just beyond the second inflection of the inhibition curve after it flattens. The arbitrary choice of an inappropriately high concentration of competing drug may produce an artifactually low estimate of nonspecific binding. Since nonspecific binding may be somewhat saturable, a low-affinity binding site may be indicated artifactually.

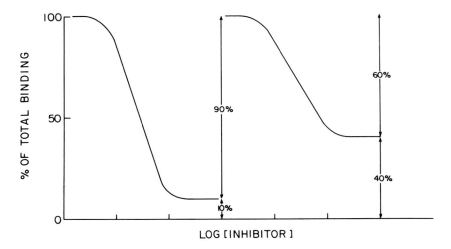

Figure 2. Two theoretical competition curves for two different competing drugs against a single radiolabeled ligand. On the left, the competing drug is capable of competing for up to 90% of the total binding; on the right, the competing drug competes for only 60% of the total binding.

After establishing the incubation time to steady state and estimating the affinity by kinetic determinations, saturation studies may be carried out. Several ligand concentrations above and below the K_d (index of affinity) estimated from kinetic studies should be used. Care should be taken with concentrations below the K_d to allow for sufficient incubation time to achieve steady state. From the saturation studies, K_d and B_{max} (concentration of specific binding sites) may be estimated by a variety of graphic methods described below. The affinity constants, K_ds, determined by saturation studies should be similar to those estimated from kinetic studies.

An important step in defining the ligand-binding assay for a specific receptor is to demonstrate that the specific binding is stereospecific for the pharmacologically active isomer.

2. Quantitative Assessment of Binding Data

Saturation binding data may be analyzed graphically by any of several similar methods to determine K_d and B_{max}. Theoretical Klotz plots are depicted in Fig. 3, and theoretical Scatchard and Eadie–Hofstee analyses are illustrated in Fig. 4. Zivin and Waud (1986) published a computer program for analysis of Eadie–Hofstee plots that permits an estimation of variance for the data derived from individual saturation studies. Their analysis provides a useful check on the reliability or inherent error in the derivation of K_d and B_{max} from saturation studies.

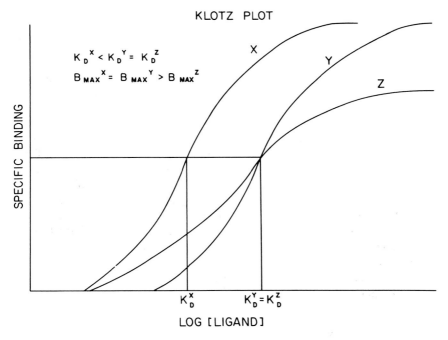

Figure 3. Three theoretical Klotz plots for ligands *X, Y,* and *Z.*

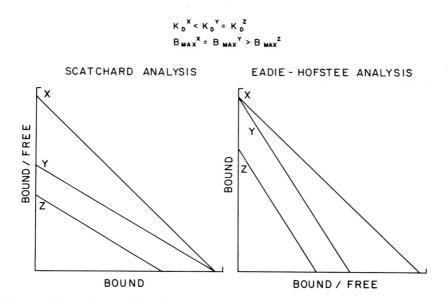

Figure 4. Three theoretical Scatchard and Eadie–Hofstee analyses for ligands *X, Y,* and *Z.*

3. Rank-Order Inhibition to Establish Pharmacological Specificity and Potency

A key step in the development of a ligand-binding assay for a particular neurotransmitter or drug receptor is the demonstration of the pharmacological specificity of the ligand. First, the capacity of other drugs or neurotransmitters to compete for a specific binding site must be determined experimentally. For example, a ligand specific for dopamine receptors should be displaced by lower concentrations of dopamine than of norepinephrine, epinephrine, acetylcholine, serotonin, etc. Second, the relative potency of compounds within a receptor-specific drug class should demonstrate a rank order potency for ligand binding site competition that is equivalent to their rank order of pharmacological effect. For example, the specific binding of the radiolabeled antipsychotic drug spiperone should be displaced by lower concentrations of the pharmacologically potent antipsychotic drug fluphenazine rather than by the less potent drug chlorpromazine. By the examination of the capacity of other drugs or neurotransmitters to compete for the specific binding site of a radiolabeled ligand, one may define the pharmacological specificity and potency of the ligand for a specific receptor site.

D. Analysis of Quantitative Data

1. Preparation of Standards

The use of radioisotopically labeled standards is necessary for the performance of quantitative receptor autoradiography. A variety of methods for making standards have been employed, including the introduction of varying concentrations of isotope into tissue paste and the impregnation of plastic polymers with radioisotopes. Commercially available standards are now of sufficient quality and isotopic concentration range to obviate the need for investigators to make their own standards. It is important to assess critically the calibration of commercially available standards. Each laboratory should independently calibrate its standards for tissue-equivalent concentration of isotope. Our method for calibrating standards has been published in detail elsewhere (Geary and Wooten, 1985a).

2. Densitometer versus Video Camera Coupled with Computer

The data from early quantitative receptor autoradiographic studies were collected by the use of microdensitometers. Although highly accurate and reproducible, such data collection procedures are cumbersome and labor intensive. With the introduction of video cameras coupled to computers, the rate of data collection should theoretically be greatly increased. However, the densitometric accuracy of any video camera system should be carefully validated with an accurate manual densitometer.

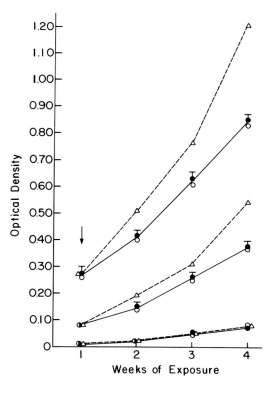

Figure 5. Noncovariation of image generation (optical density) rate curves for tritium and carbon-14 sources. Filled circles are for tritium in tissue; open circles are for tritium in plastic; and open triangles are for carbon-14 in plastic. All three sources produced equal optical density values at 1 week of exposure to LKB Ultrofilm (see arrow). The carbon-14 source differed significantly from both tritium sources at 2, 3, and 4 weeks of exposure time ($P < 0.05$, $P < 0.01$, $P < 0.01$, respectively, by Student's t-test). The two tritium sources covaried with exposure time. Reprinted by permission of authors and publishers (Geary and Wooten, 1985a).

3. Limitations for Comparisons among Isotopes

Because the rate of image generation on x-ray film or nuclear track emulsion may vary among isotopes, it is important to use standards containing the same isotope as that used to label the ligand being employed in the binding assay. Figure 5 illustrates the noncovariance of image generation for a tritium source and a carbon-14 source. Thus, in performing quantitative autoradiographic studies with tritium-labeled ligands, tritiated standards should be employed.

4. Film Response for LKB Ultrofilm and SB-5 X-Ray Film

Figures 6 and 7 illustrate the response of LKB Ultrofilm to tritium and SB-5 x-ray film to carbon-14, respectively. The linear range of LKB Ultrofilm optical density (OD) response is from about 0.08 to 0.80 OD units, whereas the linear range of SB-5 x-ray film is from about 0.01 to 1.1 OD units. Densitometric readings from below or above this range are subject to error because of either instrument limitations (low OD values) or film saturation (high OD values). Optical density values outside the linear range should be

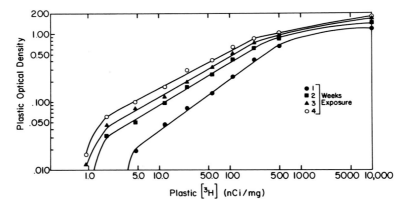

Figure 6. Relationship of tritium concentration in nine different plastic standards to optical density (OD) produced by exposure of these standards to LKB Ultrofilm for 1, 2, 3, or 4 weeks. Data are mean OD values of triplicate sets of homogeneous tritium plastic sources. All regression lines had correlation coefficients of $r \geq 0.995$ ($P < 0.01$). Reprinted with permission of authors and publishers (Geary and Wooten, 1985a).

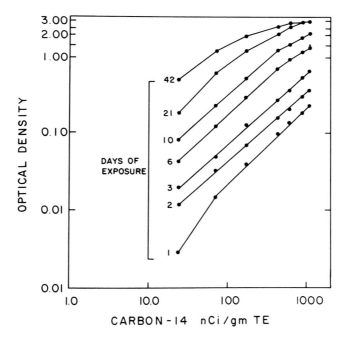

Figure 7. Relationship of carbon-14 concentration in seven different plastic standards to optical density produced by exposure of these standards to SB-5 x-ray film for 1, 2, 3, 6, 10, 21, and 42 days.

rejected in quantitative studies. In order to minimize loss of data from insufficient or excessive image generation, great care should be taken in selecting exposure times for experiments.

5. Correction for Tissue Autoabsorption of Tritium

Measurement of isotopic decay is affected by quenching phenomena inherent in the isotopic source material. When using tritium-labeled radioligands, the autoradiographic images generated are primarily influenced by the specific, regional brain tissue concentration of lipids. Thus, there is a discrepancy between the actual tissue concentration of tritium and the quantity of signal detected by x-ray film or nuclear emulsion, the magnitude of which varies directly with the lipid concentration of the specific brain region under consideration. Several methodological approaches have been employed to correct for this regional quenching of tritium-generated images. We have developed a series of regional quench corrections for rat brain by comparing $[^3H]$-2-deoxyglucose images of control brain sections generated from rats receiving $[^3H]$-2-deoxyglucose *in vivo* with adjacent sections from which lipid was extracted by *in vitro* incubation in chloroform (Geary and Wooten, 1985b). No tritium was lost from or redistributed in the tissue during chloroform extraction. In general, correction of gray matter autoabsorption amounted to about one-third of the value from unextracted sections, whereas white matter autoabsorption correction required an approximate doubling of unextracted tissue images. The fractional autoabsorption related to chloroform-extractable lipid was a constant percentage of the OD of the unextracted image for a given brain region. This was independent of the absolute concentration of tritium when data were taken in the linear range of the OD versus tritium-concentration curve. Table I summarizes some regional quench values for tritium in the rat brain. These values may be applied to autoradiographic data derived from any tritium-labeled radioligand in rats of similar strain, age, and weight.

6. Consideration of Isotope Source Thickness

Because the principal β emission from tritium is relatively weak, only tritium in the most superficial tissue (2–3 μm) adjacent to the x-ray film or emulsion is detected. Variations in tissue section thickness have little effect on autoradiographic images generated with tritium. Thus, in the routine use of tritium-labeled radioligands for quantitative autoradiography, variation in tissue section thickness is not a source of error. In contrast, carbon-14, which possesses a more potent β emission, is inclined to produce variable images if tissue section thickness is not uniform. Studies using carbon-14 in biological materials with thicknesses less than the "infinite" path length require uniformity of thickness of tissue sections. Calibration data must likewise be ob-

**Table I. Rat Brain Regional Quenching Coefficients
for Tritium**[a]

Brain regions	Percentage increase in OD after chloroform extraction	n
Motor cortex	32 ± 5	5
Cingulate cortex	36 ± 11	3
Occipital cortex	30 ± 4	3
Head of striatum	39 ± 10	5
Globus pallidus	61 ± 8	3
Diagonal band	46 ± 5	3
Nucleus accumbens	39 ± 6	3
Lateral hypothalamic area	61 ± 11	3
Lateral septal nucleus	40 ± 8	3
Basolateral amygdala	33 ± 7	3
Lateral habenula	50 ± 9	3
Mammillary nucleus	58 ± 5	3
Substantia nigra (PC)	35 ± 3	3
Substantia nigra (PR)	57 ± 6	3
Cerebellar gray matter	35 ± 3	3
Corpus callosum (genu)	118 ± 20	3
Cerebellar peduncles	151 ± 30	3
Choroid plexus	4 ± 6	3

[a] For a more complete listing, see Geary and Wooten (1985b).

tained under uniform thickness conditions. For example, analysis of 20-μm-thick sections in carbon-14 studies would require highly reproducible section thickness and standards calibrated against 20-μm-thick tissue sources. Figure 8 illustrates the phenomena described above.

III. TYPES OF EXPERIMENTS USING QUANTITATIVE FILM AUTORADIOGRAPHY

A. Mapping

The most common application of quantitative receptor autoradiographic methods is the anatomic mapping of receptor types in the brain. Figure 9 illustrates a mapping study of [^{3}H]-naloxone binding sites in the rat brain at serial rostrocaudal levels. The images consist of total and nonspecific binding at a naloxone concentration of 3 nM. A series of calibrated standards are present on the left margin. Densitometric data derived from the tissue images and standards allow for quantitation of [^{3}H]-naloxone binding sites in any brain region that can be anatomically resolved by the densitometric analysis.

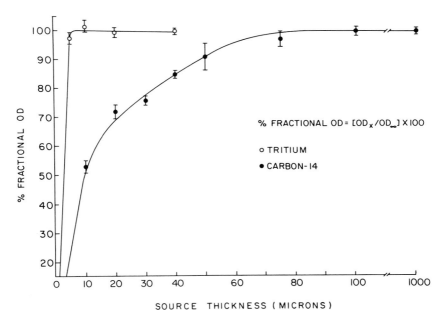

Figure 8. Comparison of image density generated by varying section thicknesses of a uniformly labeled tissue source of tritium versus carbon-14. Section thicknesses of greater than 5 μm produced no variation in the tritium-generated image, whereas section thicknesses of up to 70 μm resulted in changes in image density from a source with a single homogeneous carbon-14 concentration.

B. Regional Saturation

By incubating a series of adjacent sections in varying concentrations of tritium-labeled radioligand and coexposing the sections to x-ray film with calibrated tritium standards, regional saturation studies to determine K_d and B_{max} can be carried out in multiple brain regions simultaneously. Figure 10 depicts a saturation experiment using [^{3}H]-ouabain with seven different isotope concentrations. In order to obtain valid OD data, sections exposed to lower ligand concentrations (upper left side of figure) required reexposure to film for a longer period of time to produce images on the linear portion of the tritium concentration versus film OD response curve. Standard analyses of film data are performed as described in Section II.C.

C. Regional Specific Inhibition

The capacity of a specific inhibitor to interact with a binding site in a regionally selective manner is amenable to quantitative autoradiographic analysis. For example, examination of the capacity of a μ-selective opiate ligand to compete for brain binding sites defined by the nonselective radio-

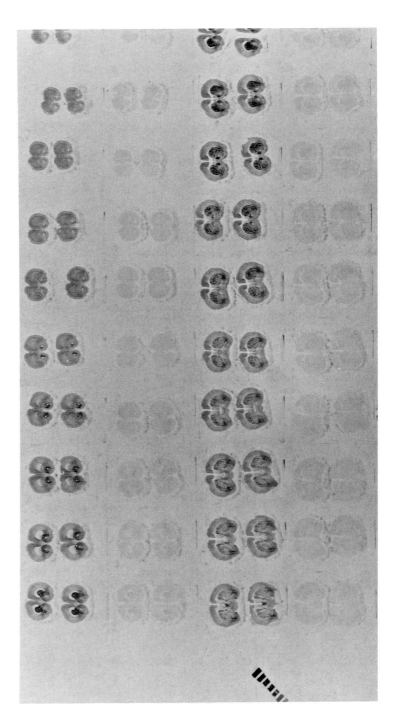

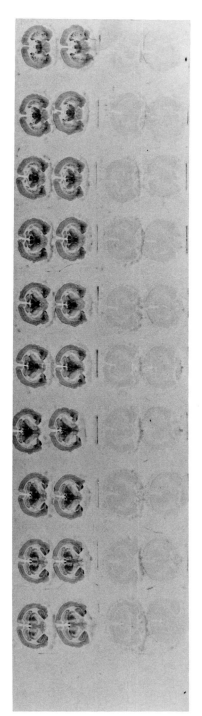

Figure 9. Total and nonspecific autoradiographic images of [³H]-naloxone binding at serial rostrocaudal levels of rat brain. Note the seven calibrated tritium standards on the left side of the figure.

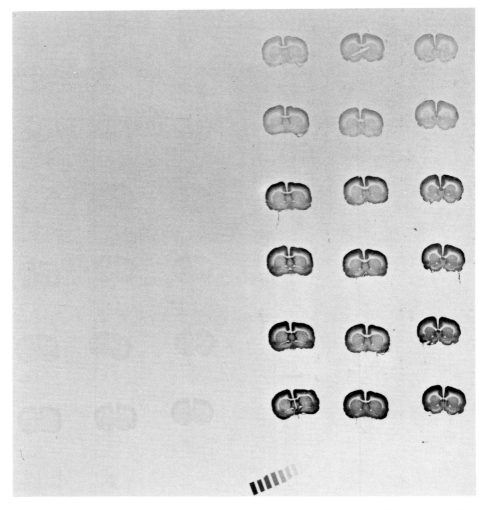

Figure 10. Total and nonspecific autoradiographic images of groups of triplicate sections of rat brain exposed to seven different concentrations of [³H]-ouabain.

labeled opiate ligand naloxone might reveal relatively higher densities of μ-specific receptors in one brain region compared to others.

D. *In Vivo* versus *in Vitro* Labeling

In order to determine if incubation of tissue sections *in vitro* with a radio-labeled ligand produces the same regional binding as that which occurs physiologically, the same radiolabeled drug can be administered *in vivo* and its disposition determined autoradiographically.

IV. SUMMARY OF ADVANTAGES AND LIMITATIONS

A. Advantages

One of the principal advantages of quantitative receptor autoradiography as an anatomic method is the capacity for highly accurate and reproducible quantitation. Not only can the density or number (B_{max}) of binding sites be estimated, but the biochemical property of affinity (K_d) may also be estimated. These properties then allow for meaningful studies of regulation with quantifiable end points to be approached experimentally.

Another major advantage of this method is the property of biochemical specificity afforded by studies of saturation and competition for binding sites by other specific ligands. Thus, anatomic localization and a high degree of neurochemical specificity are both possible by the use of this method. Furthermore, a powerful set of techniques can be utilized by combining classic anatomic techniques such as degeneration stains and tract-tracing methods with quantitative receptor autoradiography.

B. Limitations

Perhaps the principal limitation of quantitative receptor autoradiography in its present form is the lack of fine anatomic detail, largely because of the use of frozen tissue in this method. Furthermore, since most of the radiolabeled ligands are reversibly bound to their binding sites, it is not feasible to dip the labeled sections into liquid emulsion because such a procedure would result in the removal of varying amounts of ligand from the specific binding sites. Thus, the use of tritium-sensitive x-ray film or apposition of labeled sections to emulsion-coated coverslips places a major limitation on the fine anatomic resolution that may be attained by this method. Some investigators have circumvented this problem by using very high-affinity ligands; quantitative electron microscopic autoradiography has actually been accomplished successfully with soluble, reversibly bound ligands (Hamel and Beaudet, 1987).

A methodological alternative to quantitative receptor autoradiography now exists when a high degree of anatomic resolution is sought. Monoclonal antibodies have been developed for several receptors, thereby permitting their high-resolution immunocytochemical localization (Strader *et al.*, 1983; Schoch *et al.*, 1985; Triller *et al.*, 1985).

Another limitation inherent in this method is that one localizes and quantifies binding sites that are by inference "receptors." Since the method contains no assessment of receptor function, the interpretation of quantitative receptor autoradiographic studies *vis-à-vis* receptors is always subject to question and caution. Nevertheless, there is a high probability that appropriately defined specific binding sites are receptors in most cases.

V. FUTURE APPLICATIONS

The rapid development of quantitative autoradiographic methods was evidenced in the study of brain receptors and is now being seen in the study of drug and neurotransmitter receptors in other tissues (Mendelsohn, 1984).

With the advent of specific radiolabeled suicide substrates for enzymes, quantitative autoradiographic methods provide a way to localize and quantify enzymatic activity (Pegg *et al.*, 1982).

Specific antibodies bound to brain antigens, e.g., substance P, can theoretically be localized and quantified by the use of either tritiated primary antibodies or tritiated secondary complexes, e.g., biotin–avidin (Hunt and Mantgth, 1984). Thus, the capacity to quantify immunocytochemical studies is potentially available. The development and quantitative validation of such methods would then allow quantitative radioimmunoassays by autoradiographic approaches.

Techniques to perform "high-resolution" quantitative autoradiography on diffusible tritium-labeled receptor ligands are available (Duncan *et al.*, 1987). The capacity to study the cellular localization of radiolabeled drug and transmitter binding sites would be a major technical development in neuroanatomical methodology.

Rapid developments in molecular biology with gene cloning have already yielded preliminary autoradiographic studies of the localization of mRNA in brain tissue using radiolabeled cDNA probes (Gee *et al.*, 1983). Pursuit of such quantitative methodological approaches may lead to new understanding of gene regulation.

Thus, the study of quantitative receptor autoradiography evolved powerful methods potentially applicable to a wide variety of neurobiological investigations. The capacity for highly accurate quantification is virtually unique to this technique as compared to other neuroanatomical techniques.

VI. CONCLUDING REMARKS

In some instances, there is a high anatomic correlation between the regional distribution of nerve terminals specialized to release a specific neurotransmitter and the receptors specialized to bind this neurotransmitter. For example, the terminal distribution of dopaminergic axons and dendrites in the striatum, nucleus accumbens, and substantia nigra is matched by a similar selective distribution of dopamine receptors (Boyson *et al.*, 1986). In such instances receptor autoradiography provides a useful independent representation of the distribution of dopamine systems in the brain.

Numerous other examples exist, however, of apparent mismatches between the distribution of nerve terminals specialized to release a specific neurotransmitter and the receptors for that transmitter. For example, McLean *et al.* (1986) have elegantly detailed a host of apparent mismatches in various brain regions between terminals specialized to release endogenous opioid peptides and opiate receptors. Much speculation has been offered to explain such mismatches: perhaps there is "long-distance" communication between neurons that are not anatomically apposed, or perhaps receptors are expressed by some cells that are not often occupied by their specific ligands *in vivo* and are therefore not frequently utilized. Further studies are necessary for a clear understanding of the significance of such apparent anatomic "mismatches." Clearly, in some instances, the anatomic distribution of a receptor does not appear to describe a biochemically specific functional system.

REFERENCES

Alexander, G. M., Schwartzman, R. J., Bell, R. D., Yu, J., and Renthal, A., 1981, Quantitative measurement of local cerebral metabolic rate for glucose using tritiated 2-deoxyglucose, *Brain Res.* **223**:59–67.

Boyson, S. J., McGonigle, P., and Molinoff, P. B., 1986, Quantitative autoradiographic localization of the D1 and D2 subtypes of dopamine receptors in rat brain, *J. Neurosci.* **6**:3177–3188.

Duncan, G. E., Stumpf, W. E., and Pilgrim, C., 1987, Cerebral metabolic mapping at the cellular level with dry-mount autoradiography of [³H]2-deoxyglucose, *Brain Res.* **401**:43–49.

Geary, W. A., and Wooten, G. F., 1983, Quantitative film autoradiography of opiate agonists and antagonists, *J. Pharmacol. Exp. Ther.* **225**:234–240.

Geary, W. A., and Wooten, G. F., 1985a, Quantitative film autoradiography for tritium: Methodological considerations, *Brain Res.* **337**:99–108.

Geary, W. A., and Wooten, G. F., 1985b, Regional tritium quenching in quantitative autoradiography of the central nervous system, *Brain Res.* **336**:334–336.

Gee, C. E., Chen, C. C., and Roberts, J. L., 1983, Identification of proopiomelanocortin neurons in rat hypothalamus by *in situ* of cDNA–mRNA hybridization, *Nature* **306**:374–376.

Hamel, E., and Beaudet, A., 1987, Opiod receptors in rat neostriatum: Radioautographic distribution at the electron microscopic level, *Brain Res.* **401**:239–257.

Hunt, S. P., and Mantgth, P. W., 1984, Radioimmunocytochemistry with [³H]biotin, *Brain Res.* **291**:203–217.

Kuhar, M. J., and Yamamura, H. I., 1975, Light autoradiographic localization of cholinergic muscarinic receptors in rat brain by specific binding of a potent antagonist, *Nature* **253**:560–561.

McLean, S., Rothman, R. B., and Herkenham, M., 1986, Autoradiographic localization of μ- and δ-opiate receptors in the forebrain of the rat, *Brain Res.* **378**:49–60.

Mendelsohn, F. A. O., 1984, Localization of angiotensin converting enzyme in rat forebrain and other tissues by *in vitro* autoradiography using ¹²⁵I-labeled MK 351A, *Clin. Exp. Pharmacol. Physiol.* **11**:431–436.

Palacios, J. M., Niehoff, D. L., and Kuhar, M. J., 1981, Receptor autoradiography with tritium-sensitive film: Potential for computerized densitometry, *Neurosci. Lett.* **25**:101–105.

Pegg, A. E., Seely, J., and Zagon, I. S., 1982, Autoradiographic identification of ornithine decarboxylase in mouse kidney by means of α[5-¹⁴C]difluoromethylornithine, *Science* **217**:68–70.

Penney, J. B., Frey, K., and Young, A. B., 1981, Quantitative autoradiography of neurotransmitter receptors using tritium-sensitive film, *Eur. J. Pharmacol.* **72**:421–422.

Schoch, P., Richards, J. G., Häring, P., Iakacs, B., Stähli, C., Staehelin, T., Hafely, W., and Möhler, H., 1985, Co-localization of GABA$_A$ receptors and benzodiazepine receptors in the brain shown by monoclonal antibodies, *Nature* **314**:168–171.

Strader, C. D., Pickel, V. M., Joh, T. H., Strohsacker, M. W., Schorr, R. G. L., Lefkowitz, R. J., and Caron, M. G., 1983, Antibodies to the β-adrenergic receptor: Attenuation of catechol-amine-sensitive adenylate cyclase and demonstration of postsynaptic receptor localization in brain, *Proc. Natl. Acad. Sci. U.S.A.* **80:**1840–1844.

Stumpf, W. E., and Roth, L. G., 1966, High resolution autoradiography with dry-mounted, freeze-dried frozen sections. Comparative study of six methods using two diffusible compounds [³H]estradiol and [³H]mesobilirubinogen, *J. Histochem. Cytochem.* **14:**274–287.

Triller, A., Cluzeaud, F., Pfeiffer, F., Betz, H., and Korn, H., 1985, Distribution of glycine receptors at central synapses: An immunoelectron microscopy study, *J. Cell Biol.* **101:**683–688.

Unnerstall, J. R., Niehoff, D. L., Kuhar, M. J., and Palacios, J. M., 1982, Quantitative receptor autoradiography using [³H] Ultrofilm: Application to multiple benzodiazepine receptors, *J. Neurosc. Methods* **6:**59–73.

Zivin, J. A., and Waud, D. R., 1986, Analysis of one-component saturable systems such as ligand binding, enzyme kinetic, uptake, and transport data, *J. Pharmacol. Methods* **16:**1–22.

13

Processing and Analysis of Neuroanatomical Images

MICHAEL T. SHIPLEY, JESUS LUNA, and
JOHN H. McLEAN

I. BACKGROUND

Today, neuroanatomists have an almost bewildering array of techniques that are being used to study the organization of the nervous system along dimensions that were not even conceived 10 to 15 years ago. Brain circuits are no longer viewed as wiring diagrams interlinking classical brain structures but rather as subpopulations of neurons differing along morphological and neurochemical lines having interconnections with other equally specific subpopulations of neurons in multiple other brain structures. No longer are neural circuits "excitatory" or "inhibitory." Neurons may contain several transmitters/modulators, and the actions of modulators may depend on the moment-to-moment status of their target cells. The levels of these neuroactive molecules may vary with the animal's functional, humoral, or develop-

MICHAEL T. SHIPLEY • Department of Anatomy and Cell Biology, Division of Neurobiology, and Department of Neurosurgery, University of Cincinnati College of Medicine, Cincinnati, Ohio 45267.   JESUS LUNA and JOHN H. McLEAN • Department of Anatomy and Cell Biology, Division of Neurobiology, University of Cincinnati College of Medicine, Cincinnati, Ohio 45267.

mental state. On the postsynaptic side, multiple receptor subtypes are well established for many transmitter systems; these link presynaptic inputs to a growing multitude of channel types and second messenger systems, which may or may not have direct actions on the genome or gene products of the target cell. Methods for studying these phenomena in brain sections are now available, and there are exciting possibilities to apply similar techniques to *in vitro* brain-slice preparations to study functioning neuroanatomy.

Clearly, there has been a revolution in the development of neuroanatomical methods.

As recently as about 10 years ago there was not only a limited range of neuroanatomical techniques but an equally obvious poverty of analytical tools. Basically, neuroanatomists had microscopes. Optics had improved, fluorescence was used to look at monoamines, and a few heroic souls had linked various computers to microscope stages to accomplish charting and/or cell counting. By contrast, the analytical tools of the neurophysiologist were awesome. Rapid progress in the development of software and a parallel decline in the cost of hardware had put into the hands of the neurophysiologist the ability to execute elaborate experiments, store and analyze streams of high-speed data, and modify ongoing experimental contingencies, on line, as a result of data analyzed from previous experimental runs. Neuroanatomists could only sit by their microscopes and wonder what Freud would have made of computer envy. Neuroanatomists were keenly aware of the fact that they were entirely dependent on their interaural computers to perform complex pattern recognition tasks, density analyses, and spatial comparisons; to render these analyses into communicable schematics required hours of eye strain and tedious charting using a camera lucida or overhead projector. The product of this laborious process still had to be redrawn with messy ink pens, labeled, and photographed for a journal. And, when it was all said and done, the result was only a picture. To derive quantitative information about fiber lengths, branching patterns, staining density differences, and grain densities required so much time and effort that only a few laboratories could afford to generate quantitative morphological data on neural structures. Neuroanatomists were keenly aware that meaningful principles of neural organization, development, and plasticity were likely to involve changes in axonal and/or dendritic lengths and branching, but to detect biologically significant differences involved rates of data collection and analysis that were unrealistically slow in terms of the inexorable 3 to 5-year cycle of grant funds. As a result, neuroanatomists were generally impelled to concentrate on short-range goals, which usually meant qualitative rather than quantitative analyses.

It is the purpose of this chapter to indicate that much of this is beginning to change. The preceding chapters demonstrate eloquently that poverty of techniques is no longer a primary constraint to unraveling the organization of the nervous system. The goal is to suggest that equally impressive progress in data analysis may be expected in the near future so that advances in neuroanatomical techniques can be paralleled by such advances in analytical tools that neuroanatomy can grow as a quantitative, hypothesis-testing discipline.

II. ORGANIZATION OF THE CHAPTER (AND SOME DISCLAIMERS)

Image analysis in neuroanatomy is still relatively new and is likely to mean different things to different people. Here, we discuss a few basic concepts about image processing and image analysis. These concepts are enlarged on in the next two sections where basic hardware and software matters are discussed. Next, a few examples are given of the ways in which image processing and image analysis are being used on neuroanatomical problems in the authors' laboratory. Throughout, comments are made about limitations and pitfalls of image processing and analysis.

Before we move on, some disclaimers are necessary. As will become obvious, image processing and image analysis are achieved by the use of various kinds of hardware and software. The senior author is neither a computer/video engineer nor a computer scientist. This disclaimer is intended to serve as a warning and an encouragement. The warning is that this chapter does not deal with engineering and technical issues except in the most general way. What the author knows of these matters is the result of having read several excellent books and articles by some of the pioneers and experts in this field (Allen and Allen, 1983; Allen *et al.*, 1981a,b; Inoue, 1986). The contributions of these individuals are only beginning to be appreciated by the biological community. They were the true innovators. The encouraging part of the disclaimer is that if someone with the low level of engineering and computer literacy of the author can benefit from image processing and analysis, then surely this technology holds promise for many. Clearly, it helps to have someone around who actually knows what he or she is doing, and the second author has been that person.

The other disclaimer is that this chapter, unlike many of the previous ones, cannot offer protocols of techniques that can be used immediately in your work. The world would clearly be a better place if all programs ran on all machines, but until that day, the counterpart of a staining protocol—the source code of a program—is of little utility unless the users have the same hardware and operating system. What we present instead are examples of application programs written for this laboratory's system. The examples serve to illustrate the kinds of applications that are achievable with this technology and are offered with the belief that people will be able to do the same things with different systems. In fact, this is already happening.

The final disclaimer is that as this chapter is being written it is already becoming obsolete. Few areas of technology are changing as rapidly as the video camera and microprocessor fields; the growth of image-analysis/processing hardware and software is almost certainly at the bottom end of an exponential curve. Today's accomplishments are likely to be regarded as trivial and primitive compared to the state of the art when this is read. Nonetheless, there are some applications that are likely to remain as basic tools although they will be done with higher-speed, higher-resolution equipment and probably more refined algorithms.

III. IMAGE PROCESSING AND IMAGE ANALYSIS

These two terms are sometimes used interchangeably by neuroscientists, but it is useful to distinguish two generally different goals that are achieved primarily by processing and by analysis.

The goal of image processing is to modify the quality of an image. Generally this is to improve the quality so that certain features of the image can be better detected or visualized. In a sense, adjusting a microscope to give Kohler illumination is a kind of image processing in that optimal adjustment of the illumination to the optics improves the resolving power of the system and optimizes the contrast of the image. Similarly, selection of the appropriate color filter for a given photographic film can optimize the contrast of certain elements in the image.

A key feature of most image-processing/image-analysis systems is to take the image viewed in the microscope into a computer using some kind of video camera. As is detailed later, this process involves several steps; many of these steps are actually or potentially under the control of the user. Thus, there are several ways in which the image can be selectively modified by the choice of the video camera and/or by manipulating the electronics of the camera so as to modify its transfer function. One of the earliest and still most powerful uses of video in microscopy, pioneered by Allen (Allen and Allen, 1983; Allen *et al.*, 1981a, b), is to manipulate the black level and gain of a TV camera to selectively amplify a certain range of brightness in images viewed with phase or differential interference contrast optics or asymmetric illumination. The ability to modify the image information transferred through the TV camera offers many possibilities for visualizing features that are nearly unresolvable by conventional light microscopy, and the reader is strongly encouraged to read the excellent papers by Allen and in Inoue's (1986) book, *Video Microscopy*, which is essentially the Bible of video microscopy.

Signals from the TV camera are typically fed to a computer through a video analogue-to-digital converter (A/D). The system used in the authors' laboratory has two stages of image processing subsequent to the video camera. The video signal is fed to a digital video processor so that the image from the TV camera can be further manipulated in "real time," i.e., the image can be continuously modified on a frame-by-frame basis so that, for example, the contrast of the image can be changed (enhanced) at sufficient speed that the enhancements are made on a "live image." The user can scan the microscope slide by moving the *X* or *Y* controls of the microscope stage or change the focal depth by adjusting the focus control on the microscope, and the selected contrast enhancements "follow" the changing scene. Additional kinds of image processing are to sum or integrate several frames so that weak signals in noisy video images can be detected or to subtract a previously stored video frame from the current frame, a technique often used to achieve "background" subtraction, or to subtract two frames to enhance features that are different in two focal planes of an image.

The devices used to achieve these processing functions can differ and are discussed later. The point to be made here is that, in general, all of the foregoing manipulations, from adjusting the microscope or the TV camera or using a video processor, are employed chiefly to improve the quality of the image or to selectively enhance the contrast/detectability of a certain class of features or range of contrasts in the image. In general, however, image processing does not provide an analysis of the information in the image. It does not say how many objects there are or anything about their geometries, their densities (degree of staining or labeling), where they are, etc. Information of this kind is achieved by techniques of image analysis. Image analysis then involves a set of operations designed to extract information about a selected class of features in an image.

Notwithstanding this distinction, it should be obvious that the image processing and image analysis are frequently like hand and glove. Before objects or features can be measured, they must be discriminable; one must be able to distinguish the desired features from background, artifact, or other features before they can be analyzed. Image processing offers powerful techniques for improving the quality of microscope images and the detection of objects of interest. However, it does not take the next steps, which are the identification and measurement of objects. The selection of a class of objects/features and the extraction of quantitative information about the members of the class is image analysis.

There are good reasons for stressing this distinction. For one thing, some applications may only require image processing. The use of Allen video-enhanced contrast microscopy (AVEC) is a good example. It may be the case that one's basic problem is visualizing some features in a brain section or cell culture to see if they are present or not, or simply noting their spatial distribution relative to other objects. For example, one may wish to visualize and observe the behavior of growth cones in a culture system, or antibodies to two different transmitter-specific molecules may be used with two different fluorochromes in a colocalization study. The object of the colocalization experiment may be simply to look at the differential and overlapping distributions of the two populations. In such a case the biological significance of the experiment may be whether or not there are double-labeled cells, i.e., an essentially qualitative issue. Image processing alone can greatly facilitate the visualization and, hence, the interpretation of such material. However, the experimenter may be testing a hypothesis about the relative proportions of single- and double-labeled neurons and/or their size, shape, clustering, or whether the proportions change with developmental state or by physiological/pharmacological manipulation. In such cases image analysis techniques could be used to search the image, identify the neurons, and extract the desired quantitative data. This example is given because it is important to keep in mind that the biological question should motivate the techniques used and not the other way around.

Another reason for stressing the distinction between image processing and image analysis is that when one is choosing a system, this distinction may not be made clear by the vendors of equipment. It is very easy to be dazzled by equipment that can suddenly turn weakly stained fibers into clear, sharply delineated ones or turn dimly fluorescent neurons into Golgilike profiles. At this stage, one tends to be very vulnerable to statements from salesmen like, "Oh, yes, we're developing the measuring routines right now, and it will be no problem." The overwhelming impact of how much improvement in the visualization of microscopic images can be achieved by image processing is likely to blind one temporarily to the fact that if you can see your favorite features that much better, you probably very soon will want to use that improvement in visualization to test some hypothesis about quantitative differences among the objects. At this stage you may be panting to sign a purchase order. However, this is a good point at which to stop, back away, and start thinking long and hard about what you are likely to want to be doing 2 or 3 years down the road with the ability to see things you have been straining to get at for the last 2 or 3 years! Image analysis will almost certainly be in your future, and it is worth getting that capability up front.

In summary, it is useful to distinguish between image processing and image analysis. The goal of image processing is to enhance the visibility or detectability of certain aspects of an image; the goal of image analysis is to select and measure specific features/objects in an image. For most neuroanatomical applications both techniques are likely to be needed.

IV. A SYSTEMS OVERVIEW OF IMAGE PROCESSING/ANALYSIS

As noted, earlier, image processing and image analysis involve the use of specialized hardware and software to enhance and extract quantitative information from images. Before we discuss hardware and software in some detail it is useful to take a systems overview of an image-processing/image-analysis system. For illustrative purposes we will discuss the system used in the authors' laboratory. All of the elements of such a system may be necessary for many applications, and some specialized applications may require additional pieces of hardware and/or software. Because the applications discussed in the final part of this chapter were developed for such a system, its description will serve as an example of one that has reasonably broad utility.

There are four basic kinds of components in an image-processing/image-analysis system for neurobiological application: (1) *input devices*, (2) *image processor*, (3) *image analyzer*, and (4) *output devices*. The block diagrams of Fig. 1 illustrate the major flows of information between these components. The lines indicate that the most general flow is from an input device to the image processor to the image analyzer to an output device. In addition, there is, in our system, a major link between the image analyzer and the input devices:

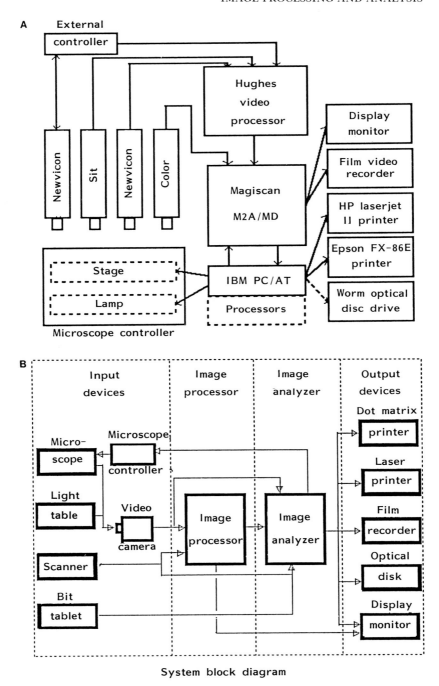

Figure 1. Block diagrams of image-processing/analysis system. A: Flow diagram of the image-processing/analysis used in the authors' laboratory. B: Systems input/output diagram of a general image-processing/analysis system.

image analyzer software is used to control the *X, Y,* and *Z* (focus) stepping motor controls of the microscope stage as well as the lamp brightness. Other lines indicate that in some applications one or more components may be omitted. In an extreme case the electronics of the video camera may be manipulated so as to provide a degree of image enhancement that is visualized and interpreted from a monitor; in this case the image processor and analyzer are bypassed. The early video-enhanced microscopic techniques of Allen (AVEC; Allen *et al.,* 1981 a,b) were based on such an approach, although today it is common to have some stage of video processing and/or analysis between the camera output and monitor.

Image processing and image analysis may be performed by the same device. In the authors' experience, the combined image-processing/image-analysis devices available in today's market do a better job of either processing or analysis but usually do not do both optimally. This reflects the historical fact that most manufacturers initially addressed either processing or analysis markets. With the emergence of applications such as neuroanatomy where both functions are needed, they have endeavored to play catch-up on one or the other, but the initial specialization usually is better developed than the secondary function. This situation will doubtless change in response to market growth. In the long run, single systems with a common machine language, operating system, and high-level-language programming library would be optimal, and that will almost certainly happen. In this chapter the image processor and image anlayzer are treated as separate devices.

Let us now consider in a little more detail the kinds of devices that comprise the four stages of a system.

V. INPUT DEVICES

The three kinds of input devices most commonly used in neuroanatomy are (1) the bit tablet or digitizer pad, (2) the video camera and a light table, and (3) the video camera and microscope.

A. Bit Tablet

One of the earliest ways of entering positional information about brain sections into a computer was through a bit tablet. A bit tablet is a flat plate on which one places a photo, drawing, or projected image of a preparation. An *X,Y* coordinate grid is incorporated into the plate in one of several ways. The regularly spaced points in this grid are addressed to the computer through an interface. With a photo, drawing, or projected image on the plate, the user traces the boundaries of desired regions, for example, the outline of sections, nuclear boundaries, and/or the locations of cells, with a cursor. The boundaries and/or object points are assigned locations based on the nearest *X* and *Y* coordinates in the tablet grid and entered into the computer. Many bit tablet manufacturers supply software that runs under the operating systems of the most commonly used personal computers. This software will store and file the point sets that define the drawn outlines and perform a range of analytical operations related to morphology.

The advantages of bit tablet systems are price and relative simplicity of operation. Since many investigators have a PC, the additional cost of a bit tablet and software is modest. If the user is already acquainted with PC software, little effort is required to be up and running quickly with the bit tablet programs. The disadvantages of such systems are that the data input is very slow; i.e., it is entirely manual and is limited by the size of the tablet and the scheme used to record the grid points. The major limitation of the bit tablet, however, is that one cannot obtain information about contrast, i.e., density. Such systems also have no facilities for image processing, i.e., improving the quality of the image being analyzed. Still, bit tablets are useful for morphometric analysis, and a bit tablet input to any image analysis system is a useful way to enter point set data from photographic material such as electron micrographs. Because these systems are relatively inexpensive and useful, they should be considered even in laboratories where larger, more sophisticated systems are available. For some applications they may be just as efficient as a video-based system and can relieve the workload on the larger machine.

B. Video Camera and Light Table

In this case, a video camera is equipped with an appropriate conventional camera lens and positioned over a light table. Photos or drawings placed on the table's surface are illuminated from above, and x-ray films or other forms of transparencies, e.g., photo negatives or polyacrylamide gels, are transilluminated by a uniform light source below the table surface. The image is scanned by the camera and led to either the processor or analyzer. For image data such as photos, x rays, gels, etc., the light table is the most practical way to enter an image into the processor/analyzer because photographs, x-ray films, and gels are very large compared to a microscope slide.

In some applications the range of gray value differences that are of experimental significance may be very great. As will be discussed shortly, most video cameras have a limited dynamic gray range of between six and eight bits, which corresponds to 64 to 256 different gray levels. An x-ray film can register more gray level differences than this. It may be necessary to discriminate as many gray levels as the film can register, but when it is, there will clearly be some loss of gray-level information if the film is imaged with a video camera that does not resolve the desired number of gray-level differences. In this case, an alternative is to use a scanning densitometer. Such devices scan a transparency and measure the optical density, point by point, much as the beam of the video camera scans the photosensitive target surface, although the scanning densitometer scans much more slowly—on the order of hours versus 1/30 of a second for a video frame. This slow speed may be inconvenient and is a major disadvantage (another is cost) of scanning densitometers. Use of such a scanning input device should be considered only in applications where all other efforts to extract gray-level information of satisfactory resolution fail. It is possible with sufficient computer image memory, for example, to extend the gray-level resolution achievable with a video camera by inputting the data two or more times under different levels of illumination such that the total gray range of the image is encompassed by combining two video frames, each limited to half of the gray-level range. In this way seven bits of gray level (128 gray levels) can be obtained from a six-bit (64-gray-level) camera. It may not be possible to view the entire density range in one computer image, but the optical density information stored in image memory can be analyzed. Notwithstanding, in situations where the primary material to be imaged contains a wide dynamic gray range that will routinely contain significant biological data, the scanning densitometer may be the data input device of choice. The key issue, though, is significance. Vendors of imaging systems often make a bigger deal out of gray-level dynamic range than may be warranted by either the biological application or the camera system.

C. Video Camera and Microscope

The most versatile input device for neuroanatomical material is a video camera coupled to a microscope. To date, most of the applications in this laboratory have involved light microscopy (LM) of various kinds, but image analysis systems can be configured with an interface to an electron microscope.

1. Optics

In a light microscope video system the quality of an image is fundamentally limited by the optics and illumination system of the microscope. Although it is frequently stated that video microscopy can be used to resolve objects beyond the limits of optical resolution, this is often taken to mean that optics are not critical. This is a misconception. To the degree that video can be used selectively to enhance contrast of an image, improving the microscope's optics and illumination system generally permits video enhancement techniques to work even better. Therefore, image processing and analysis cannot substitute for lack of optical quality and shoddy microscope alignment. There are situations where the requirements of an experiment impose certain compromises of optimal optics, and these are familiar to most neuroanatomists. For example, it is seldom possible to have the optimal correction for flatness of field and the highest numerical aperture in fluorescence optics without considerable, sometimes unacceptable, loss of fluorescent intensity. In such cases, the need for light forces one to compromise to some degree the extent to which other corrections can be tolerated in the objectives. In such cases, image processing will help. For example, if flatness of field or working distance is the primary consideration and dictates some compromise in the amount of light transmitted through the objective, it may be possible to use a SITCAM (see Section V.D) and integrate several successive video frames with image processing to boost the fluorescent signal. Thus, experimental requirements may necessitate some compromises in some optical quality, and image processing can be used to compensate to some degree. However, the fundamental fact is that if one can use optimal optics and illumination from the outset, then the final image, even with image processing, will be better. Moreover, it is always useful to bear in mind that the use of image processing will entail some trade-off of its own, although it may sometimes take a while to recognize it. In the example given above where a SITCAM and frame averaging are used to offset the loss of light resulting from the use of a long working distance lens, one obvious trade-off is temporal resolution. In order to average frames, several frames must be taken, and it takes 1/30 sec to capture each frame; if 30 frames are required, then the scene must be imaged for at least 1 sec. If the specimen fades in that time, or if it absorbs too much thermal energy from the illumination source, 1 sec may be unacceptably long. Clearly, in such situations if the optics or illumination can be improved to give a significant increase in light transmission, less averaging and therefore shorter exposure times will be needed. Therefore, in general, the better the illumination and optics, the better will be the result of all subsequent stages of processing and analysis.

In addition to the optics and illumination there are other features that contribute to the choice of an optimal microscope for video microscopy. With a microscope, the TV camera is placed in the optical path in much the same way as a photographic camera. Generally, this is done by a standard coupling called a "C-mount," one end of which screws into a ring centered around the camera face plate; the other end inserts into the camera microscope port. This means that it may not be possible to capture a video image and simultaneously take a photomicrograph. Microscope manufacturers are beginning to recognize the growing use of video microscopy and are introducing microscope bodies that incorporate both a photo camera and TV camera port. In this laboratory we have used the Nikon Microphot FX, which has both camera ports and, in addition, has the camera electronics built into the base of the microscope. This microscope thus has separate video and photo ports, economizes space (image analysis and processing systems tend to grow and take up space), is very well designed for video applications, and is moderately priced.

2. Stage and Focus Control

Another important feature in a microscope used for image processing and analysis is motorized control of the stage movements and the focus mechanism. Specific applications that utilize these features are described later, but basically this provision affords the opportunity to let the image analysis system control the region of the specimen being imaged. Thus, one can develop software to let the system scan, find, and record certain features in an image or build up a composite digital montage of a larger area. As will be illustrated later, this is especially useful in neuroanatomy because, frequently, one needs to depict and quantitate features in a certain subregion of the brain but also needs to indicate the context of that region by its relationship to other structures in the section. In order to have sufficient optical magnification to resolve a field of labeled cells or fibers, for example, it may be necessary to use a microscope objective that limits the field of view to a small region. With appropriate software and a motorized stage, however, one can resolve objects at high magnification and then rescale and reposition them to their appropriate size and location in a lower-power overview of a larger region. Alternatively one can build up a low-power "montage" image of several contiguous higher-magnification images. With appropriate software, detailed, accurately scaled "line drawings" can be extracted and printed out with a high-resolution laser printer. Aside from the qualitative visual information in the line drawing, accurate quantitative date, e.g., fiber lengths, cell size, number and staining density, for user-defined subregions (e.g., nuclei, cortical layers) may be collected simultaneously.

3. Illumination

It is also very helpful if the image processor/analysis system software can control the microscope lamp, particularly in applications where the optical density of certain regions or features in the specimens is to be measured. Examples of such applications are given later, but for now one can think of receptor autoradiography where grain density is to be related to receptor–ligand binding sites, histochemistry where the density of staining may be related to the activity of the molecule of interest, or voltage/ion-sensitive fluorescent dyes, where a change in fluorescent intensity is related to a change in membrane voltage or ion concentration. In such applications the goal is to measure the optical density of certain features or objects in an image. Optical density is the reduction in light transmitted through different points in the image; measurements of optical density are dependent on several factors that influence the transmission of light from the source of illumination, in this case the microscope lamp, to the TV camera. One important variable is the intensity of the lamp. Most manufacturers do not invest a lot of effort and expense in the design and construction of the microscope illuminators. In general, they are poorly regulated; fluctuations in line voltages are frequently detectable as changes in source illumination. Moreover, the control of lamp intensity is poor. Typically one has a rather crude analogue meter of the DC volts or current applied to the lamp; this is a poor indication of lamp intensity and is inadequate for achieving constant day-today illumination levels for measuring transmission (i.e., density) differences. Clearly, therefore, a more stable lamp current source is needed as well as more accurate ways of adjusting and equating lamp intensities from one set of measurements to the next.

The image analysis system used in this laboratory has a microscope controller interface that accepts signals from the host computer to control the microscope stage and focus stepping motors and in addition provides a reasonable well-stabilized lamp current source that can be adjusted and regulated by software commands. With such a system it is possible to monitor and achieve control of the illumination levels used in optical density measurements. For example, in the simplest case one may have a neutral-density step filter on a microscopic slide placed in the optical path. The programs we have developed for measuring densities have a routine in which one can adjust the lamp output so that the optical density measured through the density standard is compared to the readings taken at a previous time. Thus, the lamp can be adjusted independently of filament age, etc., to give a consistent output from one densitometric experiment to another. The user can consult a record file in the computer's memory to recall the illumination condition used in previous experiments measuring the same kind of experimental material.

With fluorescent lamp sources it may not be possible to control the illumination level by adjusting the current to the lamp, but with the same software approach just described, it is possible to use neutral-density filters to regulate the light reaching the TV camera so that fairly uniform fluorescent illuminator levels can be achieved across experiments. The lamp calibration software routine also helps one monitor changes in the fluorescence illumination level with lamp use.

The main point is that density measurements made by the image analysis system are measurements relative to the image source. The microscope, its optics, illuminator, and filters all contribute to the measured density. It is essential, therefore, to thoroughly understand potential sources of error and variance in making density measurements, and it is very useful if the image analysis system itself can be used to monitor and adjust critical variables such as lamp output in accordance with stored standard values. This saves set-up time, and the software can be configured so that measurements are not made until a set of calibrations have been performed. This in turn helps the user (especially new users) remember that density measurements require calibrated conditions.

4. Filters

A final factor that significantly influences the quality and contrast of the image is wavelength. An important characteristic of a video camera is its spectral response; i.e., at constant light intensity the output of different cameras varies significantly and systematically with the wavelength of the light.

Different types of video cameras have different spectral response characteristics. Some cameras may be maximally sensitive to wavelengths around 650 nm and be progressively less sensitive to longer or shorter wavelengths. This characteristic is especially important in densitometric measurements as differences in the intensity of staining with many chromagens are also accompanied by potentially significant wavelength shifts. Therefore, densitometric measurement with a black-and-white video camera should be done under monochromatic illumination.

Some video cameras have significant sensitivity in the near infrared range. Unless near-infrared cutoff filters are used, these wavelengths can distort the video image by causing a flaring in areas of low optical density. Because of this contrast the video image may be reduced, and resolution of edges may be compromised. The Newvicon camera, which is very popular and useful in many image-processing/image-analysis applications, has considerable sensivity in the near-infrared range. Its performance in most light microscope applications is greatly improved with the use of a near-infrared cutoff filter (we use a Schott KG-3).

Because video cameras are differentially sensitive to different wavelengths, there is usually some provision in the image processor and/or analyzer to linearize the camera's output across the visible spectral range. Knowledge of the spectral characteristics of the camera, however, can be used to advantage in detecting or suppressing the visibility of a class of stained objects by using very narrowly tuned chromatic filters in the microscope. A device that has proven very useful in our laboratory is a continuously variable half-wavelength interference contrast filter. Examples of the results obtained with this filter are given later (in Section VII. B) where one can essentially blind the video camera to a population of dark-blue-stained neurons while selectively enhancing the visibility of silver grains over the field, and in a second video image of the same field one can selectively enhance the blue neurons while suppressing the grains. Thus, knowledge of the camera's spectral response and judicious color filtering of the microscopic image prior to its reaching the video camera can sometimes provide a powerful type of image processing.

Another issue is uniform illumination. Each video frame is essentially a quantitative report of the brightness of each point along the horizontal and vertical scans that comprise the frame. Ideally, with no specimen on the microscope stage, the video frame should be uniformly bright at all points, as there is no specimen there is nothing to modulate the light reaching the camera face. If one tries this experiment, however, the result is usually not ideal. Typically, the center region of the image is brighter than the peripheral parts because of a lack of uniformity of illumination across the field. In our laboratory the bright center area is called the "hot spot". With the use of small, bright tungsten halogen lamps to give very intense spectrally optimal light in most of today's research microscopes, the hot-spot problem can be severe. The hot spot degrades image processing and analysis in numerous ways. For example, unless the hot spot is recognized and either minimized or corrected, it will cause significant error in densitometric readings. Secondly, the hot spot can take up precious bits in the gray-level digitation and compromise the ability to resolve significant gray-level differences in the specimen. These are certainly not the only examples that could be given.

In image analysis, the hot spot falls into the category of problems called shade correction. There are computational ways to minimize or partially correct for nonuniform illumination. However, computational corrections often entail compromises of their own that are not always made obvious to users by the machine manufacturers. In general, the more severe the hot spot, the less satisfactory are computational solutions. Therefore, great effort should be made to minimize the hot spot at the level of the microscope. Fortunately, one can develop software routines that help in this task. For example, in our system a pseudocolor display is used. Bright, distinctive colors are assigned to the gray values at the brightest and darkest parts of the image. The hot spot can be visualized while the microscope and illuminator are continuously adjusted and minimized.

Many factors contribute to uniformity of illumination, including the alignment and adjustment of the lamp, the field and condenser diaphragms, and the type and positioning of diffusion filters. There is also a significant interaction between these factors and the microscope objective, as the objectives may differentially transmit light at the center and the periphery of the lens. Hot spots are more difficult to minimize at lower objective magnification, because field size relative to lamp size is greater at low magnification and there is more field to illuminate uniformly. In this laboratory, hot-spot minimization is viewed as partly a physical problem (i.e., optics, lamps, diffusers, etc.) and partly a metaphysical problem (i.e., rampant trial and error!). Milk-glass diffusers are useful, and in some cases we have used various home-made plastic plate diffusers positioned between the field diaphragm and the condenser to increase scattered light in all parts of the field. With experience one develops various tricks that work more or less with one's particular microscope, objectives, and lamp. This effort is very much worthwhile, however, because it can minimize the need for computational "hot-spot" or shade correction at subsequent stages. One should first try to use physical means to optimize illumination uniformity and then turn to image processing and computational solutions to deal with further hot-spot problems arising from the objectives, subsequent lenses, filters, and video camera. Again, the message is that the more image quality is optimized at the microscope level the more effective will be subsequent stages of image processing and analysis. Figure 2 shows the results of various techniques to correct for "hot-spot" shading.

D. Video Cameras

Video camera technology is a vast field. This chapter can only touch on a few of the features of video cameras that are germane to their use in neuroanatomical image processing and analysis. A very elegant and far more rigorous and complete discussion of video cameras has been provided by Inoue (1986), and the present authors strongly recommend that anyone contemplating image analysis consult that excellent source.

Here we concentrate on the types of video cameras that are commonly used in image processing and analysis in several laboratories. Video camera technology is changing rapidly; the cameras we use today may soon be superseded by better devices. We first discuss why different applications require different cameras. Then we discuss enough about video camera function to indicate how users can modify camera characteristics to achieve some kinds of image improvement. Finally, we make a few remarks about new video technologies that hold promise for neuroanatomical applications.

There are two different classes of vacuum-tube video cameras that are used in two broad categories of applications in neuroanatomy. One class of camera is generally called by its various manufacturers as a low- (or ambient-) light-level camera. A second class of cameras are often referred to as very-low-light-level cameras. This terminology is not universally used, nor is it particularly easy to keep repeating, so we will simply call the first type a general camera and the second one a silicon-intensified target camera or SITCAM, for short. Purists will probably be offended by this simple dichotomy, but it is useful. General cameras are provided by a number of excellent manufacturers. We use both a Newvicon Model 68 and Model 70 supplied by DAGE-MTI, Michigan City, Indiana. Cameras in this class have broad utility. They are used in most brightfield microscopic and light-table applications where applying enough illumination to view the specimen is no problem. A SITCAM (or otherwise intensified camera) is needed in applications where the light level is much lower, either because the signal to be imaged is inherently weak (e.g., weak fluorescent immunostaining or fluorescent retrograde dye labelling) or where the illumination of the specimen must be kept low in order to limit fluorescent fading or toxic effects of the radiant energy in the light. Obviously the distinction between "low light range" and "very low light level" is entirely relative. In some image-analysis/processing applications, for example, astronomy, it may be necessary to detect down to the photon range. Specially intensified cameras called ISITS (intensified silicon intensifed cameras) have been developed. The use of these ultrasensitive cameras in neurobiological experiments has been very limited to date, but it is not hard to imagine that techniques will be developed for monitoring the activity states of specific molecules in *in vitro* systems where the biologically relevant signal range may be in the tens of photons level.

It might reasonably be asked, why not buy the most sensitive camera available and use it in all applications? The answer to this question is essentially, "Because there's no free lunch." The high sensitivity of SITS and ISITS is achieved at the expense of several tradeoffs, the most significant of which are (1) higher noise, (2) lower resolutions, (3) narrower gray-level dynamic range, (4) greater fragility, and (5) greater cost. Some of these problems can be mitigated by image processing, for example, noise. Noise in a SITCAM can be seen by eliminating all light to the camera. Under these conditions a general camera will produce a uniformly black image; a SITCAM dark image is not uniformly black but is instead a kind of gray snowy picture that is constantly changing. For those old enough to remember the early days of black-and-white television reception, the dark image of a SITCAM has a similar snowy appearance. This represents randomly fluctuating output of the camera tube, which derives from the highly photosensitive nature of the material used on the camera face target surface and/or the high degree of electronic amplification used in the camera. Such a camera will detect weakly fluorescent neurons that are simply below the sensitivity range of a general camera. The labeled neurons will appear as a signal brighter in general than the average value of the fluctuating noise, but the image of the labeled cells is improved significantly by frame averaging or frame integration using a video image processor. Since the camera noise is on a point-to-point basis, fluctuating randomly between higher and lower levels, if one sums up the point values in the image over several successive video frames, the labeled cells, which constitute a relatively invariant signal, will build up an increasing video signal while the nonlabeled background will tend to average out to some uniform gray level much lower than the cells (Fig. 3). This is precisely what is done in video frame averaging in an image processor. Thus, the "noise" level tradeoff in a SITCAM can be minimized; remember that the tradeoff here is time; several frames, each requiring 1/30 sec, must be grabbed to effect the noise reduction.

The other tradeoffs of SITCAMs are less malleable. SITCAMs have less spatial resolution—fewer points of "pixels" per frame. More importantly, they also cannot resolve as wide a range of gray levels; thus, if the cells vary considerably in their labeling intensity and if the camera sensitivity is optimized to detect the most weakly labeled cells, many of the more strongly labeled cells will saturate the camera; i.e., all cells above a certain intensity will look the same, and difference among those cells will be obscured. When cells saturate the camera they will also saturate some neighboring pixels and thus appear larger and less contrasting; therefore, their areas will be inaccurately measured. SITCAMs are also more delicate—exposure to too bright a light can damage the tube, and the tubes have generally a shorter life than general cameras. And, they are more expensive. However, SITCAMs are indispensable in very-low-light-level applications, and if treated carefully, paying attention to their performance, characteristic optima, and with the judicious use of image processing, they are an excellent investment for a wide range of important applications in neuroanatomy. Ideally, then, a neuroanatomy image analysis facility would have at least one general camera and one SITCAM. At the time of the writing of this chapter a few vendors are beginning to advertise solid-state (CCD) cameras equipped with a special early stage of photonic amplification (microchannel plate) and a cooling device to reduce camera noise. Such devices may be capable of providing both high sensitivity and wide gray-level dynamic range. Cooled CCDs have been put to good use in imaging biological structures but previously have been relatively expensive. Newer devices are beginning to appear to be in the same price range as SITCAMs and offer great potential for the kinds of image analysis/image processing discussed here.

A video camera consists, in principle, of a target surface that is sensitive to photons and some kind of device that can read the response to photons at points on the target surface. In general, the sensitivity and range of the target are a function of the photosensitive material used in the target and currents used to bias or activate the target. The point-to-point resistance or charge of the target is a function of the photons hitting those points. Thus, a steady-state image optimally focused on the target produces a two-dimensional array of charge or potential differences. In closed-circuit TV cameras (CCTV; most commonly available video cameras are CCTV), these point-to-point differences are read by an electronically controlled scanning beam. The standard is to sweep the beam along a line (by convention, called a horizontal line) and scan the surface of the target with a series of such horizontal lines, each a fixed distance below the previous horizontal line (vertical deflection), until the desired number of lines are read. United States standards are based on 60-cycle alternating line current for timing, such that the desired number of horizontal scan lines are achieved in 1/30 sec. This is actually done in two passes: A set of "even lines" is read in 1/60 sec, and a set of "odd lines" is read and "interlaced" with the even lines in 1/60 sec; the resulting set of interlaced "odd" and "even" lines constitutes one full video frame that requires 1/30 sec to read. The resulting set of odd and even, vertically offset, horizontal scans is analogous to one opening and closing of a camera shutter. Thus, one video frame is a snapshot of the charge distribution on the target during a 1/30 sec epoch, which is, in turn, proportional to the photons falling at each point. An important difference with a photographic snapshot is that a video picture is actually made up of the points that were sampled during their fraction of the 1/30 sec. A video picture, thus, is not an instantaneous snapshot in the sense of a camera but is a report of the instantaneous reading of each successively scanned point. The output of the video camera is then typically fed to the input stage of the image processor or image analyzer (Fig.1). This input stage may or may not contain an additional stage of amplification, but its major function is to convert the incoming analogue signals to digital signals.

There are several ways in which the characteristics of the camera can be adjusted to improve the quality of or selectively enhance certain features in the video image. Some characteristics are inherent in the design of the camera and become constraints once the user has selected a certain camera. Probably the two most significant of those characteristics are the size of the camera target or face plate and the physical composition of the target, as these generally set the absolute limits on resolution, sensitivity, and dynamic range of the camera.

A family of general cameras referred to as vidicons enjoy widespread use in video microscopy. These cameras are moderately priced and provide good resolution (600–1000 lines; 1-inch target face), a reasonably broad dynamic range, a γ near 1.0, and a relatively low dark current (1.0 nA). Probably the two most commonly used general cameras are the Chalnicon and Newvicon vidicons. Several manufacturers now provide such cameras as two separate components: the camera tube and associated electronics and a separate control module, which allows the user to modify certain camera operating characteristics; e.g., gain, γ, black level, positive or negative polarity, bandwidth, and aperture. Optimal use of these controls requires an understanding of the camera's electronic characteristics. When optimizing the settings of these externalized controls, it is very useful to have a two- or three-trace oscilloscope to monitor the signal from the TV camera as it is modified by the camera's electronic controls. The oscilloscope does not display the TV image but rather the line scan signal. Typically the horizontal trace of the oscilloscope is synchronized to the horizontal scans of the camera, and the vertical deflection of the oscilloscope trace displays the intensity changes along the horizontal scan. This allows one to assess the degree to which adjusting, e.g., the gain of the camera, influences the amplitude of the composite video signal. Excessive gain increases may cause clipping (saturation) of the highest amplitude (the brightest points in the image) or lowest amplitude (darker points) in the signal. This is readily appreciated in the oscilloscope trace but may not be so obvious when the image is viewed on a video monitor. The same is true for other modifications of the camera electronics; thus, the use of an oscilloscope to monitor the output of the camera is highly recommended.

Optimal adjustment of the camera can significantly enhance microscopic images. This fact was first appreciated and put to excellent use by Allen in a technique that has widely become known as Allen Video Enchanced Contrast (AVEC) microscopy (Allen and Allen, 1983; Allen *et al.*, 1981 a,b). This powerful technique was further developed by Inoue and his collaborators (Inoue, 1986). The technique has many variants, and readers are strongly encouraged to consult the original books and papers on this subject. The basic principle, though, is relatively straightforward. In a phase-contrast image the object of interest has very little inherent contrast; i.e., the object has very limited gray range. The principle used in AVEC is to optimize the range of the camera for the range of gray in the image. First, the black level of the camera is adjusted so that the darkest points in the object of interest approach the lowest output of the camera. Next the gain of camera is increased so that the brightest points in the object just approach the maximum (saturation).

The result of this is that the minimal and maximal outputs of the camera encompass the range of intensities in the interesting parts of the image. As will be described below, one can also achieve a degree of contrast enhancement through image processing by manipulating the assignment of gray values in the digital look-up table. However, this is different from video contrast enhancement because look-up table manipulations create differences between adjacent gray values by separating gray-value assignments; video enhancement creates differences by amplifying the gray-level differences over a limited range of the image gray values. Subsequent to video contrast enhancement, additional image improvement can be obtained with video processing to subtract scattered light not associated with the image plane.

VI. IMAGE PROCESSING

Image processors are devices used to modify a video image with the general goal of improving the detectability or discriminability of selected features in the image. As with most instrumentation the features of the image

Color Figures

Figure 2. Hot-spot and shade correction. A: Pseudocolor image of a blank microscope field to illustrate nonuniform illumination. Microscope lamp has been adjusted to give optimally flat illumination under Kohler conditions. Note that center is most intense (white), and the intensity falls off toward the periphery. B: Same as A, except that a milk-glass filter has been placed between the field diaphram and condenser; this improves the flatness of the illumination. C: Hot spot in A has been corrected by subtraction of blank-field frame (A) from a live image of the blank field. This results in excellent hot-spot improvement, but a small hot spot at center remains because of slight continuous variation in lamp current that is accentuated at the very center of the field. D: Hotspot correction using milk-glass diffuser in B with background subtraction of C. This results in uniform illumination throughout the field. Such conditions are optimal for densitometric measurements.

Figure 3. Analysis of fluorescently labeled neurons using SITCAM, frame averaging, and frame addition. A: Video image of neurons retrogradely labeled by fluorogold using a SIT camera (SITCAM). Note difficulty discerning weakly labeled neurons from camera noise. B: Same image as A after 16-frame average. Note dramatic improvement in detectability of labeled neurons relative to background. C: Techniques in B used to detect and graphically plot immunoreactive neurons labeled with rhodamine (green), fluorogold retrogradely labeled neurons (blue), and double-labeled cells (white) in the nucleus paragigantocellularis (PGi) in the rostral ventrolateral medulla. D: Techniques in B used to detect Rhodabead (red) retrogradely labeled cells (injection in olfactory bulb), fluorogold (blue) retrogradely labeled cells (injections in medial septum), and double-labeled (yellow) cells in the medial anterior olfactory nucleus. Two binary image frames (rhodamine and fluorogold) were added to detect double-labeled cells.

Figure 4. A–G: Look-up table (LUT) transformations. The effect of LUT transformations on an image of immunocytochemically stained neurons. This series of transformations indicates how the detectability of neurons and their processes can be improved or degraded by various standard LUT transformations. Look-up tables illustrated are (A) linear, (B) inverse linear, (C) reciprocal log, (D) reciprocal parabola, (E) parabola, (F) sigmoid, (G) reciprocal sigmoid. H–I: Contrast enhancement. H: Using the image processor contrast enhancement prior to image analyzer LUT. I: A second stage of contrast enhancement using the image analyzer LUT.

Figure 5. Contrast enhancement. A: Video image of Nissl-stained section through the olfactory bulb. B: Same image showing gray-level histogram of only the part of the image that contains the section. Note that histogram in A preferentially reflects the contribution of the area surrounding the section, whereas in B, the histogram shows only the gray levels within the section. C: Contrast enhancement using the gray-level histogram from B. Nissl image is optimally enhanced. D: Contrast enhancement selectively applied only to the right half of the olfactory bulb based on analysis of the gray-level histogram (not shown) of the gray values in the enhanced subregion in the section.

Figure 6. Analysis of intracellular calcium. A–B: Video images of cells loaded with fura-2 under two fluorescence wavelengths. C: Image created by the pixel-by-pixel ratio of images in A and B. This ratio image depicts the intracellular levels and distribution of free Ca^{2+}. D: Pseudocolor applied to image in C to aid visualization of Ca^{2+}. E: Two panels from an experiment showing change in free Ca^{2+} following stimulation of cultured fibroblasts by conditioned media. (These figures courtesy of Dr. Eric Gruenstein, University of Cincinnati Medical Center.)

Figure 7. Gray-level segmentation used to identify immunocytochemically stained neurons. A: Unprocessed video image and gray-level histogram of a field of neurons stained for tyrosine hydroxylase (TH) using ABC–DAB immunocytochemistry. B: Contrast enhancement and look-up table transformations used to selectively enhance neurons in A. C: Gray-level segmentation (see Fig. 8) used to identify neurons. Note that some small background points and the processes of some of the neurons are also detected by the thresholding. D: Object detection after binary operations were used to eliminate small points and to thin, break, and erode dendrites. E: Frequency histogram of neuronal areas (note areas expressed in pixels, not micrometers). F: Bivariate histogram showing X,Y location of each neuron and a bar of height proportional to the area of the neuron (area expressed in pixels).

Figure 9. Pseudocoloring to represent staining density. A: Video image of section through rat lumbar spinal cord stained for cytochrome oxidase. Sciatic nerve on the right side was stimulated intermittently for 20 min. B: Standard rainbow pseudocolor look-up table: white–red, most intense staining; green–blue, least intense. C: Red palate used to create user-defined pseudocolor table. User may select shade of red from any one small rectangle and apply that color to part of the gray scale in the video image. D: User-defined pseudocolor table. Vertical bar at left represents the entire 256 gray scale, darkest at bottom and brightest at top. User-selected colors have been applied to different ranges of gray scale in order to pseudocolor CO-stained section of spinal cord. This color table is entirely arbitrary but could be given a name, stored in memory, and recalled for use in future analysis.

Figure 13. Use of N-ALYSIS (MARS) to create 3-D wire-frame (A–B) and projection maps (C–D) from series of coronal chartings (E). E: DIGITAL LUCIDA was used to generate a series of chartings such as the one illustrated for a one-in-four series of sections through the medulla showing neurons retrogradely labeled in the regions of nucleus prepositus hypoglossi (PrH; open squares) and nucleus paragigantocellularis (PGi; open triangles) following injection of WGA–HRP into nucleus locus coeruleus. A–B: Pseudo-3-D wire-frame representation of neurons distributed in PrH (A) and PGi (B) in a rostral-to-caudal series of sections plotted as in bottom charting. Data from individual chartings were used by MARS program to generate wire frames as described in text. C–D: Same data in A–B were used to create scale projection maps of the distribution of neurons in PrH (red triangles) and PGi (green open squares) as they would appear viewing the medulla from the top (C, horizontal projection map) and side (D, sagittal projection map). Note how projection maps provide a useful depiction of the way the two neuronal populations are distributed in the medulla.

Figure 14. Use of N-ALYSIS to analyze cholinergic receptors in olfactory bulb. A: Darkfield video image of distribution of α-bungarotoxin (α-BTX) binding sites in rat olfactory bulb. B: Conventional pseudocoloring used to color code receptor densities in A. C: Use of N-ALYSIS (ISOMETRIC) to depict receptor density distributions as a color-coded elevation map. Horizontal white line through flat color map (upper left) is used to generate a profile analysis (upper right) cutting across the olfactory bulb. D. Use of N-ALYSIS (PROFILE ANALYSIS) to analyze α-BTX (upper panel) and QNB (lower panel) binding in rat olfactory bulb. Profile analysis in right-hand panel is used to demonstrate segregation of putative nicotinic (top) and muscarinic (bottom) binding in nonoverlapping laminae of the olfactory bulb.

Figure 15. Use of N-ALYSIS to analyze density distribution of neurotensinergic fibers in rat midbrain periaqueductal gray (PAG). A: Use of N-ALYSIS (MICRODENSITOMETER) to measure density of stained fibers in different subregions of PAG. Small square "probes" (yellow) were placed in various loci of the enhanced video image of sections through PAG stained for NT-IR fibers. For each "probe" the relative density is printed directly on the screen. Large rectangle in right-hand part of PAG shows measured density in a region devoid of fibers to measure "background." B: Use of N-ALYSIS (ISOMETRIC) to depict density of NT fibers. Analysis similar to that in Fig. 14C. C: Use of N-ALYSIS (KONTOURS) to represent the densities of NT fibers in PAG. Note similarity to A and B upper left color map. In this black-and-white representation the measured densities were for entire areas and are corrected for background.

Figure 16. Use of N-ALYSIS (IN SITU) to analyze mRNA expression in cortical neurons. A: Video image of toludine-blue-stained neurons in cerebral cortex. Selective chromatic filtering and contrast enhancement were used to increase contrast of neuronal cell body staining. B: Same image as A. Selective chromatic filtering and contrast enhancement were used to filter out toludine blue and to enhance silver grains associated with *in situ* hybridization binding of antisense mRNA to the enzyme HMGCoA reductase. C: Image in A used to generate binary mask of all neurons (blue outline). Grains (red) are being detected on a cell-by-cell basis using gray-level segmentation (slider to right). D: Segmentation analysis complete, program now pauses to allow any user-defined editing. E: Analysis completed and edited for field illustrated. Neurons shown in dark blue, and grains in magenta. F: Correlation of neuronal area (abscissa) versus grain density (ordinate). Analysis indicates that in unperturbed state there is a modest correlation between neuron size and mRNA for HMGCoA, the rate-limiting enzyme for cholesterol synthesis. Cholesterol is essential to membrane formation. In this analysis there was no correction for cells cut off center.

Figure 17. Use of N-ALYSIS (MOVIE) to analyze voltage-sensitive dyes. A: Series of pseudocolored frames of frog taste papilla loaded with voltage-sensitive dye (RH 414) and stimulated with sucrose. B: Pre- and poststimulus comparison. Left frame is dye intensity prior to sucrose administration to both; right frame taken 1 sec after sucrose applied. In this analysis, the left frame is kept constant in the display, and the user steps one at a time through frames after the stimulus so that pre- and poststimulus dye intensity can be directly compared. C: Graphic analysis of changes in dye intensity in center of papilla (white outline in image frame). Graph below plots integrated intensity on a frame-by-frame basis. Note three inflections indicating response of papilla to stimulation.

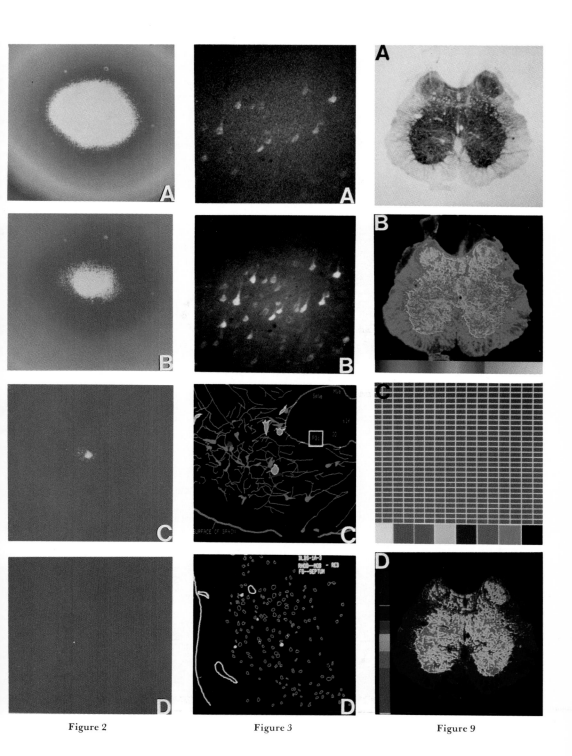

Figure 2

Figure 3

Figure 9

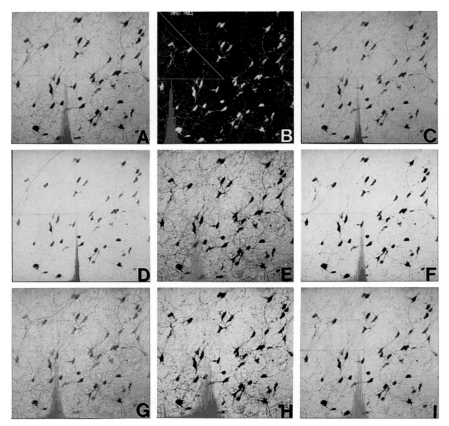

Figure 4

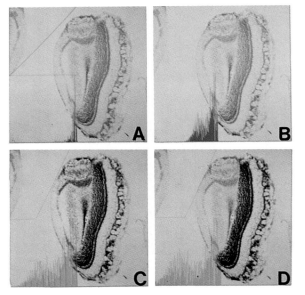

Figure 5

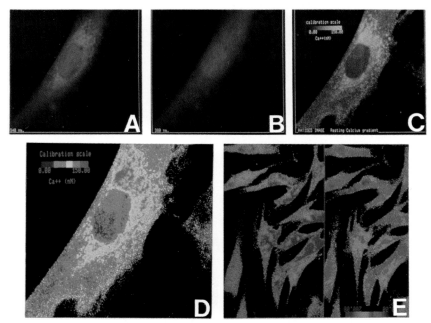

Figure 6

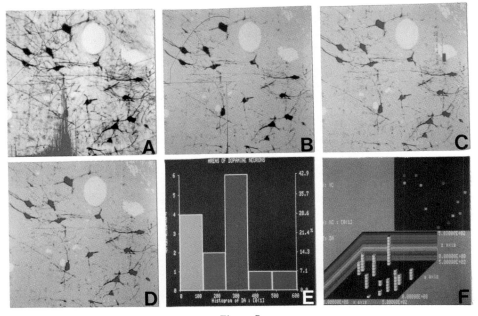

Figure 7

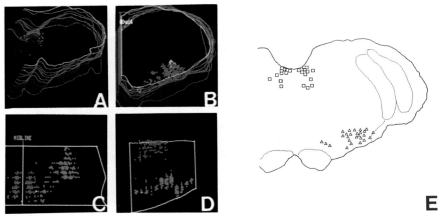

Figure 13

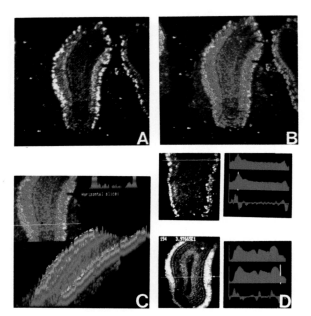

Figure 14

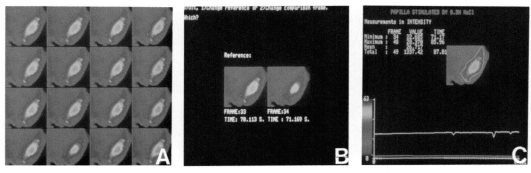

Figure 17

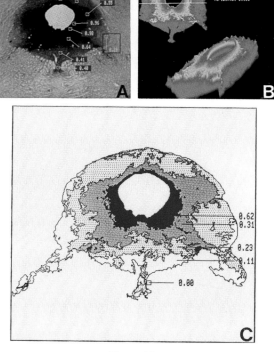

Figure 15

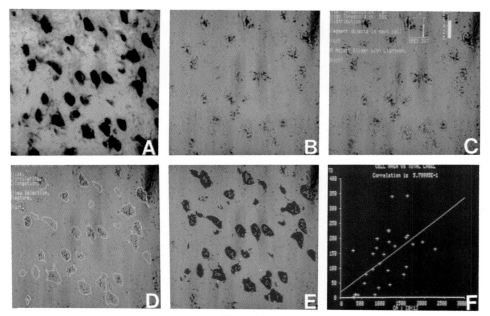

Figure 16

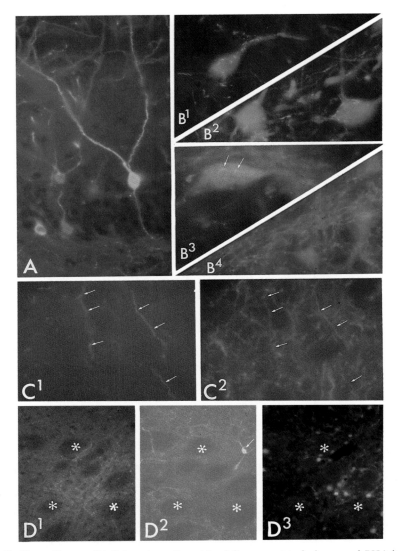

Figure 7. (From Chapter 3.) Color plate of combined fluorescent techniques and PHA-labeling. (A) Dentate granule cell labeled with PHA-L shows dendritic arborization and the axon labeled with an indirect immunofluorescence method. (B¹ and B²) PHA-L-labeled afferents (labeled green with FITC) with boutons in close apposition to true-blue-labeled substantia nigra neurons that project to the superior colliculus. The afferents, which originate in the contralateral hypothalamus, appear to make contact with the perikarya of nigrotectal neurons. (B³) PHA-L-labeled striatonigral afferent fiber (labeled green with FITC) draped across a TH-positive nigrostriatal neuron (labeled red with TRITC). Varicosities of the labeled fiber are in apparent contact with the cell body (arrow). This, however, can be verified only with the electron microscope. (B¹) PHA-L-labeled striatonigral afferents (labeled green with FITC) distributed among true-blue-containing substantia nigra pars reticulata neurons labeled by retrograde axonal transport after dye injections into the superior colliculus. (C¹ and C²) PHA-L-labeled nigrostriatal fibers (labeled red with TRITC in C¹) are shown to be dopaminergic by colabeling with TH immunoreactivity (labeled green with FITC in C²). (D¹–D³) PHA-L-labeled afferents from the prelimbic cortex (labeled green with FITC in D¹) distributed to a patch in the striatum. Somatostatin immunoreactivity (labeled red with TRITC in D²) in the same field as in D¹, showing the distribution of fibers in the striatal matrix compartment complementary to the patch into which the prelimbic cortical afferents are distributed. A single somatostatin immunoreactive neuron is located at the boundary between the patch and matrix and extends a dendrite into the patch, although its local axon collaterals are distributed in the surrounding matrix. Striatonigral projection neurons (D³) retrogradely filled from a fast blue injection in the substantia nigra pars compacta are located in the patch that receives prelimbic inputs.

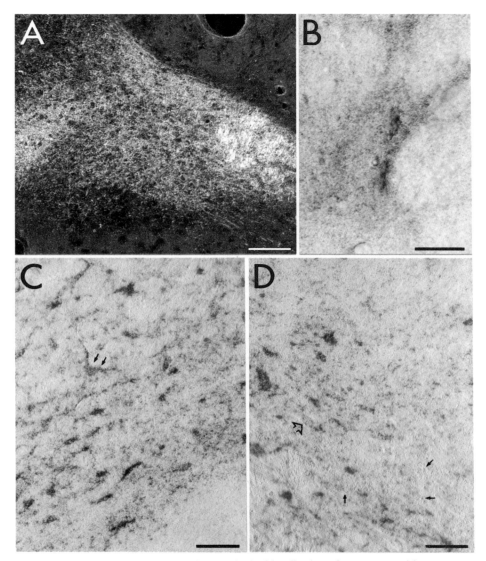

Figure 3. (From Chapter 5.) Light microscopic dual localization of transport and immunocyto-chemical labeling. A: Darkfield photomicrograph showing the autoradiographic labeling for anterogradely transported [³H]-amino acids in the medial nucleus of the solitary tract combined with PAP labeling for tyrosine hydroxylase. Amino acids were injected in the nodose ganglion 24 hr prior to sacrifice. B: Brightfield photomicrograph showing retrograde transport of HRP (brown) in neuronal perikarya of the intermediolateral column of the thoracic spinal cord com-bined with immunoautoradiographic labeling for substance P. Cervical sympathetic nerve was dipped in HRP 24 hr prior to sacrifice. C: Brightfield photomicrograph showing the retrograde transport of WGA–HRP (brown) and immunoautoradiographic labeling for TH in the ventral tegmental area 24 hr after injection of the tracer in the nucleus accumbens (black). Perikarya with only TH (single arrow) and both TH and HRP (double arrows) are evident. D: Brightfield photomicrograph showing the anterograde transport of WGA–HRP in the medial substantia nigra 24 hr following injection of the tracer in the nucleus accumbens. The anterogradely la-beled processes (small arrows) are easily distinguished from the retrogradely labeled perikarya (open arrow) and from the black silver grains indicating immunoautoradiographic labeling for TH. The autoradiographic exposure period for A was 1 month; for B–D, it was 1 week. Bar in A, 100 μm; in B–D, 50 μm.

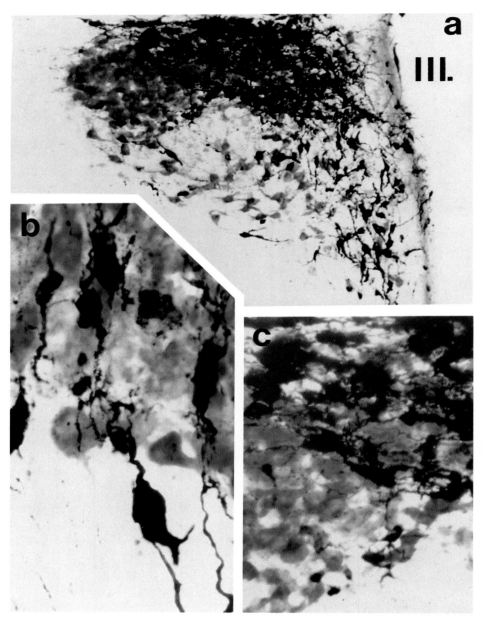

Figure 9. (From Chapter 6.) Low- (panel a) and high-power (panels b and c) color light micrographs taken from the rat paraventricular nucleus immunostained for vasopressin and CRF using the silver-intensified DAB–unintensified DAB double-immunostaining technique. The black, silver-intensified DAB-immunolabeled CRF neurons are well contrasted from the brown, single DAB-immunolabeled vasopressin neurons. (Courtesy of Dr. T. Görcs.)

processor chosen will be dictated by two primal forces: needs and budget. Here, we will describe the image processor functions we have found useful in cell and neurobiological applications using a stand-alone image-processing module (Hughes Model 794). Our image processor is a hard-wired device. It offers several useful functions that can be selected but not modified; i.e., it is not a programmable device. Its advantages include cost (cheaper than programmable systems), ease of use, and speed of operation. Its disadvantages are that its image-processing functions are fixed. In our overall system this disadvantage is offset by the fact that our image analysis system is entirely software driven and includes image-processing functions that are modifiable in software. Thus, an initial level of image processing is achieved with the fast, simple, fixed-function image processor device, and, if needed, subsequent user-defined image processing is done (although at slower speed) with the image analysis computer.

New programmable image-processing systems have proliferated in recent years and offer speed and flexibility. Typically, these systems comprise a set of customized (more or less special purpose) boards or modules that function in the environment of a host computer. Systems operating under a PC host (micro- and minicomputers) are available. Two important considerations, therefore, are the host computers that are supported by the image-processing system and the operating systems and programming languages that can be used with that host. The speed of host–image-processing system interactions and the nature of the image-processing programming language are important factors. The host computers usually run under an operating system such as UNIX, MS-DOS, or OS/2, and control of the image processer systems is done by running programs written in high-level language such as C, PASCAL, or FORTRAN. In general, FORTRAN is a less satisfactory image-processing/image-analysis language, but, because of its widespread use in other scientific applications, it has been used in some image-processing/image analysis systems; C is a much better language for many image-processing/image-analysis functions, and PASCAL also has a number of advantages. Data flow and control between the host computer and the processing boards usually flow through an interface that links through the host computer's bus. In some applications where speed is critical, it is sometimes useful to develop low-level routines written in assembly language (of the host computer). Some systems have provisions for microprogramming the hardware so that programs can be developed with additional speed in processing or analysis of images.

There is a very wide range of image-processing functions. To discuss these exhaustively or to discuss even a few in great detail is beyond the scope of this chapter. Here we will focus on a few broad categories of image-processing functions, concentrating on those that we have found to be useful in neuroanatomical applications. Clearly, that limits the discussion to the functions available in our system, and no claim is made that these are the only functions that might be useful. A general comment about image processing, especially in neuroanatomical applications, is that the selection of the image-processing functions that will optimize the detection of specific features in neuroanatomical images is largely an empirical matter. After almost 5 years of experience in image-processing/image-analysis applications, this laboratory has developed a sense for which image-processing functions are likely to produce useful results in certain kinds of applications. But this is still, for us, more of an art form than an exact science. This may reflect our failure to appreciate the relationship between image-processing theory and the characteristics of the images we work with, but I suspect we are not alone in feeling that you develop image-processing strategies by trial and error. Since at least some trial and error is necessary, it should be obvious that the speed and ease of execution and revision of a set of of image-processing functions is one of the most critical factors in devising an optimal routine for a given class of images. If it takes an inordinate amount of time to set up or execute a new function or to undo previous functions, one will try fewer variants. Therefore, when selecting an image-processing system, one should critically compare how long it takes to change parameters, chain together different functions, and undo previous steps.

A. Image-Processing Functions

In our experience, the most useful image-processing functions are contrast enhancement, contrast inversion, a few commonly used γ functions, frame averaging/integrating and frame arithmetic. With our processor system these are done at frame rate with direct analogue controls.

We will distinguish three classes of image-processing functions (1) look-up table transformations, (2) gray level operations, and (3) multiframe functions. Look-up table functions refer to the mathematical transformations used to convert analogue gray values coming in to the gray values going out. Gray-level transformations are operations that are applied uniformly to each pixel in the output image. Look-up table functions and gray-level transformations are operations that are done to a single frame or on a frame-by-frame basis. Multiframe functions are transformations that are the result of arithmetic operations involving two or more frames, e.g., subtracting one frame from another and displaying the difference image. These are among the most useful image-processing functions. To appreciate how look-up table functions work, it is useful to discuss the relationship among video cameras and output signals and digitation.

B. Digitation of Video Signals

The video signal is continuously varying analogue voltage, the amplitude of which is proportional to the intensity of light hitting the camera face plate. Because cameras have a limited gray-level range (dynamic range), it is clear the highest and lowest amplitudes represent the limits of the camera's range. The initial stage in image processing is to digitize the analogue video signal, i.e., to convert the continuously varying video amplitude signal into a set of discrete digital values using an analogue-to-digital converter (A/D converter). The two major characteristics of an A/D converter are its speed (how many times/sec it can sample the analogue signal) and its gray-level resolution. These factors determine the pixel or spatial resolution of the conversion and the smallest differences of amplitude that can be distinguished. The gray-level resolution of an ADC is measured in bits. An eight-bit A/D converter, for example, can divide the full range of analogue amplitude signals from the video camera into 256 discrete gray values. Thus, if the analogue output of the camera accurately resolves 512 gray levels and the ADC digitizes this at eight-bit resolution (256 gray levels), then the ADC would limit the number of gray values that could be distinguished in the digitized image. Vidicon cameras, however, generally can only resolve between six and seven bits of gray value from noise; SITCAMs at four to five bits, are even worse. Since most image-processing/analysis systems today have eight-bit ADCs, the gray-level resolution in most image-processing/image-analysis systems is usually, therefore, limited by the camera. Increasing the gray-level resolution beyond that of the camera provides no useful improvement in dynamic range and is much the same as the empty magnification (i.e., no gain in resolution) one obtains by placing a fixed positive magnifying lens between the object and the eyepiece of a microscope. This point is stressed because vendors sometimes make the resolution of the ADC a big selling point when, in fact, depending on the cameras that will be used and the requirements of the problem, it may not be important. Some new solid-state cameras offer much higher gray-level resolution than vacuum-tube cameras, and A/D converter resolution should be matched to their resolution.

C. Look-up Table Functions

Look-up tables are the mathematical functions used to assign amplitudes in the video signal to gray values in the output signals. The name look-up table derives from the nature of the operation: the amplitude of the analogue signal is measured, and then, by consulting ("looking up") a table of values, the digitizer assigns a gray value to that point in the image. In the case of an eight-bit ADC, the lowest amplitude is assigned a value of zero, and the highest amplitude output of the video camera is assigned 255; all amplitude (intensity) values are assigned intermediate gray values in a linear fashion. This would be a linear look-up table. In a linear look-up table the gray value assignment is determined by multiplying each amplitude measured by the same constant. At this stage it would seem obvious that a linear look-up table would result in a digitized image in which the differences between gray values in the digital image would be proportional to the intensity differences in the image. However, this is generally not true. The reason is that the input (light intensity)–output (voltage amplitude) transfer function of most video cameras generally is not linear; i.e., equal intensity differences across the intensity range do not cause equal differences in the camera voltage output. The function relating equal intensity increments to voltage output for a given camera is called the γ for that camera. Clearly, therefore, a simple linear look-up table would essentially maintain the non-linearity of the camera. This could lead to errors of measurement, for example, if one were measuring the difference in staining intensity of different objects in the image, because equal differences in staining density will not be represented by equal gray-level differences in the digital image. The most common solution to this problem is to devise a look-up table that linearizes the output of the camera and let this camera-corrected look-up table be the linear look-up table. In fact, in most image-analysis systems a camera-corrected linear look-up table is the initial (default) look-up table (Fig. 4A), unless the user specifically chooses another look-up table. The inverse linear table is essentially the negative image of the linear table; dark objects are assigned high (bright) gray values, and bright objects become dark. This works until the user decides to use a different camera. Then a linearizing look-up table for that camera must be developed and used with that camera. It is not hard to do this in a system that is software based because one need only calibrate the camera image-processing/image-analysis ADC throughput with a standard (usually a set of neutral-density filters or a slide with calibrated neutral-density increments). By reading the outputs for equal incremental inputs one can construct an input/output (I/O) curve; a look-up table that is the reciprocal of this I/O curve will linearize the new camera (all of this, of course, assumes that the A/D converter is both linear and constant, but this can be calibrated and corrected for as well).

Assuming that the camera and A/D converter are linearized, enhancement of some images may be achieved by using a non-linear look-up table. For example, a commonly used alternative to the linear look-up table is the log function in which assignment of gray values from the video analogue signal is made by a log function rather than by multiplying by a constant. As can be seen in Fig.4C, with the reciprocal log function the gray-value assignments for equal intensity in the low-intensity range also results in a greater gray-value separation in the digital image, and the gray-level assignments for equal increments in the high-intensity range also result in smaller gray-level differences. Thus, if the features to be detected are dark objects against a light background (e.g., Nissl- or DAB-stained neurons), the use of a reciprocal log (Fig. 4C) look-up table will result in more resolvable differences among the dark objects. The log look-up table will have the opposite effect and will preferentially enhance bright objects in a dark field. Four other useful LUTs are the parabola/reciprocal parabola (Fig. 4D,E) and the sigmoid and reciprocal sigmoid function (Fig. 4F,G). As shown in Fig. 4, these functions preferentially enhance grays at the low and high ends of the scale and reduce the contrast of grays in the midgray range or preferentially enhance grays in the middle relative to the high and low ends.

For the kinds of look-up tables described so far, it is fairly easy to appreciate what effect the look-up table will have on the transformed image. However, look-up tables can be devised in which the resulting tranformation is not so intuitive. A useful technique for assessing the results of any look-up table tranformation is the gray-level histogram (GLH). In a gray-level histogram the abscissa is a scale of all the possible gray values the image-processing/image-analysis system can represent; in an eight-bit system the abscissa of the gray-level histogram runs from 0 (black) to 255 (white), i.e., has 256 bins. The ordinate of the gray-level histogram represents the number of pixels in the image at each gray level. For example, in the gray-level histogram of a uniformly black image, there would be one vertical bar in the 0 bin and no vertical bars in other bins; a uniformally white image would have a single vertical bar in the 255th bin; in the GLH of an image in which all gray levels from black to white were equally represented, all bins would have vertical bars of the same height. With a little experience, one can visualize and fairly quickly identify the part of the histogram that contains the gray values of the objects of interest. For example, if one looks at the gray-level histogram of a field of darkly stained cells against a light background, there will be a bimodal distribution (Fig. 4A,B). the distribution at the low end represents the cells, and a second distribution at the high end represents the background. With a stain that gives continuous variation, e.g., cytochrome oxidase, this histogram will be broader and may contain several distinct small peaks corresponding to regions with greater or lesser cytochrome oxidase staining intensity. Figure 4 illustrates how the gray-level histograms change as the result of modifying the look-up table.

The look-up tables discussed earlier were similar to each other in one important respect. The transformation was applied to each gray level in the scale. Thus, the entire range of the gray-level scale was preserved, and the look-up tables either multiplied each intensity level by a constant to arrive at its gray-level assignment or multiplied each intensity by some function such that the gray-level assignment for each intensity was weighted in some way. All intensities in the input signal are still represented in the output signal; no intensities were thrown out. However, significant contrast enhancement can be achieved by ignoring parts of the intensity range. If the objects of interest are, for example, dark cells on a light background, the information in the background is probably inconsequential. In this case one can use a look-up table that is, e.g., linear over the range of intensities encompassing the stained cells but throw out the gray-level differences in the background, i.e., assign all intensities above a certain level to the highest gray-level bin and then spread the remaining lower intensities over all the rest of the gray-level bins. In this way small differences in intensities are assigned gray-levels that are more widely separated; i.e., the contrast between adjacent intensities is enhanced. Here it is very important to note that intensity differences themselves have not changed; rather, the gray levels assigned to them are spread apart so that they can be more easily appreciated in the display.

It is likewise essential at this point to recognize that one has corrupted the data in terms of making density measurements. Contrast enhancement achieved by stretching a given range of intensities to extend over the entire usable gray-range scale (Fig. 5C) will lump certain close intensities together and provide a relative separation of them on the gray-level scale from other intensities. This is how enhancement is achieved. However, this changes the relationship between the gray levels of any two points in the image and, hence, the measured density differences of those points. The situation is similar to contrast in a photographic print. If a negative is printed on high-contrast paper, certain features in the scene are enhanced relative to others, but this is at the expense of the continuous gray tones that may have been present in the negative. There are several ways to deal with this problem. Usually, contrast enhancement is used to improve the detectability of certain features in an image, to make them stand out. Frequently this is done so that the features can be selected for measurements. For most geometric measurements contrast enhancement will not significantly distort the data; the potential problem arises, as we have seen, with density measurements. Now, in many image-processing/image-analysis systems, one can store the original unenhanced image and then create a second enhanced gray image. This enhanced image can be used to create a mask for selecting objects to be measured. The mask is essentially a binary overlay (a one-bit, one-color image superimposed on the gray image) that is used to identify the pixel subsets that are to be measured from within the entire image. One way, therefore, to deal with the enhancement–density problem is to use the enhanced image to create an object mask and then use the mask to extract the desired density information from the original image.

Another solution is to run the video image through an initial processor and obtain a gray-level histogram in the second-stage image-processing/image-analysis system using the gain setting in the initial image processor. The gray-level histogram is centered in the gray-level range of the second system. Next, contrast enhancement is performed in the initial processor. When the processed image is digitized using a look-up table in the second processor, there are no gaps in the gray-level scale (Figs. 4H,I and 5B). This separates the gray levels, but so long as the measured density information is compared to density information from images processed identically, then the ratios of the gray levels can be used to compare relative densities. If a density standard is used, for example, a radiolabeled microscale, and if the microscale is measured under identical conditions of illumination and enhancement, then the densities in the enhanced image can be directly calibrated from steps on the scale. More will be said later about density measurements; the key point here is that look-up table transformations can significantly influence density measurements. Unless the effect of the look-up table is recognized, it can lead to erroneous conclusions about the interpretation of different staining densities. Look-up tables are, however, one of the most valuable tools in image-processing/image analysis and can be used to achieve truly remarkable degrees of image enhancement. The gray-level histogram is an equally important and valuable tool for assessing the distribution of gray-levels in the image, suggesting potentially useful tables, and assessing the results of using a given look-up table. Most image-processing/image-analysis systems today are provided with preselected look-up tables, and some systems allow the user to devise custom look-up tables.

In most systems the tables and gray-level histograms apply to the entire image. In neurobiology, this if often unsatisfactory because a typical image may contain many pixels that are biologically uninteresting. For example, to visualize a given brain region at optimal magnification, a considerable fraction of the total image may lack tissue, or only a small part of the section may contain the label of interest. In such cases the gray-level histogram of the entire image will be more a reflection of the background than of the interesting part of the image. To deal with such cases (which tend to be the rule rather than the exception), we have developed programs that allow the user to delineate an arbitrary subregion of the image with a light pen and view the gray-level histogram for that region only (Fig. 5A–D). This greatly facilitates the selection of an appropriate look-up table to enhance optimally the region of interest. The look-up table is applied over the entire image, and, in our system, the look-up table is continuously applied to the live video image so that the desired image enhancement is retained at different focal planes or as one moves the microscope stage to view other parts of the field or other sections. A further refinement is to apply different look-up tables to different subregions of the same image. This technique allows selective local enhancement of different subregions in the same image but can only be done on a captured (digitized or stored) image and not on a live image (Fig. 5D). The ability to view the gray-level histogram of a local arbitrary region and to define look-up tables based on that histogram has, in our experience, proven to be an extremely powerful way to obtain optimal image enhancement in the complex images that are typical in neuroanatomy.

D. Frame Averaging/Integration

A very useful function in image processing is the ability to average or integrate multiple frames. For example, SITCAMs can be used to image very weakly fluorescent cells or reduce the illumination level to prolong the life of the fluorochrome. As noted earlier, however SITCAMs have an appreciable amount of noise. Thus, if one grabs a single frame there are likely to be regions in the image with, for example, very light pixels in regions of the image that are actually dark. In such cases averaging a few frames will be of great benefit. The camera noise will fluctuate from point to point randomly in the single frames. If several frames are averaged, the random fluctuations at each point average out. Since the fluorescent objects have a higher frame-to-frame average signal, the result of averaging will be to enhance the signal (fluorescent cell/fiber) relative to the random noise. (Any nonspecific fluorescence in the preparation will also be enhanced, as it will remain constant from frame to frame.) In our system, look-up table transformations may be applied to the averaged image so that a further degree of contrast enhancement is achieved (Fig. 3A,B).

As with many of the aforementioned image-processing techniques, averaging is not without its potential pitfalls and trade-offs. Most fluorochromes undergo some degree of fading under continuous illumination, and frame averaging involves prolonged exposure of the preparation to illumination; thus, there is some trade-off between signal-to-noise improvement and signal loss from fading. In general, the decay of fluorescent fading is probably not linear and may vary with section thickness, mounting medium, and the procedures used to achieve the fluorescent tagging, such as direct or indirect immunofluorescence, ratio of fluorochrome to secondary antibody, and the fluorochrome itself. Thus, although averaging can dramatically improve the detectability of labeled elements, its use may impact on subsequent analysis of density (fluorescence intensity) differences. However, in many neuroanatomical applications (e.g., double-label immunofluoresence and/or fluorescent tracers), only 6–12 frames of averaging produces great improvement of signal to noise and the time required to grab so few frames is generally inconsequential. Averaging techniques, thus, are very useful in double-label studies and for enhancing the detectability of weakly fluorescent signals such as those associated with some monoclonal antibodies or antibodies to cell surface molecules.

E. Addition and Subtraction of Images

Another useful set of multiframe techniques involves adding or subtracting two or more frames to create a sum or difference image. For example, suppose one wanted to compare the spatial distributions of two different cell populations or two different labels in a certain brain structure. One could stain alternate serial thin sections with different antibodies and use image analysis to map the locations of each separately, then compare the two maps. An alternative that can be used if the two sets of sections do not differ significantly in terms of shrinkage would be to frame-grab the section containing the first label, use landmarks in that image to precisely align the section containing the second label, and then add the two frames to create a composite image of the two sections. Provided the two markers do not overlap appreciably, such a technique would allow one directly to compare the two distributions. If the labeled objects are close together, and/or if the sections are too thick, then the composite may obscure the two distributions, but in many cases adding the images of adjacent sections can provide useful information.

Taking the difference between two frames also has useful applications. In a difference image only the pixels that are different in two images will be displayed when one image is subtracted from the other. The utility of this becomes obvious from a few examples. Frequently it is not possible to correct the microscope for nonuniformity in optics or illumination. Frame subtraction can often be used to help correct such problems. Fluorescent illumination frequently results in a "hot spot"; i.e., the illumination is more intense in the center than the periphery of a section. Fluorescently labeled cells in the center of the image may be "saturated" while cells in the periphery appear to be more weakly fluorescent. By taking one frame in a part of the section that is devoid of labeled cells but has uniform background fluorescence and the "hot spot" and then subtracting this frame from the frame of the field that contains the labeled cells, one can minimize the "hot spot" because it is common to the two frames while retaining the labeled cells, which are present only in the second frame. In our image processor it is possible to store the background frame and continuously subtract it from the ongoing frame so that the hot spot is automatically subtracted as one scans different parts of the field. In fact, the operations described are slightly more complicated, as it may be necessary to rescale the gray values in the difference image. But this can be done with hardware or software in our systems.

Another use of difference images is to look at changes in an image across time. If one is looking at growth cones in cultured cells, one can use difference images to analyze the parts of the growth cone that move during a given time interval. By analogy with the "hot spot" problem discussed above, the parts of the image that do not move will not be seen in the difference image, whereas the parts of the image that do move will be seen.

Neurobiologists are beginning to use voltage- and ion-sensitive dyes to measure time-varying changes in membrane potential or ion concentration in *in vivo* and *in vitro* preparations. In such cases, the objects do not move in time, but rather their fluorescent intensity changes across time. Frame-difference techniques can be used to pinpoint specific sites of intensity change. There are currently many limitations and pitfalls to the measurements of voltage-sensitive dyes. Many membrane potential changes (e.g., action potentials) are very brief events (1 msec), but it takes 1/30 sec to grab a frame or 1/60 sec to grab the odd or even lines in a frame. This is obviously too slow to record action potentials. One may be able to arrange the experiment so that the stimulus causing the action potentials is varied to occur at different points in time in relation to the onset of the frame sweep and thus build a composite image that captures the average membrane changes. But this is slow and will probably not be the method of choice. Vacuum-tube cameras with much faster frame rates and solid-state CCD cameras that can simultaneously integrate photons in thousands of separate contiguous photodiodes will probably become the optimal way to measure such rapid events. However, many interesting biophysical and ionic events may have slower time courses and may be difficult to measure with ion-sensitive electrodes. In such cases, video frame rates may not be limiting, and the advantages afforded by measuring many such events simultaneously in a large two-dimensional area may make video image processing/image analysis the method of choice.

Multiframe manipulations are not limited to addition and subtraction. It is also possible to take the ratio of two images, i.e., to divide one image by the other. Such techniques are being used, for example, with dyes that change the wavelength of their fluorescence when they bind Ca^{2+}. One frame is grabbed and stored under one filter set; then another frame is grabbed and stored using a second filter set. The ratio of the two frames creates a third frame that displays the spatial distribution of the free Ca^{2+} (Fig. 6).

Multiframe operations require that the two images to be added, subtracted, or ratioed be in perfect spatial register, because the arithmetic is done on a pixel-by-pixel basis. If one image is shifted relative to the other, then the appropriate pixels will not correspond in the resulting image. Therefore, it is essential that the specimen not move during the time it takes to capture the two frames. Physical stability of the specimen relative to the video camera is therefore critical. At high optical magnification, sources of specimen movement are numerous, so special care must be taken to ensure stability. If one wishes to add, subtract, or ratio the same image under different fluorescent filter conditions, it is necessary to ensure that there is no optical shift at the two wavelengths. One way to do this is to compensate physically by aligning the two filter sets so that there is no displacement. This is difficult, expensive, and requires that the two filters always be used in the same holder. Another solution is to use software routines to move the microscope stage to compensate for the optical displacement. The important thing is to identify factors that can cause image misalignment and take appropriate steps to eliminate or compensate so that the misalignment does not cause an error when adding, subtracting, or ratioing successive frames.

F. Gray-Image Operations: Contrast Enhancement

Look-up table manipulation and multiframe operations, when used correctly, can significantly improve the detectability of objects of interest. Many image-analysis systems also provide the user with additional operations that can be performed on digitized gray images. Generally, these are mathematical operations that are applied uniformly to each pixel in the image; such functions are called gray-image operators. Some gray-image operators are intended to filter out small sets of pixels that differ in gray value from the majority of pixels in the immediate neighborhood and are called smoothing filters. For example, a mean smoothing filter looks at each pixel in the image, takes the mean of that pixel and its nearest neighbors, and changes the gray value of that pixel to the mean. By doing this successively to each pixel in the image, regions of small gray-value deviations are smoothed out. Such operations are useful for image-analysis applications where relatively large objects or regions are sought in a grainy background. Sometimes autoradiographs have local variations in grain density that may be attributable to artifact, and these can be improved by smoothing filters, but unless one is fairly certain that the irregularities in the image are not biologically significant, it may be best to avoid smoothing because the resulting image may look nice but be corrupted. Another class of gray-image operator does the opposite of smoothing; such convolutions sample neighborhoods of pixels and apply a function that tends to emphasize contrast differences of small regions. These filters are generally known as edge or contrast filters, but the authors have found such operations to be of limited utility in neuroanatomical material. The fact that this laboratory has not found smoothing and edge filters particularly useful may be because neuroanatomical images are too complex for such filters or that we have not had the patience or insight to use them to advantage. As noted earlier, much of image processing and image analysis is still empirical; one tends in the beginning to try many kinds of operations and eventually converges on certain kinds of operations that work for one's application.

VII. IMAGE ANALYSIS

Through a combination of appropriate optics, illuminations, filters, camera adjustments, and image-processing operations, one generally achieves a considerable improvement in image quality and/or a selective enhancement of certain classes of objects in the image. The degree of enhancement may not represent the best one could get, as there are few rules or criteria for assessing what is ideal enhancement. The criterion that we use is whether the objects of interest are sufficiently detectable that one can now move to the next step of analyzing the material. As noted earlier, this is the point at which, according to our practical definition, one moves from image processing to image analysis.

Generally, in image analysis one uses a series of operations to define a subset of the objects in the image whose features one wishes to measure and/ or chart for a reconstruction. The identification results in a "binary mask." This is essentially a one-bit-deep image that is typically superimposed as a colored template on top of the gray image so that one can directly visualize whether all the desired objects and only the desired objects have been identified. The binary mask then serves to identify the X and Y locations of all the points (pixels) in the image that will be included in the measurements. Contiguous sets of binary pixels define an object. If two objects partially overlap, the binary map will often define one object, and special binary operators can be used to edit the binary mask. Once the mask is correct the full range of morphometric and densitometric measures can be extracted for the object set.

For example, suppose one has optimally enhanced (image processing) a field of immunocytochemically stained neurons such that all, or the majority of them, are clearly distinguished from the background. Now one wishes to determine how many neurons there are, their size, their shape, e.g., are they roundish or long and skinny, or their density. Such morphological questions can be answered very quickly if the boundaries of each neuron in the field are defined. The usual way to do this is to use contrast differences between the objects and the background by an operation called gray-level thresholding (also called segmentation or slicing).

In the simple case above, suppose that image processing has resulted in an image in which the neurons are very dark and the background is very light (Fig. 7A,B). In thresholding, we define a range of gray values that encompass the object set, telling the computer to identify all the pixel sets that fall within that gray-value range and ignore all the pixels that fall outside the range. To facilitate the determination of gray values to retain, one can observe a gray-level histogram of the image. If there are very dark neurons and a very light background, the histogram will indicate this with two peaks—one in the dark pixel range for the neurons and one in the light pixel range for the background. In our system one can use a slider that is displayed on the monitor (Fig. 7C). The slider ranges from the lowest to the highest gray value represented, and with the light pen one can set the upper and lower limits of the slider so that all pixels in the image that fall within the range indicated by the slider are covered with a colored binary mask (Figs. 7C and 8). Thus, one can directly and rapidly change the upper and lower threshold settings and instantly view, for any given threshold range, which neurons and which nonneuronal pixels would be recognized by that

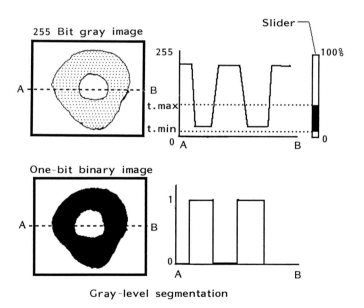

Gray-level segmentation

Figure 8. Gray-level segmentation. Upper panel: At left is the hypothesized gray image of a uniformly dense "donut"-like structure. At the right is the gray-level profile of a line A–B through the image. Dotted lines (t. min and t. max) indicate the low and high boundaries used to segment the gray image. The "slider" at far right is used to adjust t-min/t-max to set the upper and lower thesholds of the segmentation. Lower panel: The one-bit binary overlay (mask) created by the segmentation in upper panel. All of the pixels within the binary mask are taken as an object or feature. Parameters of the object can be calculated by measurement routines in the image analyses.

threshold setting. Alternatively, one can use the light pen to indicate two points on the histogram within which all gray values will be masked.

Once the upper and lower thresholds are appropriately set, all pixels under the mask are potential identified objects. Next, various so-called "binary operators" and interactive light-pen-based editing are used to remove non-neuronal features or to add neurons that were missed (Fig. 7D). "Binary operators" are functions that are used to alter binary images generally for the purpose of making the binary mask conform better to the size, shape, and location of the desired objects in the gray image. Two standard binary operators are erosion and dilation. In erosion, one pixel is removed at each point around the boundary of a binary object. Clearly this is used to reduce a binary mask that exceeds the size of the corresponding gray object. Dilation is the opposite operation and is used to increase the size of the binary object. When two gray objects partially overlap via a thin connection (e.g., two neurons with the dendritic tree of one neuron partially overlapping the cell body of the other neuron), the combined use of erosion followed by dilation can often be used to separate the overlap. Other binary operations include thinning—removing pixels around the border but always leaving a one-pixel bulge to the main mass of the objects; skeletonizing—shrinking the binary down to its one-pixel-wide backbone; and breaking nodes—separating all binary objects that are connected by only one pixel. These latter operations are often useful in fiber-mapping operations. One can also do arithmetic on binary images. Two binary images can be combined by addition, or the objects common to two binary images can be removed or selected by binary image subtraction. Other, more specialized binary operations can be created in software as required.

Binary operators are very useful in optimizing the binary mask, but in many neuroanatomical applications the gray image is too complex to define completely in a binary mask using global binary operators alone, and for this reason most systems provide for interactive editing, whereby the user can remove or add binary features with a device such as a mouse, joystick, or light pen. In our software, to be discussed presently, we have developed fairly sophisticated editing routines so that one can bring thresholding, binary operators, and light-pen-based editing to bear on a given problem in a fast and efficient manner.

Once satisfied that the neurons are defined, the user now chooses measures to be made, and the computer makes the measurements and displays them on the screen or stores them in a data file. The same operations can then be performed and measures taken for successive microscopic fields. Appropriate identifiers can be assigned to the files so that one can keep track of the case, the slide, the section, the antibody used, etc. At the end of a set of measures, statistical information can be obtained from the data in the file (Fig. 7E,F). Software routines allow one to sort the data into subsets, e.g., all neurons larger than 25 μm^2.

In the example given, dark-separated neurons on a low-background field, the analysis was simple and straightforward. In our experience such examples are not in the majority because neuroanatomical material is generally complex. Even in the case of finding immunocytochemically stained neurons, it is seldom possible to select unambiguously all the neurons in a field by gray-level thresholding alone, even with heroic image processing. There are several obstacles. (1) Frequently the background has local variations. The neurons throughout the image are more intensely stained than their local background, but the staining intensity of neurons in one part of the section may be fairly close to the background staining in another part of the section. Thus, the local signal-to-noise ratio of neurons to background may be fairly constant, but there may be enough global variance to cause problems with global gray-level thresholding. In general, algorithms for dealing with local variations in signal-to-noise base line are not yet very efficient. (2) A second problem is that neurons may be so closely clustered that their somata and/or dendritic processes overlap. In this case, gray-level thresholding will result in merging two or more neurons as one object. To the degree that dendrites and/or local axonal processes are well stained, this problem is worse (Fig. 7A). Both of these problems are exacerbated by increased section thickness. Overlap is reduced in thin (5-to-10-μm) sections, but antigen retention and antibody penetration can be a problem with the cryostat-mounted sections; the lower temperature necessary for such thin sections also introduces problems of freeze artifact that can cause loss of antigenicity and/or distortion of cell morphology. Thus, if one wishes to estimate the absolute numbers or proportions of antigenically homogeneous neurons, the use of thin cryostat sections may lead to errors in quantitation. However, comparison of such material with a few stained sections under more optimal conditions (e.g., 30-μm floating sections) can indicate whether there will be significant quantitative errors in the cryostat material. Thus, the processing of the material can sometimes be modified to optimize image analysis. In general, however, we have found that the dictates of the experiment or the reagents constrain the degree to which one can optimize the material. Therefore, we have found it useful to develop software that facilitates a more interactive analysis of neuroanatomical material.

Key features of this software are (1) use of image-processing/enhancement routines that operate on real-time images so that images are continuously enhanced through changing focal planes and across changes in viewing field; (2) routines that allow the delineation of object sets or the reconstruction of objects that are much larger than the field being viewed; (3) routines that allow multiple, independent object sets to be defined so that one can keep track of cells/fibers in different subnuclei or cortical layers; (4) routines that measure densities in arbitrarily defined regions; (5) utilities that keep track of the microscope/lamp conditions used in a given set of density measurements so that identical conditions can be duplicated for similar measures in future experiments; and (6) routines that facilitate use of the light pen for rapid on-screen interactive editing.

The software we have developed is generally useful for charting, measuring objects, and creating neuroanatomical reconstructions of a wide variety of anatomical material. Chartings and reconstructions are printed out in publication-ready format on a laser printer with text, graphics, and quantitative information about the features in the reconstruction. Our software is strictly born out of our needs and the range of complexities and limitations of the kinds of neuroanatomical/neurobiological data we deal with. Thus, the routines are more specialized than those in off-the-shelf image-analysis systems and are doubtless ideosyncratic. The software appears, though, to have proven generally useful to others working on the same kinds of problems.

The organization of this section essentially follows the sequence of our software package NEUROANALYSIS, which has been shortened to N-ALYSIS. N-ALYSIS goes from general procedures such as calibration and image processing through various subprograms developed to deal with specific kinds of neuroanatomical problems. Examples from published and unpublished work are used to illustrate the application of the software. Finally, a few examples from more specialized programs are presented.

A. N-ALYSIS

N-ALYSIS is organized around a series of menus and submenus. At each stage in the program the image being processed or analyzed can be passed forward or backward to other menus in the program. One need not pass through the menus in any particular order; thus, if a specific analysis is to be performed one can go directly to the appropriate menus in the program.

N-ALYSIS *Main Menu*

    CALIBRATION
    VIDEO SETUP
    PSEUDOCOLOR Output Table
        Write/Read Gray-Image(s) to/from
          Disk
        Gray-Level Operators
        Line Gray Profile Analysis
    DIGITAL LUCIDA
        Reconstructions
    ISOMETRIC Plot
    KONTOURS
        Microdensitometer
        Results

1. CALIBRATION

This program contains a set of routines for using an optical micrometer slide to calibrate the dimensions in an image. The user images the micrometer scale, uses the light pen to indicate on the screen two points defining a calibrated distance on the scale, and then types into the computer the actual distances in micrometers between the two points. The computer reckons how many pixels there are between the two points and then calculates the micrometers per pixel. Thus, one can calibrate X and Y distances for the total magnifications of the specimen.

This calibration is called the scale factor for that magnification. If one uses the same set of objectives and intermediate lenses from experiment to experiment, one can calibrate each objective once, store the resulting scale factors in a file, and then, when measurements in the image are made, only tell the computer which objective is being used, and the computer will apply the appropriate scale factor to the measurements taken. In essence, the computer makes all measurements in terms of pixels and then multiplies the pixels by the scale factor for that objective. As will be noted below there is an alternative way of calibrating X and Y distances that does not require keeping track of the objectives being used but rather calibrates with respect to stage motor movements. However, in situations where the same setup is used routinely from experiment to experiment, it is very useful to recall the calibration parameter from a file in the computer at the onset of a given day's analysis. This part of the program also contains provisions for calibrating density measurements.

2. VIDEO SETUP

This program is used directly with the video camera or in conjunction with the image processor. VIDEO SETUP contains a number of routines to modify the LUTs, calibrate the illumination of the microscope, perform shade corrections, apply pseudocolor, etc. VIDEO SETUP operates on live (framerate) images fed directly from the camera or from the image processor. The program is used to optimize microscope setup and image processing for subsequent analysis. The program also contains routines for positioning the stage and adjusting the focus using the light pen and the monitor screen.

With the light pen the user can delineate local regions in the image and examine the gray-level histograms of those regions (Fig. 5). Contrast enhancement with either the image processor or modifications of the video look-up table in the image-analysis computer is used to optimize the contrast of user-defined regions (Figs. 4 and 5). The contrast enhancement appropriate for that region of interest is then uniformly applied to all parts of the live image. The enhancements continue to be applied even if the user repositions the stage or the focus. Thus, if one optimizes the contrast of, e.g., PHA-L-labeled fibers in one part of the specimen, the same contrast enhancement will continue to be applied as one follows the fibers throughout the section plane and thickness. At any point in VIDEO one may digitize the image, "copy" it into memory, and continue with further processing.

On quitting VIDEO, one can store the image in memory and/or retain all of the VIDEO SETUP parameters and move to another part of the N-ALYSIS program so that additional processing/analysis can be done on either the stored image or the same image in real time.

3. PSEUDOCOLOR

The next program in the menu (one need not go through these programs in any set order) is a set of routines that allow the user to define and use any arbitrary pseudocolor look-up table; i.e., the user can assign colors to different gray values or ranges of gray values. A few standard pseudocolor look-up tables are also provided. These standard tables are typical of those used in many processing/image-analysis systems. The darkest grays are assigned shades of blue (darkest blue for darkest gray), followed by green, yellow, orange, and red; white is sometimes assigned to the last gray value on the scale (Fig. 9B). Such "rainbow" pseudocolor tables are useful and intuitive in the sense that the most intensely stained or labeled areas are bright reds/oranges ("hot") and low or nonlabeled areas are blues and greens ("cool").

Sometimes one wishes to assign colors to only certain parts of the gray range, and/or one may wish to lump the gray values in the image into a few ranges. In addition, one may wish to use only a few colors that differ markedly in hue. Standard look-up tables do not easily allow this, so we developed alternative approaches.

In one approach, the light pen and a gray-range slider similar to that described above for gray-level segmentation or thresholding are used to assign colors to ranges of gray values (Fig. 9C,D). The user selects a color, and the color is applied to the gray values in the image that fall within the upper and lower boundaries defined with the light pen using the gray-scale slide. This approach is especially useful in the system that has 256 gray levels. Once the user is satisfied with the "custom" pseudocolor look-up table, the program has a provision for naming and storing that particular look-up table into a memory file so that it can be used with similar experimental material in future applications.

4. DIGITAL LUCIDA

The next program in N-ALYSIS is called DIGITAL LUCIDA. DIGITAL LUCIDA began as a simple program for creating multicolor graphic reconstructions using the video microscope image as a template. The program grew to have increased graphics capabilities and also to allow one selectively to process local regions of a stored gray image and to extract measurements based on drawn and/or segmented regions. It is a kind of video *camera lucida*, morphometrics package all rolled into one, and it is one of our workhorse programs.

With a conventional *camera lucida* the image being viewed in the microscope is generally very dim and fairly difficult to see. In DIGITAL LUCIDA the reconstructions are done on enhanced live video images. In our system the image is viewed on a 26-inch high-resolution monitor. This large monitor makes it very easy to delineate small features with the light pen. As different sets of objects and features are reconstructed, one can change the image processing to markedly and selectively enhance those particular features. For example, one can initially enhance Nissl staining to delineate architectural features and then change the processing to enhance retrogradely labeled or immunocytochemically stained neurons. As noted earlier, the enhancements are applied at frame rate (1/30 sec) so that the image is continuously enhanced throughout changes of focal plane and as the stage is moved. A second critical difference between DIGITAL LUCIDA and a conventional *camera lucida* is that the features in the reconstruction can be simultaneously measured, so that there are quantitative data about the reconstruction. Thus, the reconstruction of neuroanatomical images with DIGITAL LUCIDA is both easier and more accurate because the material is optimally enhanced and the resulting reconstruction yields a quantitative analysis of the features in the reconstruction.

In the graphics portion of the program one can use the light pen to draw selected features in either a live or stored processed image. Different features can be drawn with lines of different colors. In addition, the user can select the thickness of the line and can choose among a solid line, dashes, or a dotted line with different spacing between the dots/dashes. This allows one to create multicolored drawings of neuroanatomical material or to represent features with different kinds of outlines (line thickness; dotted–dashed) (Fig. 3C,D). The features in the image need not always be delineated by the light pen. As noted earlier, one can frequently use thresholding (segmentation) or a combination of thresholding and light-pen interactions to delineate objects. Thus, DIGITAL LUCIDA has thresholding routines in addition to its light-pen mode.

The colored graphics can be photographed on 35-mm slides using a video recorder and used in lectures or to generate color prints for posters or manuscripts (Fig. 3C,D). If one wishes to create a black-and-white line drawing for a manuscript, one can simply create the drawing with lines of one color and indicate different features by varying the thickness or style of line of different shapes and sizes (Fig. 10).

DIGITAL LUCIDA also has icons and text. Thus, one can represent, for example, labeled neurons with squares, circles, or triangles (upright or inverted). The user selects the desired symbol, specifies its size (and color) and then deposits the symbol over each chosen feature (e.g., retrogradely labeled neurons) in the video image. The icons can be open outlines or filled symbols, so that one can represent a large number of different features in the same drawing (see Fig. 13). Additional primitives allow one to create straight lines, arrows, pointers, grids, geometric figures, etc., and text, letters, and numbers so that regions and features can be labeled. The graphics part of

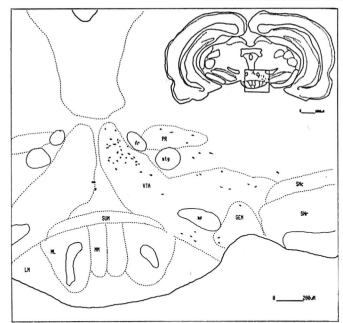

Figure 10. Use of N-ALYSIS (DIGITAL LUCIDA) to chart retrogradely labeled neurons. Upper right-hand corner shows low-power charting created in DIGITAL LUCIDA for purposes of providing ventral midbrain–caudal hypothalamic area (square) charted at higher magnification in the rest of the reconstruction. WGA–HRP injected into nucleus of horizontal limb of the diagonal band. Retrogradely labeled cells are plotted in their precise location; each neuron's size is to scale (5-μm accuracy).

the program also has provisions for creating graphic drawings to summarize anatomic information (Fig. 11A). We have also created an icon for a calibration bar so that one can position a calibration bar of any arbitrary length in any part in the image, and the calibrated length of the bar is automatically calculated and printed on the screen beside the bar (Figs. 10 and 11B). Another set of routines allows one to solidly fill discrete outlined parts in the drawing or to fill regions with dots of various densities (we call this PARA-FILL). This feature is useful for indicating zones of differential terminal labeling. By varying the density of the dots one can graphically illustrate gradients of labeling (see Fig. 15C).

The finished drawings are printed out directly on a laser printer. If high-quality glossy paper or mylar sheets are being used, the resulting printout is suitable as original illustration material for a manuscript; i.e., the printouts do not have to be rephotographed.

Additional utilities allow one to enclose the reconstruction with a frame and to select one of several sizes for the hard-copy printout; multiple reconstructions can be stored in memory and then recalled selectively and placed at any location in the display to create multifield reconstruction montages. Alternatively, one can make a montage from the individual hard copies and

A

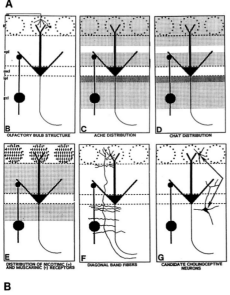

B

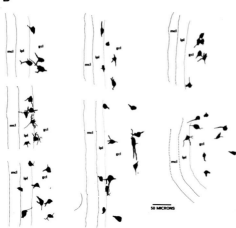

50 MICRONS

Figure 11. Use of N-ALYSIS (DIGITAL LUCIDA) to make schematics (A) and to reconstruct neurons (B). A: Graphics utilities in DIGITAL LUCIDA to create schematic of the organization of cholinergic markers in rat olfactory bulb (M. T. Shipley, unpublished data). B: DIGITAL LU-CIDA used to reconstruct AChE-positive/ChAT-negative neurons in rat olfactory bulb. Reconstructions of neurons in eight different fields illustrate the consistent laminar localization, size, and morphology of candidate cholino-ceptive neurons in rat main olfactory bulb (Nickell and Shipley, 1988).

photograph the ensemble; the advantage to this is that somewhat greater detail can be achieved by plotting each image at the full 512×512 resolution of the image-analysis system. With the advent of 1024×1024 resolution systems, the details of multifield reconstruction will increase fourfold.

In neuroanatomical reconstructions a major problem is accommodating both the resolution and the scope of the image. For example, suppose one wishes to reconstruct the precise distributions of immunocytochemically stained fibers (and measure the fiber lengths) in a fairly large section through the brain. In order to resolve individual fibers with sufficient detail to threshold and/or delineate them accurately, the optical magnification needs to be fairly high, ×40 or greater objective. However, at such optical magnification one can only view a small fraction of the anatomic field on the display at one time because the scope of the image is limited by the field size of the objective. Clearly, one could use DIGITAL LUCIDA, as described above, to sequentially reconstruct a series of contiguous fields, print out each field, and make a montage of the resulting printouts. This would still result in manifold reduction of time and effort compared to making a *camera lucida* drawing, inking the drawing, and making a photographic reduction. Moreover, the reconstruction made with DIGITAL LUCIDA would also compute the total lengths of fibers and/or number of crossings of fibers per unit area or volume of the section.

Although the resolution-versus-scope problem can be overcome by montaging, the number of applications involving this kind of problem led us to develop a modified version of DIGITAL LUCIDA called EXTENDED DIGITAL LUCIDA in which the montage is created directly in the computer's memory as the microscope stage moves sequentially to each successive part of the total field. The complete reconstruction is made only at the end of the mapping (Figs. 10 and 12). EXTENDED DIGITAL LUCIDA also has provisions for moving the stage in a systematic way so as to minimize the number of regions that must be viewed in a high magnification. This is accomplished by first viewing the region at low magnification and using edge-finding routines or the light pen to delineate the overall area of interest. Next, the user determines which optical magnification and which image-processing routines optimally resolve the desired features at higher magnification. Next, at that higher optical magnification, the system's overall magnification is automatically determined by a routine that uses stage movements to calibrate a magnitude scale factor.

In stage movement calibration, the stage is moved by software routines so as to position an arbitrarily chosen object in the image to lie at the center of a cross hair positioned in the lower left corner of the screen; next, the stage controller is used to position the same object in a cross hair in the upper right-hand corner of the screen. The computer then calculates the numbers of X and Y stage motor steps that were required to move the object along the diagonal from the first to the second cross hairs. The pixel distance along the field diagonal is fixed, and now the system knows how many micrometers the stage moved to position the specimen from the first to the second cross hair. The Pythagorean formula is used to compute the micrometers per pixel and thus the overall calibrated magnification.

Next, the system reckons how many such high-magnification frames will be required to encompass the region delineated in the initial low-magnification view and then moves the stage to the first region. The thresholding and/or the light pen is used to make a binary reconstruction of that part of the field. When the first field has been reconstructed, the system moves the stage so that the next part of the field is viewed. All previously chosen image enhancements are automatically applied to each subsequent subfield so that no time is lost. A useful feature of the program is that each time the stage moves to another part of the field, the reconstruction moves with it, keeping

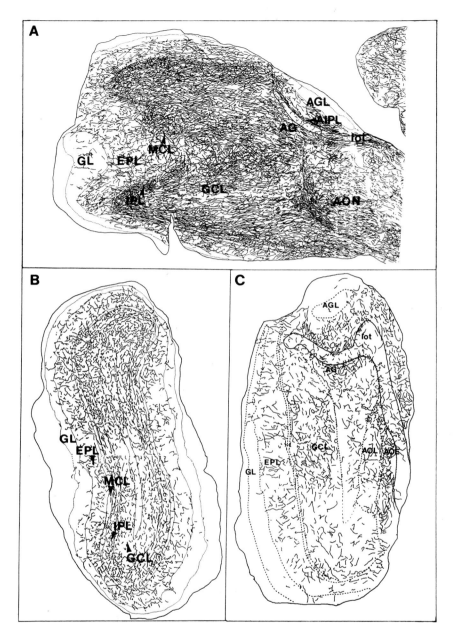

Figure 12. Use of N-ALYSIS (EXTENDED DIGITAL LUCIDA) to chart fiber distributions. A: Sagittal
25−μm sections through rat olfactory bulb stained for dopamine-β-hydroxylase immunoreactivity. Fibers and olfactory bulb layers were reconstructed from high-magnification (×40), real-
time enhanced video images. Numerous ×40 fields were reconstructed, stored in memory, and
printed out as a composite reconstruction. Several extended reconstructions were montaged to
produce the final reconstruction. With new software printouts the entire image can now be
reconstructed in one composite image. B−C: Reconstructions similar to that shown in A for
10-μm cryostat sections. (From McLean *et al.*, 1988).

in register with the underlying video gray image. Part of the previous field and the corresponding parts of the reconstruction remain in the new field so that the user has continuity of the new and the previously viewed field. By moving successively from one part of the field to the next, the user creates a composite reconstruction of areas much greater than could be encompassed in one viewing at the desired objective magnification. Because the scale of the drawing is determined in the stage movement calibration subroutine at the outset, the magnification of the reconstruction is known; then, the user can use the light pen to define two points anywhere in the finished reconstruction, and a calibrated scale bar is automatically added to the reconstruction. Various graphic symbols, text, etc. can be appended to the reconstruction using the graphics routines in the program so that a final publication-quality printout can be obtained. The reconstruction is stored in the computer memory, and, when completed, a hard-copy printout is made on the laser printer (Figs. 10 and 12).

We have used this program to reconstruct immunocytochemically stained fibers in the rat olfactory bulb at different stages of postnatal development and have automatically extracted information about total fiber length and/or fiber density (length per unit area or volume) for all of the cytoarchitectonic layers (McLean and Shipley, 1987a,b). This information was used to estimate the developmental growth rates of fibers of each layer. A significant result of this study was the demonstration that serotonergic fibers reach a fairly constant average density in all layers except the glomerular layer by the first to second postnatal week. By contrast, serotonergic innervation of the glomerular layer, a site of continuous synaptic turnover, continues to increase well into adulthood. This observation was simply not obvious from visual inspection of the material. Thus, image processing/image analysis allowed us to rapidly generate precise, elegant reconstructions that are more than just "pretty pictures"; the reconstructions yielded complex morphological data about differential growth rates of serotonergic fibers in different layers of the same cortical structure. This, in turn, led to a new biological hypothesis that serotonergic fibers in the glomerular layer of the olfactory bulb may be involved in modulating synaptic turnover and/or stabilization.

This example was chosen because it indicates the ways in which a classically tedious and time-consuming problem in neuroanatomy—section charting/reconstruction—can be done much more easily and more accurately with the aid of image analysis. Of equal importance, the information portrayed visually in such chartings can be elevated from impressionistic to quantitative statements that are capable of supporting new hypotheses or helping to choose among alternative hypotheses. This is not meant to demean the importance of reconstruction/charting alone to illustrate critical information about neuroanatomical patterns and organization. Because our knowledge of the complexity of the brain's structural and chemoanatomical organization is still increasing at a rapid pace, and we have probably only scratched the surface of molecular neuroanatomical diversity in the CNS, the need to portray such information in visual abstractions is obvious. Visual reconstructions will continue to be a critical tool in neurobiology for the foreseeable future. The interaction between such abstract visual data and trained neuroanatomical minds will remain essential to progress in neuroscience. However, there is an obvious need to reduce the time and effort required to generate such analyses. Image analysis has the potential to do this and at the same to introduce a powerful degree of quantitation that, if not abused (measurements for their own sake), can vastly increase the experimental repertoire of the neuroanatomist.

5. Maps and Reconstructions (MARS)

One of the most frequently encountered problems in neuroanatomy is how to represent distributions of features (labeled cells, terminal fields, etc.) through a series of anatomic sections. This is generally referred to as charting or mapping. In DIGITAL LUCIDA we have the ability to generate highly accurate, detailed reconstructions of a single section. A series of charted sections can be arranged into the kinds of sequential montages frequently used by neuroanatomists to portray the distribution of labeled cells, fibers, or histochemical–immunocytochemical staining gradients with DIGITAL LUCIDA. Quantitative information about numbers and sizes of cells, fiber length/dendrites, or staining density can be generated for the charted sections.

However, it is also possible to use the data from a series of chartings to obtain additional insight about the three-dimensional distributions of specific elements in the brain. Two ways of doing this in MARS are three-dimensional (3-D) wire frames and projection maps.

a. Wire Frames. In 3-D the individual charted sections generated in DIGITAL LUCIDA are aligned such that the sections are displayed as a pseudo-3-D perspective view of the sectioned solid object. The viewing angle can be selected by the user. This kind of representation is usually called a wireframe representation in computer graphic systems. To enhance the 3-D effect, pseudocolor can be used so that foreground sections are color coded to appear closer than background objects. Examples of such pseudo-3-D mapping are shown in Fig. 13A,B in which two populations of medullary neurons labeled by retrograde transport from the nucleus locus coeruleus are depicted. The detail achieved in these displays is limited by the pixel resolution of our system (512×512). Finer details could be achieved by transferring the point-set data from each section to a graphics computer capable of higher resolution (1024×1024 or greater), a development currently underway in our laboratory. The benefits of doing such wire-frame 3-D modeling in a graphics computer environment go beyond resolution. Several computer-aided design (CAD) systems have specialized software for removing hidden lines, smoothing contours, connecting points, shading, real-time rotation, perspective shrinking, etc. As these CAD systems can now be put together at relatively modest cost if one already has the host computer, it is expected that auxiliary graphics hard- and software will become common-place in neuroanatomical image-analysis facilities.

Nothwithstanding the esthetic allure of such 3-D renderings, there are alternative ways of representing the distributions of features through a series of brain sections that may even make one's point more clearly.

b. Projecting Maps. One such alternative used in MARS is the projection map. In this kind of map, individual coronal sections are plotted using DIGITAL LUCIDA. These chartings are used in MARS to create projection maps in the sagittal and horizontal planes. In order to generate sagittal and horizontal projection maps from coronal sections, the user needs to specify fiduciary points in each coronal section. For example, in the horizontal and sagittal medullary projection map shown in Fig. 13C,D, the midline of each section was determined by internal anatomic landmarks, and the lateral, dorsal, and ventral limits of the sections were determined by having the computer construct, for each section, the minimal rectangle, two sides of which are parallel to the midline, that just encloses the hemimedulla. The magnification of the section was previously calculated in DIGITAL LUCIDA; the user need only specify the section interval distance, and the program will automatically scale the calibrated locations of the boundaries and all features in each section and plot the projection maps. Thus, with a series of sections plotted in DIGITAL LUCIDA, no additional effort is required to generate projection maps in the two planes orthogonal to the section plane. Several different populations of features may be simultaneously plotted on the same maps, either using different colors (as in Fig. 13C,D) or using different geometric symbols for black-and-white hardcopy printout.

Although such projection maps lack the initial esthetic impact of 3-D wire frames, they may actually make it easier to discern patterns of distributions when several different populations of cells are plotted in the same map.

6. ISOMETRIC

ISOMETRIC is the first of a set of routines for analyzing density information, i.e., for analyzing how different parts of an image differ in terms of staining or labeling intensity.

In a transmitted-light microscope image, different parts of the field will generally differ in the amount of light passing through the specimen. Each point in the image has X and Y values that define its spatial location and a Z value that represents its depth in the focal plane. In addition, each point has an I value (intensity), which is the transmittance at that point. The intensity scale is divided into as many gray levels as the system can resolve. Since the hardware limiting factors of resolution are the camera and the A/D converter, the I scale typically is 64 (for a six-bit machine), 256 (eight bit), or higher. Thus, for an eight-bit machine each point in an image will have an I value of 0–255; 0 means no light is passing through the specimen, and 255 means that the maximum amount of light is passing through and typically means that that point is saturated, i.e., there is an indeterminate amount of light outside the dynamic range of the system. The *I* value, thus, represents the amount of light passing through the specimen. In many typical neuroanatomical problems one wants to know the intensity of the staining; i.e., one wants to know how much the staining reduces the light, and this is usually refered to as the density. Density, thus, is essentially the reciprocal of intensity.

As noted, intensity or density may be referred to some absolute value or, in most practical situations, to some relative value, e.g., the ratio of the density of a given point to the least dense points in the image. In many neuroanatomical experiments, absolute density values are hard to obtain because they require some independent means of measuring changes in the variable (e.g., antigens stained by an antibody) in order that differences in the staining can be systematically related to differences in the amount of the variable present in the section. In receptor autoradiography, one typically uses a standard scale so that grain density in the tissue can be compared with grain density in a calibrated area of scale. This is generally not yet possible with antigens or histochemical stains, so one must usually resort to relative measures of staining intensity and make some tenuous assumptions about linearity. Occasionally one can obtain correlative radioimmunoassay data, but this only partially addresses the issue of linearity or lack thereof in a staining-density curve.

Notwithstanding, in immunocytochemical staining such density measures can provide an indication of variations in antigen expression levels as long as the underlying assumptions and the limitations to such measures are clearly recognized and understood.

With these important questions in mind, it is reasonable to consider ways in which densitometric data can be quantified and/or depicted. ISOMETRIC is one way of analyzing such data. This analysis is really an extension of a kind of analysis with which most neuroanatomists are already familiar—color coding of densities in receptor autoradiography. In this case a pseudocolor lookup table is used to assign different colors to regions of different grain density so that one can gain an appreciation of the spatial distribution of receptor densities in a brain (Fig. 14A,B). In ISOMETRIC the idea of density color coding is simply carried one step further. The computer transforms the flat two-dimensional gray image by tilting it and representing high-density regions as peaks and lower-density regions as valleys (Figs. 14C and 15B). In other words, density is represented by elevation on an artificial image that represents a perspective view of the original flat image. This is similar to the way that cartographers represent elevations. On a flat map, mountain ranges are typically shown as various shades of browns, oranges, and reds while plains are beige, valleys green, and sea level is blue. Alternatively, elevation data can be represented in a perspective drawing in which elevation is represented by shading, interposition, etc. We have developed ISOMETRIC to allow us to represent anatomic staining densities in the same way. This pseudo- or perspective 3-D mapping of densities provides a dramatic visualization of the distribution of densities in a region. This density—elevation mapping can be displayed with continuous variations in gray tones corresponding to elevation, or colors may be used to further highlight the variations in elevation.

Such isometric maps of density have the same problems of other perspective maps, chief among which is that high elevations in the foreground obscure lower elevations in the background; i.e., valleys may be hidden by mountains. This can be overcome. We typically use both a flat color-coded map and an elevation map side by side so that one can observe whether interesting regions are hidden. In addition, we have developed routines so that the user can take a cut through the elevation map and view it end-on (Figs. 14C and 15B). The cut can be made as any straight or curved arbitrarily drawn line. The combination of these maps and cutting procedures allows one to precisely analyze subtle variations in density in any anatomic subregion of the section. A series of such perspective maps of equally spaced sections through a brain structure can convey a powerful visualization of the distribution of some entity (receptors, labeled fibers) throughout the 3-D volume of a neural structure. We have used this kind of analysis to illustrate how immunocytochemically stained neurotensinergic (NT) fibers are distributed throughout the midbrain periaqueductal gray (PAG) (Shipley *et al.*, 1987) (Fig. 15B). In this example, we were able to treat fiber-density data very similarly to receptor-density data. By imaging the stained fibers at a relatively low magnification below the level of resolution of single fibers, it was possible to map the heterogeneous density distribution of NT fibers throughout PAG. We have also used this program to map transmitter receptor densities (Fig. 14C) and AChE and cytochrome oxidase histochemical staining density distributions.

7. KONTOURS

The major goal of KONTOURS was to develop a way of representing density distributions in a series of anatomical sections using black and white line drawings in order to avoid the expense of publishing such data in color.

In KONTOURS, the image may first be processed in order to highlight the density distribution in the desired part of the image. If processing is used, all subsequent fields, must, of course, be subjected to identical processing as they are analyzed. Next, the program subdivides the image into regions of equal density range. The program draws boundary lines of different color around regions whose density falls within a predetermined range of the scale. The user decides how many intervals of density are desirable. Typically three to seven intervals are appropriate. If four intervals are chosen, the program draws boundary lines around all regions in the image where the per-pixel density falls between 0 and 24% (most dense); then it draws a different colored boundary line around regions where the per-pixel density is 25–49%, and so on. The program has been designed to find "holes in donuts"; i.e., suppose the 0–24% density range defines several areas some of which have within them regions where the density is in the 25–49% range; in such cases the program draws an interior boundary line that excludes the less-dense areas (Fig. 15C).

The resulting analysis displays the original gray image with four sets of colored boundary lines that divide the image into four sets of regions of equidensity from 0 to 99% of the density scale. These isodensity boundary lines are superimposed on the original anatomical gray image so that the user can visually assess whether dividing the images into four equidensity regions is informative or whether it might be better to try fewer or more subdivisions.

When KONTOURS is applied to a section containing immuno- or histochemically stained cells or receptor autoradiographic anterograde labelling, the equidensity mapping frequently results in the delineation of areas that correspond to the boundaries of known anatomic subdivisions, e.g., nuclei, cortical layers, etc., indicating that the variable of interest is differentially or preferentially localized to specific anatomic regions. However, the equidensity mapping is incredibly accurate and objective, and therefore it frequently identifies contours that result from various kinds of artifact in the section (e.g., holes, bubbles, specks of dirt, etc.). As a result, the equidensity parsing may be noisy. One way to deal with this is to generate less noisy histological material. Still, we are only human, and having done the best we can, we blame the reagents and try smoothing filters in the initial processing stages to eliminate small artifacts. Unfortunately, such smoothing can result in the blurring of density contours that are not artifacts, so smoothing operations may not work. Thus, we have developed ways of interactively editing the isodensity images. One very useful tool is simply to remove all boundary lines within all or any given part of the density range that fall below a selected size range. One can view the effect of using a given size filter, and, if inappropriate, one can return to the original equidensity boundaries and try again. Generally, rejecting equidensity boundaries below a certain size range cleans up such images nicely, and so long as one reports with the data that regions smaller than x μm^2 were not considered, the analysis can be objectively evaluated by the reader.

At this stage the program has still not achieved the major goal of eliminating color because the four different equidensity regions are bounded by four colors. To eliminate the need for color, we developed a set of routines that allow one to fill different regions of equidensity with dots of different spacing (Fig. 15C). Typically, we solidly fill (dots of zero spacing) the areas of greatest (0–24%) density, fill with dots spaced 1–2 pixels apart the next densest area, dots spaced 4–6 pixels apart for the next area, and leave the least-dense area unfilled. Finally, all the color planes are collapsed to one color, and the image is printed out on the laser printer. The resulting maps have a half-tone quality and convey density distribution in an accurate, visually effective, and inexpensive fashion.

Another routine in the program allows one to measure and annotate the average density of each equidensity area in the map (Fig. 15C). In addition, one can correct the density measures for the contribution of background. For example, one can use the light pen to delineate an arbitrary region in the image that is devoid of actual staining. In such a region the only contribution to measured density will be background staining and the attenuation of transmitted light resulting from the thickness of the section. If the average density measured in such a region is subtracted from the measured densities in all other parts of the image, then the corrected density in those parts of the image will reflect only the contribution of the staining. After correction for background, it is legitimate to take the ratios of corrected densities in different parts of the image as an indication of the proportional staining in those areas, and by making certain assumptions about linearity of the staining, one may infer that one region has, for example, three times the amount of the variable being stained as another. The relative densities of similar regions in different sections can also be compared if the density in comparable-background areas is normalized.

This kind of analysis can be especially useful, for example, if one has a manipulation that changes in receptor or antigen density in a specific subregion of the brain. For example, one might make a localized lesion to deplete fibers or up-regulate receptors in a given nucleus. Now one could process a normal brain (or use the contralateral half of the lesioned brain) to measure the background-corrected densities in the affected and unaffected areas in the normal and experimental brains. The ratios of the corrected density measures in an unaffected part of the brain allow one to normalize for variance in staining between the normal and experimental brain. Having corrected for variance of staining from technical factors, one can then ratio the corrected measures of density in the affected area of the brain and draw reasonable inferences about the degree to which the lesion changed the density of fibers or receptors in the area of interest.

8. Microdensitometer (MDENS)

MDENS is a simple, useful program for measuring densities. In MDENS the user can directly measure the average raw or corrected density in arbitrarily defined regions of the image. In one mode the light pen or keyboard is used to define a box, rectangle, or circle of arbitrary size. A region so defined is displayed as a binary outline so that the user can determine if its size and shape are appropriate. This outline now constitutes a "probe" that can, using the light pen, be rapidly placed at any number of locations in the image (Fig. 15A). Each time the "probe" is placed somewhere in the field, the numerical value of the average density enclosed by the "probe" is printed on the screen and connected by a line to the center of the region outlined by the "probe."

In this mode the densities in various regions of a section can be sampled in a manner analogous to a punch sample for biochemical assay. With this analysis, one can compare densities in different parts of the same section or in the corresponding parts of different sections.

In a second mode, the user arbitrarily defines the size and shape of the "probe" by drawing it on the screen with the light pen. This is very useful when one wants to sample the same anatomic subregion in successive sections.

The density measures can be corrected for background/section thickness as in the other density programs.

9. Profile Analysis

Profile analysis is a graphic method for analyzing the gray level or density distribution in an anatomic section. By analogy with KONTOURS, the density at each point in the image is considered to be an elevation. With the light pen, a straight or arbitrary line is drawn somewhere in the section, and the computer generates a histogram. The abscissa of the histogram represents the pixels located successively along the line; at each point along the abscissa a vertical line is erected the height of which is proportional to the density of that pixel. Profile analysis thus shows the density profile along any cut through the section (Fig. 3D). As with the other density programs, there are routines for subtracting the average background from the profile.

A profile analysis accurately reports density differences in neighboring pixels and is thus very sensitive to factors that cause local fluctuations in density. For example, if the section is being analyzed at a magnification at which blood vessels are greater than one pixel wide, the staining variable, e.g., autoradiographic grains or immunocytochemical stain, will generally not be present in the lumen of the vessel. A line drawn through the section that intersects vessels will generate a profile that has very low density values randomly distributed in regions where the average density over the tissue may be high. In this example it would be desirable somehow to smooth the histogram to eliminate the "vascular noise." The program provides two ways of doing this. Since vessel holes will generally not have an appreciable linear extent in a thin section, one can draw the profile line and specify that the line be converted to a strip n pixels wide. At each point along the line the densities of series of lines n pixels wide, perpendicular to and centered along the profile line, will be determined, summed, and divided by n to give the average density for that point in the profile strip. Usually three-, five-, or seven-point line width will effectively eliminate small random variations in density.

This smoothing procedure may not work well if the actual density distribution is changing rapidly at right angles to the profile line. For example, in a highly gyrated cortex, if one were to draw a profile from the pia to the white matter, a three- to five-pixel strip might be too gross and blur density differences in adjacent cortical layers. In such a case, it might be better to average along the line. In this smoothing procedure the density of each point along the abscissa of the profile would represent the average of the pixel in the image represented by that point and the one, two, or more nearest neighbors on either side. This is a running average, which is less sensitive to variations perpendicular to the profile line than the previously described orthogonal average.

The rest of this program contains utilities for analyzing the line profile. One can, for example, request that the maximum and minimum density be identified, and a binary cursor will appear on both the profile and the point in the image of maximum and minimum density (Fig. 14D). Similarly, one can pinpoint all the inflection points or all the points where the inflection exceeds a certain value, e.g., one standard deviation. Such analyses allow one to determine if points of significant change in the staining/labeling density profile correspond to anatomic features in the section.

10. Organization of N-ALYSIS

The subprograms of N-ALYSIS have now been briefly described. The final point to be made about the program is its flexibility. One may have gotten the impression from the description that each subprogram is a more or less exclusive option, whereas in fact the program has been designed so that only parts of each subprogram may be used and then the image can be further analyzed by other subprograms until the desired analysis is complete. This gives the user considerable flexibility, and with a little experience and imagination, one can begin to approach entirely new kinds of material/problems with a new analysis.

This was one of the original goals of our program development. We did not want to be tied down to certain fixed, specialized analyses that might somehow subtly inhibit us from tackling new kinds of neurobiological problems or new labeling techniques. We think we have been reasonably successful, as we have not yet encountered a situation in which we avoided the use of a new technique because we did not have a way of analyzing it. When existing software was not appropriate, new routines were developed and integrated with the more general tools of N-ALYSIS. Below are given a couple of examples of this kind where new, special purpose programs were developed using some existing routines from N-ALYSIS and additional routines to deal with unique aspects of the problem at hand. The two examples are the analysis of *in situ* hybridization data and the analysis of time-varying changes in the intensity of voltage/ion-sensitive dyes.

B. IN SITU

It is actually fairly easy to obtain a relative quantitation of *in situ* hybridization data, and although we have not yet done so, it should not be much of a problem to devise an external standard for calibrated quantitation. In our efforts to date, we have used an antisense mDNA probe directed against the message for HMGCoA reductase, the rate-limiting enzyme for cholesterol synthesis (in collaboration with Dr. Sohaib Khan, University of Cincinnati). We are investigating whether this message is regulated by events that are associated with increased membrane synthesis (e.g., neural development, regeneration).

So far we have used tritium-labeled antisense probes. The developed autoradiographs are counterstained with toludine blue. In the IN SITU program, the field of interest is imaged under either bright- or darkfield illumination. For the purpose of example we describe the program's operation under brightfield conditions. The goals of our analyses so far have been to measure grain number/density on a per-cell basis, to correlate grain density with the locations and/or morphological features (size, shape, etc.) of the cells, and to compare such data from two populations of cells—normal and manipulated.

The field is first processed to enhance the detectability of cells. We use chromatic filters to selectively pass the blue range and contrast enhancement to further selectively enhance the stained cells (Fig. 16A). Next, a combination of gray-level thresholding and interactive light-pen editing is used to create a binary mask to identify all cells and to separate those that partially overlap (with thinner sections overlap is reduced). This binary mask is stored in memory. Next, the chromatic filter and contrast enhancement settings are selectively adjusted to suppress the blues and enhance the contrast of developed silver grains (Fig. 16B). At this point the focus may need to be adjusted slightly so that grains are as sharp as possible. An autofocus routine may be used for this. Next, thresholding is applied, and the detected grains are identified in a second binary mask. Local thresholding is sometimes done interactively, as the chromatic filtering and digital contrast enhancement used to suppress the blue counterstaining may create local variations in background grays (Fig. 16C,D). The binary mask of the grains is then stored in memory.

Next, the two masks, the one for the cells and the one for the grains, are recalled and displayed simultaneously in two different colors superimposed on either the cell or grain gray image (Fig. 16D,E). This gives the user an opportunity to assess visually the accuracy of the two detection analyses and further edit any obvious artifacts, overlaps, and any cells/grains that were missed.

At this stage it is possible to write the results to a file so that there is a record of the number of grains within the boundary of each cell. It is also possible to calculate the number of grains that lie outside of cells and the total area of the field not covered by cells. By dividing the number of grains lying outside of cells by the total area not containing cells, one has a simple measure of the average background grain. This average background can be used to correct the measured grains per cell. One can list the corrected grains per cell, calculate the mean, variance, etc., in grains per cell, or generate histograms to correlate grains per cell on the basis of size, shape, location, etc. (Fig. 16F). Usually one performs the grain-per-cell analysis over several microscopic fields before analyzing the results in statistical or graphic form. It turns out that this same program is also excellent for analyzing [^{3}H]-thymidine cell birth dating or steroid receptor binding data, as the raw data from these kinds of experiments are similar to *in situ* data.

C. MOVIE

MOVIE is a program developed to grab and store a series of frames at frame rate (25 full or 50 half frames per second in our system). Basically the image-processing/image-analysis system is used as a digital movie camera. In this mode, the movements of objects could be tracked, but the principal use of the program to track time-varying changes in the gray levels of stationary objects, i.e., changes in intensity, rather than changes in spatial location. The program is being used to detect and analyze changes in the fluorescence intensity or absorption of a family of dyes that signal changes in membrane potential. The preparation—cultured cells, a tissue slice, or an *in vivo* preparation—is loaded with the dye of interest, placed on the microscope stage, and imaged via the camera.

The resting intensity level of a dye-loaded preparation is usually high enough to be detected by a Newvicon camera. The problem is that typically the fluorescence intensity or absorbance changes are modulated by only 2–4% when the membrane potential changes by a physiologically significant amount. Thus, one is required to detect a change of only a few gray levels. Various strategies are being tried to improve the detection of such small changes. First, the black level and gain of the camera are adjusted to the range of the signal where the intensity change occurs. The signal is further enhanced in the image processor. Second, the image is being measured and continuously subtracted from a stored image taken under "background" conditions, i.e., where no physiological stimulus is applied to the preparation. This difference image is rescaled and contrast enhanced to expand the range around the difference image. A series of frames of such difference images are grabbed at frame rate and stored in memory.

The program is designed to allow the user to capture a predetermined set of frames before a stimulus in order to have a set of prestimulus images; then the stimulus is applied, and frames are captured continuously from the onset of the stimulus, or a set of frames is taken followed by a pause and then the next set of frames, and so on. The limit to the number of frames is the system RAM image memory (an optical disk will increase the stored frame capacity). The number of frames stored can also be increased by reducing the size of each frame. By reducing the frame from 512×512 to 128×128 pixels, the number of stored frames can be increased by 16 times; the obvious trade-off is that a correspondingly smaller part of the field is analyzed.

MOVIE also contains a number of utilities for analyzing when and where intensity changes occurred in the field. A simple way is to apply a pseudo-color look-up table to the images and search the array of images for frames when the pseudocolor distribution changes (Fig. 17A). This can be tedious, and if a large number of frames are stored, they cannot be viewed simultaneously. A second kind of analysis is to view one frame taken under prestimulus conditions and, adjacent to it, step one frame at a time through all the frames taken during or subsequent to stimulation (Fig. 17B). This side-by-side comparison of pseudocolored images facilitates the identification of frames where there are changes. Frames so identified can be earmarked and subsequently recalled from memory and displayed as a static array or as a dynamic display with the pseudocoloring applied sequentially at a selectable speed across the array from one frame to the next to generate a dynamic sequence. Alternatively, the frames may be viewed one at a time at a variable rate of speed, like a movie film, so that one can observe dynamic changes.

All of these are techniques that can be used to alter the display so that the user can better detect patterns of intensity change. This allows the observer to interpret changes in terms of the anatomic organization of the preparation.

A more focused analysis (after the user knows generally where and what to look for) is to use the light pen to delineate a region of suspected intensity modulation in a single frame and then have the computer calculate the intensity per unit area (average intensity) for that subregion in all subsequent frames. The resulting average intensity of the identified region can then be plotted graphically to indicate the frame-to-frame intensity changes in the region of interest (Fig. 17C).

The use of voltage-sensitive dyes is still in its infancy, and many issues such as the best dye for a given preparation, optimal preparation, and best ways of delivering stimuli so that changes can be detected at the relatively slow rate of frame capture dictated by standard scan rates are still being explored. Much progress is expected with the advent of faster, more sensitive cameras. The general kinds of software developed in MOVIE should provide a point of departure for capturing, detecting, and analyzing membrane-potential-related events in living cell, tissues, and possibly *in situ* brain structures. Among the most exciting applications of voltage-sensitive dyes are the studies of the salamander olfactory system by Kauer and co-workers (Kauer, 1988).

VIII. FACTORS IN CHOOSING AN IMAGE-PROCESSING/IMAGE-ANALYSIS SYSTEM

There are many factors to consider when choosing an image-processing/image-analysis system. Two critical factors are budget and intended use. Some laboratories have limited resources to commit to imaging equipment, and some laboratories are not primarily involved with visual data. When resources are absolutely limited, there are three general tacks one can consider. One is to form a group of users, pool resources, and buy a system that has the capabilities to service many applications. A second possibility is to purchase a system that can be expanded later as resources and needs increase, and a third possibility is to put something together from scratch, i.e., buy some boards and write software. The authors have seen a few home-grown systems that are useful; however, we have seen far more where the boards were bought and little was ever accomplished. Building one's own system is a tremendous undertaking.

When resources are less limited, the possibilities are more numerous. There are a number of commercially available systems that offer image processing and image analysis. Currently, most systems are stronger in image processing than analysis. This is because, generally speaking, processing is a hardware, board-based technology, whereas analysis is software based. Software-based technologies are a double-edged sword. On the one hand, software is intrinsically more malleable than hardware; i.e., one will seldom tamper with a manufacturer's boards to alter their performance, but, in principle, one can develop new software to tackle new problems in image analysis. On the other hand, the software in most systems is intimately tied to the hardware of the system, the input, frame-grabbing, and processing boards (data boards), as well as to the host machine and its operating system. Thus, software developed for one vendor's system will generally not run on another system even if the host and operating systems are the same, because the interface to the data boards and memory may be quite different.

In order to develop new and different application software, most manufacturers have developed a library of routines in some high-level language, e.g., PASCAL or C. These higher-level commands allow application software to be written without concern for that system's host and data-board interactions. This library is the absolute key to any system. If the library is rich and well structured, programmers with little background in image analysis can work with biologists to develop new application software. However, if the library is not comprehensive, or if the high-level language is not optimal for image-analysis application software, development will be very slow and tedious. Manufacturers will generally not release the source code for their application software, so when developing new code one generally must start from the library. The library, thus, is the key to whether one can easily develop new applications or not. The brutal fact is that few commercial systems offer the range of software needed for the kinds of applications discussed in this chapter. Our software was developed in house using the manufacturer's library. In retrospect, we were lucky to have chosen a system with an excellent library, and even with that, our current software has taken approximately 4 person-years to develop.

There are certain features that contribute to the power and versatility of a library. Some of these are the ease with which one can execute routines like "first blob–next blob"; i.e., how do you go about finding the defined features in the image? Another critical feature is how easy is it to define an arbitrary region of interest in which to define objects? Many systems work with the frame concept; i.e., the user defines a rectangular frame somewhere in the image, and features are detected and analyzed in that frame. However, the vast majority of the applications discussed in this chapter make use of the ability to define an arbitrary region—the shape of a brain section or a substructure, e.g., a nucleus, the hippocampus, the caudate—and the analysis is targeted on that region alone. Arbitrary region analysis is a critical feature that is seldom found in libraries.

Another key feature to look for is the ease with which one can delineate objects in the live video image. Many systems require that the live image be grabbed before analysis can be commenced. Thus, if one wishes to follow a feature, for example, a stained fiber, that continues outside the viewing field or passes in and out of the focal plane, it may be necessary to repetitively go back and forth between the live and the digitized image and even to repeat the image enhancement setting each time. This is incredibly tedious, time consuming, and frustrating. Our software has been developed to allow features to be detected in live, continuously processed images. It is important to determine if a given manufacturer's system will accommodate such applications.

Another feature to look for is the device used to interact with the image. The majority of systems use a mouse; our system uses a light pen. In our experience, it is much easier, faster, and more accurate to delineate the complicated features that are typical of neuroanatomical material with a light pen applied directly to the video monitor than with a mouse that activates a cursor on the screen. A mouse is fine for pointing at windows, but it is not so great for tracking a PHA-L-stained fiber.

When considering an image-processing/image-analysis system, it is essential to test the system with one's own material and to ask to see analyses done of the sort one will want. If this chapter serves no other purpose, perhaps it will serve as a source of examples for asking if a system can do the kinds of things discussed here. Be wary of statements like, "It should be possible" or "I think we can do it." Most of these things can be done by a team of experienced programmers if the vendor's machine has a decent library. In dealing with the vendors of high-cost image-analysis systems, it is best to leave nothing to trust and to remember that all things considered, a salesman's job is to sell you his machine. If you are told that a critical piece of software can be developed for you, do not purchase the system until it is developed bug-free and rigorously tested by you in your application. The incentive to develop your software is rooted in the potential of the sale; that incentive is removed once you have signed the check.

It is also useful to visit someone else's laboratory or request the vendor to give you a list of customers doing similar kinds of things to those you will want to do. Ask how the system performs and how the vendor supports the instrument. Do they return phone calls promptly? Do they help users develop application software?

If the resources are available, a comprehensive processing/analysis system with a solid programming library is the best choice. This is because research applications are not as rigid as industrial/manufacturing or clinical laboratory applications. As researchers, we need to be able to change analyses as our knowledge increases, and we need new kinds of analyses as new techniques arise. If the vendor of a machine primarily targets industrial and manufacturing markets, then their software development may emphasize specific applications, and they may not provide useful tools for new research application development. Frequently, you will be assured that you can perform your analysis with their "General Purpose Analysis" package, but look at this very closely. The number of steps it takes to get the processing/analysis you want may be so great that you and your co-workers will grow weary (and old) making their software fit your different applications. Try very hard to sit down and go through a typical analysis, noting how quickly you move through the task. Do you have to wait for certain things to execute? Do you get rapid visual feedback, or must you adjust parameters and move to another point in the program before you can assess the results? Remember, no matter how good the system is or you are, the complexities of many applications are going to require a lot of trial and error until you hit the optimal way to do the analysis. Delays at each step in execution will inhibit your trying alternative approaches.

Assuming one generates the resources and identifies a system for which one can write new and useful codes, then image processing and analysis can be of immense benefit in neuroanatomy. The classic boundaries between neuroanatomy and other techniques of neurobiology are dissolving rapidly. Cell and organ cultures offer great promise for combined structural, chemoanatomical, and functional analyses. These kinds of approaches offer opportunities for detecting and quantifying a growing range of dynamic features of neural organization, function, and development. Imaging and the analysis of imaged data will become an increasingly important tool in neurobiology. Certain aspects of this technology will become better standardized and more accessible. We hope that this chapter communicates some of the power, excitement, and fun of this new technology.

Acknowledgments. Several individuals have made important contributions to the development of the application software presented here. Mr. Peter Hug pioneered some of the early programs that, in skeletal form, still haunt N-ALYSIS. Mr. John Foster, John Gayler, Bill Burnip, and John Keat of Joyce-Loebl, Inc., have contributed advice, expertise, and equipment. All their contributions were essential to our work, and we gratefully acknowledge their support. Mr. Jim Hamlin of Nikon Instruments has contributed equipment and has been a steadfast supporter of our efforts and a friend. Dr. Eric Gruenstein, Co-Director of the University of Cincinnati Center for Image Analysis, has likewise contributed ideas and hard work to sustain the Center's activities and growth. Drs. Robert Cardell, Jr., Harry Rudney, and Dean Robert Daniels of the University of Cincinnati College of Medicine helped with financial support for the Center in its early days. Dr. William T. Nickell, from the University of Cincinnati, has helped with hardware problems and contributed ideas for improving software and calibration routines. Ms. Sharon

Harding has provided excellent secretarial support, and Dr. Beata Frydel has shepherded much of the histology and helped with illustrations. Finally, many of our colleagues and collaborators have contributed their support, data, and suggestions for software improvement. Chief among these are Drs. Gary Aston-Jones, Larry Swanson, Michael Behbehani, and Vincent Pieribone. We thank Drs. Robert Gesteland and Heather Duncan for their critical reading of the manuscript. We gratefully acknowledge the support of: U.S. Army DAAG 29-83-G-0064, DAMD 17-82-C-2272, and DAMD 17-86-C-6005 and NINCDS-NS-20643, 22053, and 23348.

REFERENCES

Allen, R. D., Travis, J. L., Allen, N. S., and Yilmaz, H., 1981a, Video-enhanced contrast polarization (AVEC-POL) microscopy: A new method applied to the detection of birefringence in the motile reticulopodial network of *Allogromia laticollaris, Cell Motil.* **1:**275–289.

Allen, R. D., Allen, N. S., and Travis, J. L., 1981b, Video-enhanced contrast, differential interference contrast (AVEC-DIC) microscopy: A new method capable of analyzing microtubule-related motility in the reticulopodial network of *Allogromia laticollaris, Cell Motil.* **1:**291–302.

Blaha, G., Blair, W., Nickell, W. T., and Shipley, M. T., 1984, Cholinergic (CH) receptors in the rat olfactory bulb: Nicotinic (N) and muscarinic (M) cholinergic receptors are segregated and coincide with acetylcholinesterase (AChE), *Neurosci. Soc.* **10:**1183.

Glaser., E. M, Tagamets, M., McMullen, N. T., and Van der Loos, H., 1983, The image-combing computer microscope—an interactive instrument for morphometry of the nervous system, *J. Neurosci. Methods* **8:**17–32.

Inoue, S., 1986, *Video Microscopy,* Plenum Press, New York.

Kauer, J. S., 1988, Real-time imaging of evoked activity in local circuits of the salamander olfactory bulb, *Nature* **331:**166–168.

McLean, J. H., and Shipley, M. T., 1987a, Serotonergic afferents to the rat olfactory bulb: I. Origins and laminar specificity of serotonergic inputs in the adult rat, *J. Neurosci.* **7:**3016–3028.

McLean, J. H., and Shipley, M. T., 1987b, Serotongeric afferents to the rat olfactory bulb: II. Changes in fiber distribution during development, *J. Neurosci.* **7:**3029–3039.

McLean, J. H., Nickell, W. T., and Shipley, M. T., 1986, Afferent connections to the horizontal limb of diagonal band, *Neurosci. Soc.* **12:**351.

McLean, J. H., Shipley, M. T., Nickell, W. T., Aston-Jones, G., and Reyher, C. K. H., 1988, Chemoanatomical organization of the noradrenergic input from locus coeruleus to the olfactory bulb of the adult rat, *J. Comp. Neurol.* (in press).

Nickell, W. T., and Shipley, M. T., 1988, Two anatomically specific classes of candidate cholinoceptive neurons in the rat olfactory bulb, *J. Neurosci.* **8:**4482–4491.

Shipley, M. T., McLean, J. H., and Behbehani, M. M., 1987, Heterogeneous distribution of neurotensin-like immunoreactive neurons and fibers in the midbrain periaqueductal gray of the rat, *J. Neurosci.* **7:**2025–2034.

Index